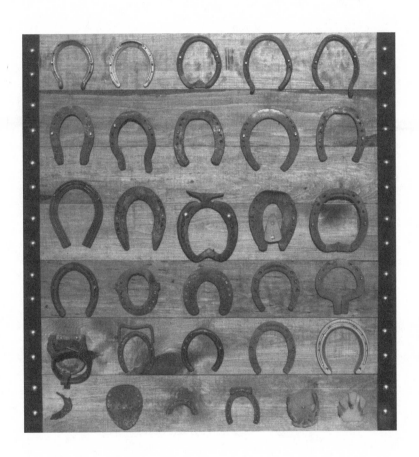

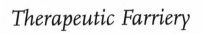

Therapeutic Farriery

Therapeutic Farriery

A MANUAL FOR VETERINARIANS AND FARRIERS

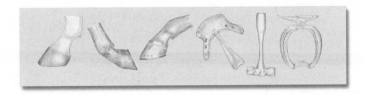

YEHUDA AVISAR

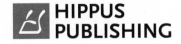 HIPPUS
PUBLISHING

San Luis Obispo, California

ISBN 978-0-9790011-0-9
FIRST EDITION

10 9 8 7 6 5 4 3 2 1

Designed and typeset by Terri Wright, Santa Barbara, California.
Copyediting by Jeanette Morris, Atascadero, California.
Cover painting, Gold Rush by Caly Garris, Scio, Oregon.
Scanning and photographic enhancement by Austin MacRae, Santa Barbara, California.
Gallery photos and drawings by Yehuda Avisar.
Printed, Smyth-sewn and bound by Thomson-Shore, Dexter, Michigan

DISCLAIMER
The author and the publisher disclaim any liability or loss incurred
consequently, directly or indirectly, from the use and application of
any information contained in this book.

LIBRARY OF CONGRESS CONTROL NUMBER 2006934919

Library of Congress Cataloging-in-Publication Data
Therapeutic Farriery
Include appendices, references and index.

1. Farriery. 2. Therapeutic farriery. 3. Corrective farriery. 4. Equine podiatry.
5. Equine lameness. 6. Horseshoeing. 7. Orthopedic horseshoeing.

Printed on acid free, 50% post consumer recycled paper.
Manufactured in the United States of America.

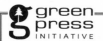

green
press
INITIATIVE

Hippus Publishing is committed to preserving ancient forests
and natural resources. We elected to print *Therapeutic Farriery*
on 50% post consumer recycled paper, processed chlorine free. As
a result, for this printing, we have saved:

24 Trees (40' tall and 6-8" diameter)
10,144 Gallons of Wastewater
4,080 Kilowatt Hours of Electricity
1,118 Pounds of Solid Waste
2,197 Pounds of Greenhouse Gases

Hippus Publishing made this paper choice because our printer,
Thomson-Shore, Inc., is a member of Green Press Initiative, a
nonprofit program dedicated to supporting authors, publishers,
and suppliers in their efforts to reduce their use of fiber obtained
from endangered forests.

For more information, visit www.greenpressinitiative.org

Copies of this book can be ordered from **www.hippuspublishing.com**

To Miri, Nitzann, Ronni and Talia

Contents

Preface

THIS BOOK IS WRITTEN FOR VETERINARIANS, FARRIERS AND STUDENTS OF both professions who are interested in the therapeutic aspects of farriery. Its aim is to increase the collaboration between the two professions by providing information common to both fields.

The first part of the book describes the development, anatomy, conformation, physiology and mechanical properties of the foot of the horse, and its relationship to other structures. This part also contains a proposed foot grading system aimed at improving communication between veterinarians, farriers and horse owners. The second part describes the locomotion and balance of the foot and the effects of farriery manipulation on the foot and limb. The third part deals with hoof care, prevention and treatment of orthopedic disorders in foals. The fourth part includes a discussion of legal aspects involving foot care procedures in horses and describes various techniques used in therapeutic farriery. The last part of the book deals with therapeutic farriery of foot disorders, abnormal foot conformation and stay apparatus injuries.

The descriptions of therapeutic horseshoes and devices in the text follow the condition for which they are commonly used, although some of them may be applied to different conditions as well. An attempt was made to include farriery methods from various sources. The dimensions provided for the construction of various therapeutic devices may be modified according to the size of the horse, available materials, and personal preference.

For convenience, the references list was placed at the end of the book in alphabetical order. A list of resources for various products described in the text is provided in Appendix A.

Throughout this work, the emphasis is on prevention of foot and limb disorders rather than relying on "fixing" problems. This approach can be achieved by adhering to proper hoof care management protocol (beginning with the foal and continuing with the adult horse), by educating horse owners about the limitations of their horses, by improving hoof quality through research and genetic selection, and by developing horseshoes that are more "horse friendly."

—*Yehuda Avisar*
San Luis Obispo, California

Acknowledgments

THE AUTHOR WOULD LIKE TO THANK Dr. Suzan Stover, University of California, Davis, for reviewing the anatomy chapters, and Professor Hans Geyer, University of Zurich, Switzerland, for reviewing the chapter on hoof quality.

Many of the photos that appear in the text are works of the late Mr. Charles A. Heumphreus, who was the farrier at the School of Veterinary Medicine, U.C. Davis.

The author would like to thank the following associations, publishers and institutes for providing material for the manuscript: Journal of Veterinary Diagnostics, Compendium of Continuing Education for the Practicing Veterinarian, American Association of Equine Practitioners, Oxford University Press, American Scientist, Euroscience (The Veterinary Quarterly), Equine Veterinary Journal, Australian Veterinary Journal, Thompson Veterinary Health Care Communications (Veterinary Medicine), American Veterinary Medical Association (American Journal of Veterinary Research and Journal of American Veterinary Medicine Association), Dover Publication, Thompson Publishing Services, Florida Museum of Natural History, Gainesville and the American Museum of Natural History, New York.

—*Yehuda Avisar*

Part 1 The Foot

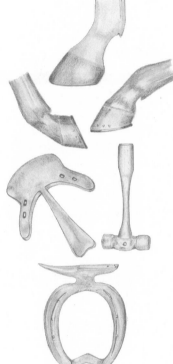

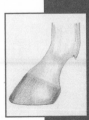

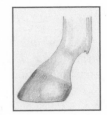

Chapter 1

Development of the Horse's Limb

ADAPTATIONAL CHANGES

THE EVOLUTIONARY HISTORY OF THE HORSE is a complex process that includes branching and extinction of different horse-like species throughout its course. This process, which lasted 55 million years, resulted in the development of a single genus, *Equus* (MacFadden, 2005). The ancestors of the modern horse, *Equus caballus*, underwent radical evolutionary changes that included increase in body size, elongation of the limbs and development of compound teeth. These adaptations enabled the horse to become a "grazing animal that lives and feeds on open grassland" (Storer et al., 1974).

Among the earliest known ancestors of the horse was *eohippus*, a small creature that lived in the Eocene epoch (◆ fig. 1.1). Eohippus was about the size of a whippet. It had padded feet with four functional toes on the foreleg and three on the hind leg (Simpson, 1951). Reconstruction of fossilized remains of eohippus revealed that it was a fast-running animal. In order to maintain this running ability while increasing body size, later ancestors went through several adaptation changes (Hildebrand, 1982). These changes include permanent raise of the wrist (knee) and the heel (hock), which increased the effective

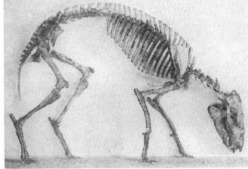

A

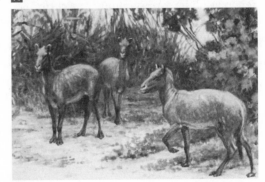

B

◆ **Fig. 1.1.** Early ancestor of the horse, eohippus. A. Skeletal fossil. B. Reconstruction based on the skeleton, note the padded feet. (Reprinted by permission from from Simpson, G.G. 1951, plate XX, courtesy of the American Museum of Natural History Library (items #32650 and 312630), painting by Charles R. Knight.)

3

length of the limbs. This allowed greater stride length and more ground coverage for each contraction of the muscles. Simultaneously, the strength and rigidity of the leg bones increased. In the forearm, the radius and ulna fused together; the stouter radius formed the shaft. In the gaskin, the tibia and fibula fused, and the fibula tend to become vestigial (Simpson, 1951).

The joints of the limbs, except those of the shoulder and hip, became pulley-like, with restricted motion to the fore-and-aft plane. The muscles facilitated simple requirements of flexion and extension of joints, while rotation (pronation and supination) were lost. Restricted motion of the limbs was essential for prevention of dislocation of joints during motion in the heavier ancestors (Hildebrand, 1982). Elongation of the limbs and restriction of joint movement to one plane allowed the horse to become an efficient runner at moderate speed for a prolonged time (Hildbrand, 1959; Hildbrand, 1982).

Another important change was the shifting position of the heavy leg muscles from the lower limb upward. This adaptation provided a biomechanical advantage that reduced fatigue during motion (Hildebrand, 1982). Evolvement of long tendinous attachments connects the muscles to the lower limb. Each tendon with its corresponding muscle formed a *musculotendinous unit* responsible for flexion or extension of the limb. In addition, each digital flexor tendon has a powerful check ligament that evolved to guard its muscle against excessive tension (Simpson, 1951). The check ligaments of the hind limbs are less developed (page 8).

DEVELOPMENT OF THE FOOT

EARLIER ANCESTORS OF THE HORSE had a padded foot fitted with several toes; the phalangeal bones carried weight similarly to the way dogs bear weight. The evolvement of this foot into the present day foot represents a radical change in mechanical type, characterized by a transition from a *pad-footed type* into a *spring-footed type* horse (Simpson, 1951) (♦ fig. 1.2). The horse's foot evolved in unity with the limbs and body. This process began with the loss of one front toe in *Mesohippus*, with both fore and hind feet ending with three toes; the side toes became smaller and probably carried less weight. The protective pad was still present in Mesohippus hooves. During the evolvement of *Merychippus*, the side toes were much smaller and did not reach the ground in resting position. Each of the toes ended in a well-developed small hoof. Merychippus was standing on the extreme tiptoe, and the pad may already have become a vestige; the central toe was associated with complex ligaments that become part of a spring mechanism. The actual toe reduction evolved in *Pliohippus*, which carried weight on a big central toe that ended in a large hoof capsule similar to that of Equus (Simpson, 1951). Other evidences of adaptational changes are the *splint bones* that present in *Equus* as remnants of the second and fourth metacarpal/metatarsal bones of its ancestors.

The evolvement of the hoof capsule along with the suspensory ligament, flexor tendons and check ligaments resulted in a spring-foot type horse that was quite different from its ancestors (♦ fig. 1.3). Being single-toed places the horse family within the order *Perissodactyla*, which includes animals with odd numbers of toes (Ellenberger et al., 1949; MacFadden, 2005).

The functions of the encapsulating hoof include protection of the foot, interdigitation with the ground and absorption of shock. Present day feral horses show that the hooves are adapted to seasonal environment of snow, ice, mud and arid conditions. The horny hoof capsule not only protects the inner structures of the foot from physical trauma and environmental hazards, but it also allows the horse to kick. The unique shape of the hoof allows it to dig into the ground during motion and to propel the horse efficiently, whereas the physiological characteristics of the horn allow it to deform during impact and absorb shock.

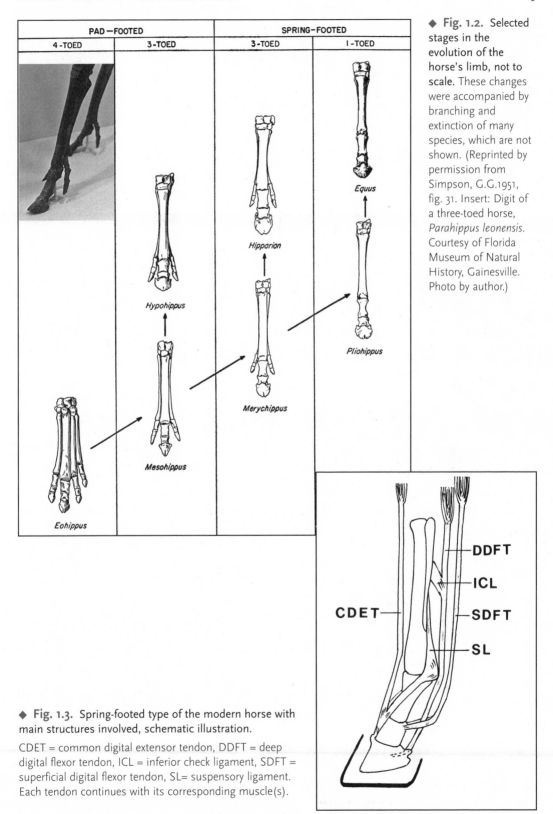

◆ **Fig. 1.2.** Selected stages in the evolution of the horse's limb, not to scale. These changes were accompanied by branching and extinction of many species, which are not shown. (Reprinted by permission from Simpson, G.G.1951, fig. 31. Insert: Digit of a three-toed horse, *Parahippus leonensis*. Courtesy of Florida Museum of Natural History, Gainesville. Photo by author.)

◆ **Fig. 1.3.** Spring-footed type of the modern horse with main structures involved, schematic illustration.

CDET = common digital extensor tendon, DDFT = deep digital flexor tendon, ICL = inferior check ligament, SDFT = superficial digital flexor tendon, SL= suspensory ligament. Each tendon continues with its corresponding muscle(s).

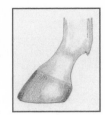

Chapter 2

The Stay Apparatus

THE *stay apparatus* (SA) IS A SYSTEM OF muscles, tendons, ligaments and bones that passively support the limbs and enable the horse to stand with little or no muscular effort (Sisson and Grossman, 1953). During motion, the stay apparatus participates in shock absorption (Smithcors, 1961c) and in the recycling of spring energy (Hildebrand, 1982; Hildebrand 1987). The main structures involved in the stay apparatus of the horse's limbs include the suspensory ligament, the flexor tendons and their check ligaments, and in the hind limb, the patellar locking mechanism. For topographical and directional terms, see chapter 3.

 THE SUSPENSORY LIGAMENT

THE *suspensory ligament* (SL) LIES BETWEEN THE deep digital flexor tendon and the cannon bone; the ligament originates from the palmar aspect of the carpal and cannon bones in the foreleg, and from the plantar area of the cannon bone in the hind leg (♦ fig. 2.1). The ligament descends and splits into two branches at the distal third of the cannon bone; each branch inserts on a *sesamoid bone* at the fetlock joint. The branches continue obliquely as

extensor branches and join the *common digital extensor tendon* on the front of the digit. The SL, sesamoidean bones and sesamoidean ligaments form a strong sling behind the fetlock joint. This sling or *suspensory apparatus*, supports the fetlock joint (Smithcors, 1961a) and prevents its collapse (Bradley and Grahame, 1946).

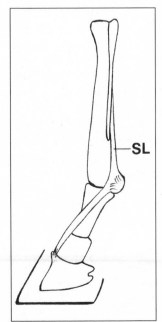

♦ **Fig. 2.1.**
The suspensory ligament (SL) and one extensor branch, schematic illustration.

SL

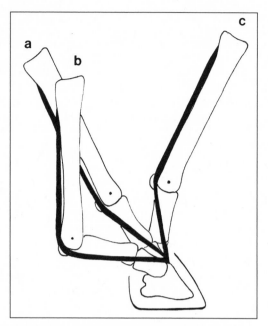

◆ **Fig. 2.2.** Ligamentous spring mechanism, schematic illustration. The position of the fetlock is shown during impact (a), midstance (b) and breakover (c). The suspensory ligament supports the fetlock during the first half of the stance phase; as weight is shifted forward, the ligament bounces the horse forward. (Reprinted by permission by the American Scientist staff, from Hildebrand, M.1987. fig. 5.)

During motion, the angled pastern, together with the suspensory apparatus, reduces the amount of concussion considerably (Smithcors, 1961c). At high speed, the fetlock extends (dorsiflexes) and the digit becomes flexed at the coffin joint. The pastern may form a 90° angle with the cannon bone, and may become nearly horizontal with the ground (◆ fig. 2.2). As the fetlock dorsiflexes, the suspensory ligament stretches. Toward the end of the support phase, the weight of the horse is shifted forward, and the ligament snaps back like a rubber band, releasing recycled spring energy that bounces the horse forward (Hildebrand, 1960). This mechanism is the hallmark of the spring-footed type horse. Schryver et al. (1978) indicated that the deep digital flexor tendon resist the extension of the fetlock joint in the lightly loaded digit dur-

ing walk. As the speed of the animal increases, the contribution of the suspensory ligament and the superficial digital flexor tendon increases.

Several factors may affect the function of the springing mechanism of the fetlock, these include the strength of the suspensory ligament, the conformation of the horse, hoof length and horseshoes. Weak suspensory apparatus may be inherited or develop from repeated insults to the suspensory ligaments. In horses with straight pastern conformation, the fetlock typically yields poorly to weight loads. Consequently, the horse becomes predisposed to injury from increased concussion forces transmitted through the bony column. In addition, the lack of springiness makes the ride on these horses uncomfortable. In horses with sloping pasterns, the opposite effect occurs. During motion, the fetlock joint becomes excessively dorsiflexed, thus predisposing them to suspensory apparatus injuries.

THE FLEXOR TENDONS AND CHECK LIGAMENTS

THE FLEXOR MUSCLES ORIGINATE at the upper limb and descend toward the digit. These muscles continued as flexor tendons at the lower palmar/plantar half of the horse's limb, which insert into the digital bones. The *superficial digital flexor tendon* (SDFT) splits at the pastern into two branches; the first inserts in the first phalanx and the second, which is much stronger, inserts into the second phalanx. The *deep digital flexor tendon* (DDFT) passes beneath the split SDFT, crosses the navicular bone and inserts in the flexor area of the third phalanx. Both flexor tendons of the forelimb and the DDFT of the hind limb have a check ligament that reinforces the tendons by joining them to the bony column (*see* ◆ fig. 1.3). The *check ligament* of the DDFT attaches the tendon to the palmar/plantar aspect of the cannon bone. Being below the check ligament of the SDFT, the check liga-

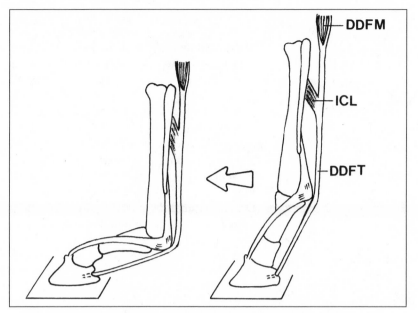

◆ **Fig. 2.3.** Function of the inferior check ligament, schematic illustration. During rest, the check ligament shares load with its flexor muscle. During loading the flexor muscles stretch (relax) until the check ligament is pulled taut. An increase in muscle load is checked (prevented) by transfer of weight from tendon to bone.

DDFT= Deep digital flexor tendon, ICL= Inferior check ligament, DDFM= Deep digital flexor muscle.

ment of the DDFT is termed the *inferior check ligament* (ICL), while the former is termed the *superior check ligament* (SCL).

During rest, the check ligaments assist the animal in maintenance of standing posture with relatively little muscular exertion (Bradley and Grahame, 1946; Shively, 1983). As weight bearing is increased, the check ligaments prevent overstretching of the digital flexor muscles by sharing more loads (Shively, 1983; Sønnichsen, 1982). At breakover, the flexor muscles begin to contract; their corresponding tendons flex the limb while tension is removed from the check ligaments (◆ fig. 2.3); the spring action of the suspensory ligament assist this part of the stance phase.

The check ligaments of the forelimbs are well developed in comparison to these of the hind limbs; this may reflect the higher load that is carried by the forelimbs in addition to the horse's inability to rest one forelimb at a time. The only time that one-forelimb bears weight at rest is when the horse is pointing with a painful limb (Smithcors, 1961a).

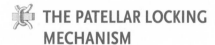 THE PATELLAR LOCKING MECHANISM

UNLIKE THE FORELIMBS, the hind limbs carry less weight and can rest alternatively (Smithcors, 1961b) by the patellar locking mechanism (Hildbrand, 1982). This mechanism relates to the simultaneous motion of the stifle and hock (◆ fig. 2.4). When the stifle extend, the hock extend too by the tendinous superficial digital flexor muscle; this structure is attached to the tuber calcis or point of the hock. Flexion of the stifle results in flexion of the hock by the tendinous *peroneus tertius* (Hildbrand, 1982). Therefore, preventing movement of one joint will result in lack of

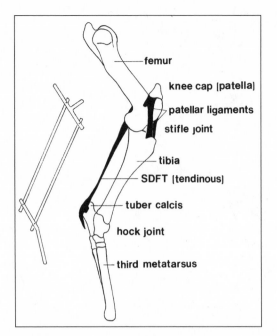

movement of the other joint. Strong ligaments connect the *patellar bone* to the tibia.
These ligaments allow the pulling of the patella by the *quadriceps* muscle over the eminence
(projection) of the femur. When the patella
situates on top of that eminence, the stifle
joint is "locked". Hence, stifle flexion is prevented (Hildbrand 1982; Hildbrand, 1987)
and the hock cannot be flexed. In this locked
position, the limb bears weight with minimal
muscular effort, thus permitting flexion of
the opposite limb into a resting position.
Once the horse begins to move, the patella
unlocks and the two joints can move freely.

◆ **Fig. 2.4.** Patellar locking mechanism. The
structures involved in this mechanism form a
parallelogram that becomes fixed when the patella
is "locked," thus movement of the stifle and hock
is prevented. See text for details. (Reprinted by
permission of the American Scientist staff, from
Hildebrand, M. 1987, fig. 4.)

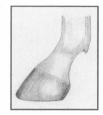

Chapter 3

Structures of the Foot

TOPOGRAPHICAL AND DIRECTIONAL TERMINOLOGY

THE FOLLOWING SECTION INCLUDES topographical and directional terms that appear in the text (Shively, 1982; Adams, 1974; Stashak, 1987) (◆ fig. 3.1).

distal. A topographical term that designates a location far from the trunk.

dorsal. Pertaining to the front part of the limb up to the level of the carpus or tarsus.

lateral. Pertaining to the outer side of the limb.

medial. Pertaining to the inner side of the limb.

palmar. Pertaining to the sole and the back part of the forelimb up to the level of the carpus.

plantar. Pertaining to the sole and the back part of the hind limb up to the level of the tarsus.

proximal. A topographical term that designates a location close to the trunk.

solar. An old term that designates the bottom aspect of the hoof.

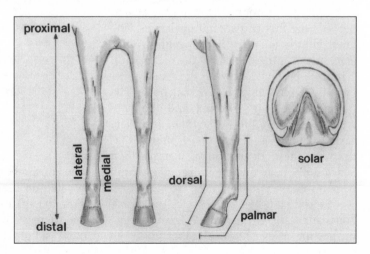

◆ **Fig. 3.1.** Topographical and directional terms of the lower front limbs. (Adapted from Stashak T.S. 1987, fig.1.1.)

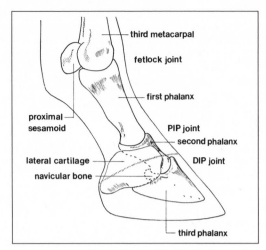

◆ **Fig. 3.2. The digit.** Note the anatomical relationships between the hoof, digital bones and lateral cartilages. (Adapted from Bradley O.C. and Grahame T. 1946, fig. 65. Some terms have been modified to modern terms.)

PIP = proximal interphalangesl (pastern) joint. DIP = distal interphalangeal (coffin) joint.

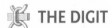

THE DIGIT

THE HORSE'S *digit* IS a homologue (equivalent) of the human middle finger. The digit consist of three main bones: *the first phalanx, second phalanx,* and *third phalanx* bones (Sack and Gabel, 1977), and a smaller bone called the navicular bone (◆ fig. 3.2). The plural of phalanx is *phalanges.* The three digital bones form two joints; the upper joint is the *proximal interphalangeal* (PIP) *joint,* or as commonly called, the pastern joint. This joint is shared between the first and second phalanges. The lower joint is the *distal interphalangeal* (DIP) *joint,* or as commonly called, the coffin joint. This joint is shared between the second phalanx, third phalanx and navicular bone. The cannon bone, first phalanx and the two-sesamoidean bones form the *fetlock joint.* The cannon bone is a common name that describes the *third metacarpal* bone or *third metatarsal* bone of the forelimb and hind limb respectively.

Supporting ligaments reinforce the digital bones and stabilize the digit. These ligaments include the *collateral ligaments* that attach the

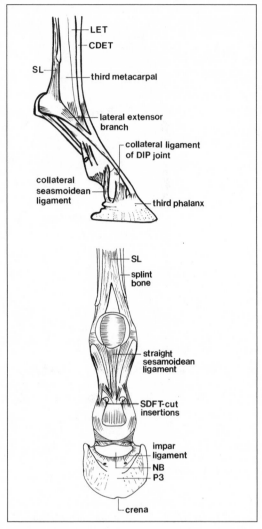

◆ **Fig. 3.3.** Ligaments of the digit, lateral and palmar views. (Adapted from Bradley O.C. and Graham T. 1946, figs. 66 and 67. Not all structures are shown, some terms have been modified to modern terms.)

LET = Lateral extensor tendon. CDET = Common digital extensor tendon. SL = Suspensory ligament. DIP = Distal interphalangeal (coffin) joint. SDFT = Superficial digital flexor tendon. NB = Navicular bone. P3 = Third phalanx.

sides of the bones, the *sesamoidean ligaments* situated on the palmar/plantar aspect of the digit, the ligaments of the navicular bone, and the extensor branches of the suspensory ligament (◆ fig. 3.3). Several ligaments attach the

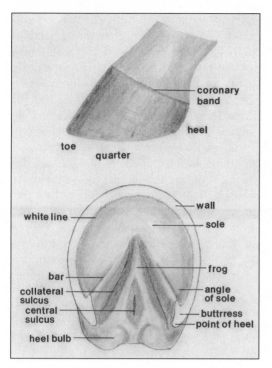

◆ **Fig. 3.4.** Topography of the hoof. Lateral and solar views. (Solar view adapted from Bradley O.C. and Grahame T. 1946, fig. 60. Some terms have been modified to modern terms.)

lateral cartilages to the digital bones (Bradley and Grahame, 1946).

THE EXTERNAL PARTS OF THE HOOF

THE *hoof capsule* IS A MODIFIED *epidermis* consisting mostly of hard keratin. The hoof wall includes the horny part of the hoof that is visible when the horse stands. The wall is divided into three regions: toe, quarters and heels. The *toe* includes the dorsal area of the hoof wall, the *quarters* include the medial and lateral sides of the hoof wall, and the *heels* include the palmar or plantar area of the hoof wall (◆ fig. 3.4). A thin layer of soft horn called *periople* covers the proximal surface of the hoof wall.

The *solar* aspect of the hoof includes the bearing surface of the hoof wall, the bars,

sole, frog, white line and portion of the bulbs of the heels. At the heels, the hoof wall turns inward, forward, and continues as the *bars*. The curved area that is formed between the heels and the bars is called the *buttress*.

The *white line*, or white zone, borders the sole and the hoof wall and forms a tight seal between the two structures. The *sole* occupies the area between the white line and frog. The sole of the domestic horse is concave and bears very little weight directly (Smithcors, 1961a), thus, during motion, it is less susceptible to impact forces (Thomas, 1998) and more protected against bruising. Ovnicek (1996) indicated that the sole of wild horses is flat, bears weight and supports the third phalanx. The *angle of the sole* is the area between the bars and hoof wall. This area is prone to bruising caused by excessive pressure. A common name for this site is the *seat of corn* (Johnson and Asquith, 1993).

The frog is a soft cornified triangular structure situated in the palmar/plantar 2/3 of the sole. It protects the bottom of the foot while permitting expansion of the hoof wall during motion. The two grooves formed between the sole and frog are termed *collateral sulci* or commissures; the groove in the middle of the frog is termed the *central sulcus* or cleft of the frog.

THE FOOT AND ITS CONTENTS

THE *foot* INCLUDES THE HOOF and all the structures within it up to the level of the coronary band (Bradley and Grahame, 1946; Sisson and Grossman, 1953). The *coronary band* or coronet is a narrow strip that borders the hoof capsule and skin. The bones within the foot include the third phalanx, the navicular bone, and part of the second phalanx.

The *third phalanx* is an enlarged and modified bone that is similar in shape to the hoof. The bone is firmly attached to the inner portion of the hoof wall by strong laminated structures that suspend it within the foot (◆ fig. 3.5). This anatomical arrangement prevents direct weight bearing by the third pha-

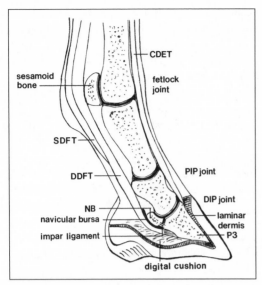

◆ **Figure 3.5.** Longitudinal section of the digit.
(Adapted from Bradley, O.C. and Grahame, T. 1946,
fig. 61. Some terms have been modified to modern
terms.)

P3 = Third phalanx. NB = Navicular bone. PIP =
Proximal interphalangeal (pastern) joint. DIP =
Distal interphalangeal (coffin) joint. DDFT = Deep
digital flexor tendon. SDFT = Superficial digital
flexor tendon. CDET = Common digital extensor
tendon.

lanx on the sole. In the normal foot, the dorsal border of the third phalanx is parallel with the hoof wall. The solar margin of the third phalanx is not parallel to the ground. In most cases, the palmar/plantar margin is higher and slopes toward the toe. The angle formed by the solar margin relative to the ground is termed the *angle of the third phalanx*. The spatial relationship of the third phalanx to the hoof capsule is important when dealing with laminitis. The distal margins of the third phalanx are scalloped by vascular channels that transect the bone. A larger notch may appear at the center of the dorsal margin. This notch, which is described in some texts as *crena* (toe notch) is normal. Situated on the third phalanx are the insertion areas for the extensor and flexor tendons, which counter each other. The *common digital extensor tendon* (CDET) is inserted into a protrusion located on the dorsal aspect of the bone.

This protrusion is termed the *extensor process*. The deep digital flexor tendon (DDFT) inserts into the flexor area that is located at the palmar/plantar surface of the bone. A pair of *lateral cartilages* increases the size of the internal framework of the foot further. These cartilages are also termed the ungual cartilages of the third phalanx. The lateral cartilages are attached to the wings of the third phalanx, and continue backward to form a rigid framework that provides support to the palmar/plantar aspect of the foot. The proximal part of the lateral cartilages protrudes above the coronary band (see ◆ fig.3.2). The thickness of the lateral cartilages varies among horses, and may represent variations in foot conformation among horses (Bowker et al., 1998).

The space between the lateral cartilages contains a wedge-shaped structure made of fibro-elastic tissue. This structure is the *digital cushion*. The digital cushion is bordered by the DDFT dorsally, by the bulbs of the heels at the palmar/plantar area, and by the frog at the solar area. The digital cushion aids in circulation of the foot by permitting expansion and contraction of neighboring structures (Butzow, 1961; Taylor et al., 2005). It is also involved in shock absorption during motion. Bowker et al. (1998) indicated that the tissue composition of the digital cushion varies considerably among horses and this variation may be the result of environmental stimuli.

The *navicular bone* is a small boat-shaped bone situated at the palmar/plantar aspect of the DIP joint, and sharing that joint with the second and third phalanges. The navicular bone is attached into place by the navicular *suspensory and impar ligaments* (◆ fig.3.5). The bone functions as a pulley for the deep digital flexor tendon that passes around the flexor surface of the bone, and continues dorsally to insert into the *semi-lunar* crest, or flexor area, of the third phalanx (Butzow, 1961). In addition, the navicular bone protects the DDFT during motion by maintaining a constant angle of insertion for the tendon that prevents tearing of the tendon at its insertion point (Rooney, 1974a). Located between the navicular bone and the DDFT is a small, fluid-filled cavity called the *navicular bursa*. This structure reduces friction between the navicular bone and DDFT. The impar ligament forms a seal between the navicular bursa and the DIP joint (Gibson et al., 1990). Penetrating wounds that involve the navicular bursae pose a serious threat to the horse.

The Dermis

The dermal structures of the foot are called *dermis*. The dermis forms the inner layer beneath the horn and it is rich in blood vessels and nerves. The term dermis is equivalent to corium, which is an old term commonly used in textbooks.

The dermis maintains the growth of the hoof by nourishing and supporting the epidermis or horn structures. The dermis is divided into five regions: the perioplic, coronary, sole, frog, and laminar dermis (◆ fig. 3.6). A sixth region may be reserved for the terminal horn that is associated with the white line. All regions of the dermis, except that of the perioplic dermis, produce *hard keratin*. The keratin is produced by epithelial cells called *keratinocytes* that are located on the outer surface of the dermis. The *perioplic dermis* produces the periople, which is made of soft keratin. The importance of the periople is not clear although it may form a seal between the skin and hoof wall.

The surfaces of all the dermis, except that of the laminar dermis, are roughened by minute projecting structures called *dermal papillae*. Each of these papillae fits into a corresponding *epidermal peg* or socket situated on the equivalent horn. Horn growth from the papillae give rise to tubular structures called *horn tubule* (see below). Each dermal papilla is responsible for the maintenance of a single horn tubule (Pollit, 1995). Each horn tubule is made of several concentric layers of keratinized epithelial cells. The horn tubules on the outer portion of the hoof wall are smaller, more numerous and elliptical in cross section (Nickel, 1938). Normally, the horn tubules grow in the direction of hoof growth. The spaces between the dermal papillae produce less organized horn called *intertubular horn* (Smithcors, 1961a).

The Horn Tubules

The mechanical properties of the hoof wall have been attributed to the structural arrangement of the horn tubules (◆ fig. 3.7). Rooney (1974a) proposed that the structure of the

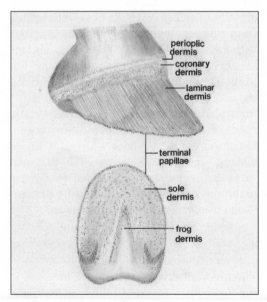

◆ **Fig. 3.6.** The dermis of the foot. Lateral and solar views. (Adapted from Bradley, O.C. and Grahame, T. 1946, fig. 56, 57. Terms have been modified to modern terms.)

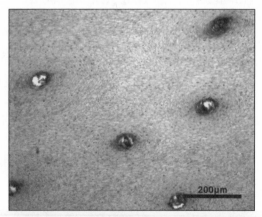

◆ **Fig. 3.7.** Microscopic cross section of hoof wall showing the horn tubules situated within the intertubular horn. (Photo courtesy of Prof. H. Geyer, University of Zurich.)

horn tubules provides elasticity to the hoof wall. Butler (1977a) proposed that the anatomy of the rigid, closely spaced, flattened horn tubules in the external portion of the hoof wall reduces evaporation loss from the hoof. Bertram and Gosline (1986) indicated that the tubular and intertubular horn form a series composite that responds more uniformly to loading in different directions. Reilly et al. (1998a) described four zones of decreasing horn tubule density from the outer toward the inner layers; these differences in tubular morphology may facilitate load transfer and prevent failure (Reilly et al., 1996), which could result in wall cracks (Kasapi and Gosline, 1998). Thomason et al. (1992) indicated that wall cracks propagate parallel to the horn tubules along the weakest plane, but they do not extend to the inner layers because of the high water content that gives high crack resistance.

The Laminar Dermis

Deep at the coronary band the dermal papillae are replaced by small plates (laminar structures) termed *dermal laminae*. The dermal laminae, which are the basic structures responsible for laminar horn growth, fit into corresponding *epidermal laminae* or epidermal ridges (Pollit, 1995). Most of the laminar horn production takes place at this laminar growth zone at the coronary band. More distally, the majority of the laminae are less productive and involved in suspension of the third phalanx within the hoof (Daradka and Pollitt, 2004). Growth of the epidermal laminae occurs from the coronary band downward, together with the rest of the hoof wall, but it is supported and nourished by dermal laminae throughout its entire length. Therefore, the *laminar dermis* includes the area of laminar growth and the area of laminar support.

Horn production at the dermal laminae gives rise to closely spaced keratinized plates of horn that form the inner part of the hoof wall. These plates are the epidermal laminae. There are about 600 *primary epidermal lami-*

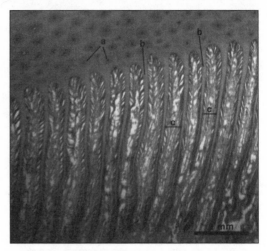

◆ **Fig. 3.8.** Microscopic cross section of the hoof wall showing horn tubules (a), primary epidermal (b) and dermal laminae (c). (Photo courtesy of Prof. H. Geyer, University of Zurich.)

nae; these laminae can be seen with the naked eye. The primary epidermal laminae are firmly attached in a dovetail fashion to corresponding plates of *primary dermal laminae*. The dermal laminae are attached to the third phalanx by connective tissue. The strength of the laminar bond is enhanced by 60-120 *secondary dermal and epidermal laminae* that branch from the primary laminae and interdigitate with each other (◆ Fig. 3.8). The large surface area created by the laminar pattern is the key to the strength of this bond (Coffman et al., 1970). This firm *laminar bond* suspends the third phalanx within the hoof (Budras et al., 1998). The dermal laminae also form a gliding surface for the hoof wall as it grows distally. Leach and Oliphant (1983b) proposed that microscopic structures called *desmosomes* maintain detachment and attachment between the dermal and epidermal layers.

The White Line

The union of epidermal laminae (situated at the inner distal surface of the hoof wall) and of *terminal horn* (produced by *terminal papillae* situated at the distal margins of the dermal laminae) forms the *white line* (Pollit, 1995;

Budras et al., 1998) (see ◆ fig. 3.6). The terminal horn is soft and relatively dark; it fills the spaces between the neighboring horny laminae (Budras et al., 1998) and forms a seal between the sole and the hoof wall (Pollit, 1995).

Budras et al. (1998) indicated that the white line serves as a barrier against ascending bacteria. Wagner et al. (2001) proposed that the white line serves as a mechanical buffer zone between the rigid hoof wall and the laminar interfaces, which permits normal hoof wall and third phalanx displacement and deformation during motion.

Blood Circulation

Blood circulation to the foot is maintained by the *digital arteries* and *digital veins* that course the lateral and medial aspects of the digit. These vessels branch at the level of the pastern into dorsal and palmar (or plantar) vessels and enter the foot (◆ fig. 3.9). Blood reaches the foot via the arteries, enters the capillaries and returns to the heart via the veins. In addition, the foot contain several areas of rich vein networks called *venous plexuses*. Venous plexuses can be found in the coronary band and in the inner surface of the lateral cartilages.

The veins of the horse's foot do not contain valves that prevent backflow of blood, thus the return of blood from the foot toward the heart is maintained by the pumping action of the foot. As weight is placed on the foot, the internal structures within it are compressed, venous pressure is increased and blood is pumped upwards. This pumping mechanism is observable following laceration injuries to the pastern, as blood spurts from a severed digital vein each time the horse bears weight on the limb (Smithcors, 1961c). Ratzlaff et al. (1985) and Bowker et al. (1998) proposed that the veins of the horse's foot might attenuate shock during motion (see chapter 8).

Blood flow to the foot may be altered in various lameness conditions. Excessive weight bearing on a supporting limb (healthy

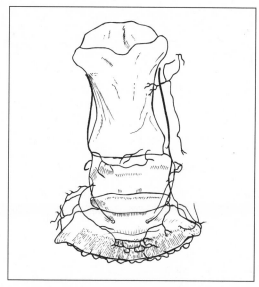

◆ **Fig. 3.9.** Blood supply to the foot, palmar view, schematic illustration. (Adapted from Bradley, O.C., Grahame, T. 1946, fig. 48.)

limb) in lameness conditions reduce circulation to the toe wall area (Redden, 2003). Low hoof angle may reduce circulation to the heel area (Colles, 1983b). Painful conditions of the foot cause an increased pulse in the digital arteries. This pulse is felt by placing the fingers against the digital arteries at a level slightly below the sesamoidean bones. An increased *digital pulse* may be an early indication for development of laminitis.

The Digital Nerves

The *digital nerves* course along the lateral and medial sides of the digit along with the digital arteries and veins (◆ fig. 3.10). At the pastern level, each nerve branches into dorsal and palmar/plantar nerves. These nerves continue to branch as they innervate the foot (Schumacher et al., 2004). Most of the nerves of the foot are sensory nerves that are involved in the production (and detection) of lameness. Other nerves are involved in *proprioceptive impulses* that are responsible for positional awareness of the feet by the horse (Smithcors, 1961c).

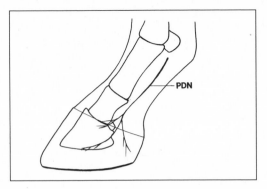

◆ **Fig. 3.10.** The palmar digital nerve (PDN) and its branches, schematic illustration. The palmar digital nerve provides deep branches to the DIP joint and navicular bursa, and branches to the heel region and sole. (Adapted from Schumacher, J., et al. 2004, fig. 10.)

Selective regional anesthesia (foot block) of the foot with local anesthetics is applied in diagnostic and surgical procedures. The palmar digital nerve (PDN) is commonly anesthetized as part of the diagnosis of navicular disease and other lameness conditions. Neurectomy or surgical transection of the palmar digital nerve is a procedure used in horses with severe chronic lameness in order to reduce pain and, in specific circumstances, maintain their usefulness.

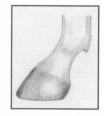

Chapter 4

Hoof Conformation

GOOD *hoof conformation* IS EXTREMELY important for proper hoof function. Hoof conformation is determined by genetic and environmental factors. Genetic factors determine the general shape of the hoof, hoof size and proportion to body weight, horn thickness and horn qualities such as toughness and brittleness. Environmental factors affect the shape of the hoof through the forces that are applied to it during contact with the ground; alteration of these forces may be caused by abnormal limb conformation, imbalance, lameness conditions, horseshoes and horseshoe adjuncts. Other factors that may affect the shape and quality of the hoof include environmental moisture and salts. The effect of the environment on hoof shape is more noticeable in horses with poor hoof quality and it can seriously impair their use. Other causes that may lead to development of abnormal hoof conformation include foot diseases, direct trauma, and injuries above the foot. Hoof conformation is commonly evaluated subjectively for the purpose of prepurchase examination, treatment of lameness, and prior to trimming or shoeing.

HOOF SHAPE AND OUTLINE

THE *hoof's shape and outline* CHANGE continuously throughout the life of the horse. These changes may be caused by the effect of wear between hoof trimming, water loss or gain, environmental stimulus or disease. Observation and evaluation of these alterations is an important part of therapeutic farriery.

The general shape of the hoof is similar to a tipped cone that was cut at the upper section. The cone-like hoof has the ideal shape for meeting stress (Rooney, 1974a; Leach in Kilby, 1982). The open area at the bulbs of the heels and the sloping hoof wall permit expansion of the hoof when it is loaded (Colles, 1989a). The bottom of the hoof is concave; deep concavity forms a structure that resists mechanical loads better than a flat hoof can. (Redden, 2003). There are breed variations in hoof shape and outline among horses, for example, a flat and thick sole is more typical to draft horses, whereas a concave and thin sole is more typical in Thoroughbred horses.

Although hooves of opposite limbs may have a mirror image of each other, the hoof is an asymmetrical structure. There are no two hooves that are alike. The curve of the hoof at the lateral quarter is wider than the curve of the medial quarter (◆ fig. 4.1). Hence, the angle of the hoof wall formed with the ground plane is slightly steeper on the medial aspect of the hoof than on the lateral aspect of the hoof (Bradley and Grahame, 1946; Mackay-Smith, 1993). Therefore, trimming the hoof in order to establish equal lengths at the medial and lateral sides will result in a hoof that is out of balance (Butzow, 1961). A study (Roland et al., 2003) on geometric symmetry of hooves in Thoroughbred racehorses showed that the lateral hoof width, measured at the widest part of the hoof, was 3 percent greater than the medial width. In another study (Kane et al., 1998), the difference was 7 percent. This asymmetry places the center point of the natural hoof slightly off center (Bradley and Grahame, 1946). However, a study on 91 fore and hind hooves from a mixed population of horses showed that the hoof *center of mass* (COM) relative to the medio-lateral plane did not vary significantly, and the hoof was symmetrical about its center plane (Arabian et al., 2001).

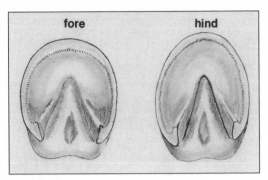

◆ **Fig. 4.2.** Solar outline of fore and hind hooves, solar view. (Adapted from Bradley, O.C., Grahame, T. 1946, fig.60.)

The *solar outline* of the fore and hind hooves is different. The outline of the fore-hoof is larger and more round, whereas the outline of the hind hoof is smaller, narrower and more pointed (◆ fig. 4.2). This difference is attributed to limb function. Blombach (1994) indicated that the round shape of the forehoof facilitates breakover at the center of the foot while the more tapered hind hoof allows the horse to pivot and push off from the medial or lateral side.

The hoof angle may affect the solar outline of the hoof as can be observed when comparing horses with long-toe low-heels to horses with short-toe high-heels (Glade and Salzman, 1985). The shape of the hoof outline tends to change between shoeings, with a tendency toward development of long-toe low-heels hoof conformation; this change results from more wear at the palmar/plantar aspect of the hoof.

The shape of the hoof may be affected by wear caused by abnormal limb conformation. Toeing-out in the barefoot horse leads to development of a hoof outline that is characterized by wear at the medial toe wall and flaring lateral quarter. The opposite changes are observed in horses that toe-in.

Several disease conditions, such as navicular disease, may alter the hoof shape and outline and are commonly accompanied by a hoof with a short outline from toe to heel caused by excessive toe wear and increased

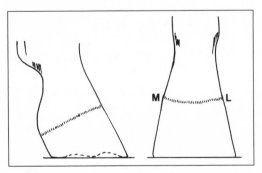

◆ **Fig. 4.1.** Hoof shape. The side view shows the sole and frog outline (broken line). The dorsal view shows a steeper medial side (M) compared to the lateral side (L).

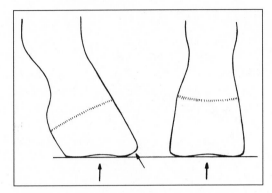

◆ **Fig. 4.3.** The effect of hard soil on hoof shape, side and dorsal views. The arrows indicate areas of increased wear. (Adapted from Rooney, J.R. 1999, fig. 3.)

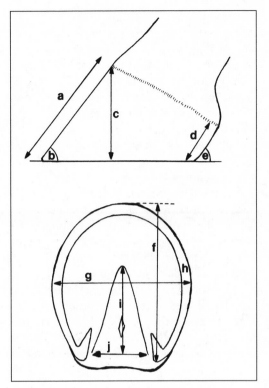

◆ **Fig. 4.4.** Hoof parameters. Side view: toe length (a), hoof angle (b), hoof height (c), heel length (d), heel angle (e). Solar view: hoof length (f), hoof width (g), hoof wall thickness (h), frog length (i), frog width (j).

growth of the heels. The solar outline of a contracted hoof may resemble that of a mule. This condition may be accompanied by *frog atrophy* characterized by increased frog ratio (page 23).

The shape of the hoof capsule in the barefoot horse may be affected by *frictional forces* created during hoof contact with the ground. The type of soil and the amount of exercise determine the degree of wear. Horses that live on soft ground roll their hooves into the ground as they move. This leaves the bearing surface of the hoof fairly level. Horses that live on hard, rocky ground, wear the center of the toe and the quarters. As a result, the toes become rolled and shorter and the quarters become arched (Rooney, 1999a) (◆ fig. 4.3).

 HOOF DIMENSIONS

THE *hoof dimensions* INCLUDE VARIOUS ANGLES, lengths and ratios measured at the hoof capsule. These measurements are used to evaluate hoof conformation and balance, and to compare hooves of different horses. Measurements of hoof dimensions include the hoof angle, heel angle, toe and heel length, hoof height, frog ratio, wall thickness, hoof width and length, and various ratios (◆ fig. 4.4).

Hoof Angle

The *hoof angle* is the angle formed between the center of the toe wall and the solar surface. Measurement of the hoof angle provides an important parameter with regard to foot balance. The data on recommended hoof angles in the literature is quite variable. Rick (1907) recommended that the feet be trimmed to establish a 53° for the foreleg and 58° for the hind legs, but he did not provided a range of optimal angles for the fore and hind hooves. Butzow (1961) indicated that the first phalanx should form an angle of about 55° with the ground. Recommended hoof angles for Standardbred horses vary between an average of 48° in the front feet of trotters, and 54° in the hind feet of trotters and pacers

(Simpson, 1968). According to Stashak, (1987) and Adams (1974) the recommended hoof angles of 45° to 50° for the forelimbs, and 50° to 55° for the hind limbs, is erroneous; these hoof angles are rarely appropriate for the conformation of the horse's individual limbs (Balch et al., 1995a). Smyth and Goody (1972) indicated that native Welsh ponies have upright feet with hoof angle of 50° to 60° compared to 45° to 50° in Thoroughbreds and half-bred horses.

Establishment of proper hoof angle relates primarily to the inclination of the horse's digit. For most horses, the hooves are trimmed at an angle of 50° to 54° for the forelimb and the 53° to 57° for the hind limbs (Butler, 1985; Balch and Metcalf, 1990).

The hoof angle of the barefooted horse may be affected by the environment. A study that compared three groups of feral horses showed that as the ground becomes harder, the hoof angle decreases. The hoof angle of the front feet ranged from 57° to 68° in horses that live on soft sand, 54° to 62° in horses that live on sandy packed sod and gravel, and 51° to 57° in horses that live on hard rocky environment (Ovnicek, 1996). Measurements of hoof angle in a different study on feral horses showed a range of 50° to 60° in the fore and hind feet (Jackson, 1997).

Variations in hoof angle can affect the horse's performance and lead to lameness. In a study of 95 Thoroughbred racehorses, successful horses tended to have a higher hoof angle, whereas lower hoof angles were associated with musculoskeletal problems that prevented racing or training (Kobluk et al. 1990). Low hoof angle has been linked experimentally with navicular syndrome (Colles, 1983b) and with strained deep digital flexor tendons (Lochner et al., 1980). A study on a group of horses with under-run heels (collapsed heels) showed that for 1° of reduction in the angle of the third phalanx, the force exerted by the DDFT on the navicular bone at the beginning of the stance phase increased by 20 percent (Eliashar et al., 2004). Abnormally high hoof angle may result in excessive strain on the common digital extensor tendon.

Heel Angle

The *heel angle* is the angle formed between the palmar/plantar aspect of the heel and the ground. Ideally, the heel should be parallel to the hoof angle. Large differences between the hoof angle and heel angle is common in horses with under-run heels. This difference is less pronounced in horses with long-toe low-heel hoof conformation.

Toe Length

Measurement of *toe length* is an important parameter of hoof balance. The toe length is measured at the center of the dorsal hoof wall from the coronary rim to the margin of the hoof wall. The *coronary rim* is a depression located approximately at the hair borderline (Balch et al., 1998a). Alternatively, the hair borderline or a constant distance below it may be used.

When toe length is established, the horse's height, weight, and type of work should be considered (Turner, 1992; Balch et al., 1995a). In addition, the length of the toe depends on whether the horse is barefoot or shod (Balch et al., 1995a). Traditionally, Standardbred racehorses are trimmed with long toes in order to increase the stride length (Simpson, 1968; Balch et al., 1991b) although this method has not been shown to be effective (Balch et al.,1994). Similarly, lengthening the toes in Thoroughbred racehorses in Japan did not result in a longer stride (Tanaka, 1998).

Bradley and Grahame (1946) indicated that the hoof wall lengths for the toe, quarter and heel form ratios of 3:2:1 for the forelimb, and 2:1.5:1 for the hind limb. Turner (1992) indicated that the length of the heel should generally be one third of the length of the toe. Due to individual and breed variations, these ratios should be used as guidelines only.

Hoof Height

Hoof height describes the general position of the foot in relation to the ground. When proper hoof angle and toe length are established, the hoof height is optimal. Because hoof height continuously changes with hoof growth and wear, maintenance of proper trimming and shoeing intervals is important.

The Frog Ratio

The *frog ratio* is the ratio between the frog width and length, measured at the widest and longest points (Turner, 1992; Kane et al., 1999). Contracted hooves have frog width that is less than 67 percent of the frog's length (Turner, 1992).

Hoof Horn Thickness

The *hoof horn thickness* is determined by genetic factors, and by growth and wear. Horn thickness may vary according to location on the hoof capsule and breed variations. The hoof wall is thickest at the toe where maximum strain is being concentrated at the breakover point. From the toe toward the heel, the horn thickness tapers gradually and then increases again at the buttress. The relatively thin wall at the quarters and heels permits normal hoof expansion (deformation) during weight bearing.

The hoof wall has to be thick enough in order to absorb concussion forces efficiently. Thin-walled hooves have limited shock absorption capability, which predisposes the horse to concussion-related lameness and hoof wall cracks; unfortunately thin hoof wall conformation is common. In addition, driving horseshoe nails in hooves with thin walls is difficult and can result in injury.

Under natural conditions, the sole sheds away regularly as the outer insensitive sole dries and become flaky. This normal shedding is accompanied by distinct shedding of the frog semiannually (Smithcors, 1961c; Balch et al., 1991b). Natural shedding of the sole and frog may be interrupted by hoof wear and by hoof trimming. Various measurements of normal hoof horn thickness, at different locations on the hoof capsule can be found in Steckel et al. (1989).

Hoof Width and Hoof Length

The *hoof width* is measured at widest part of the hoof. Since the hoof is not symmetrical, these points may not be perpendicular to the long axis of the hoof when an imaginary line connects them. The *hoof length* is a line measured from the point of the heel along the long axis of the hoof up to the level of the toe (◆ fig. 4.4).

Ratio of Hoof Wall Thickness to Hoof Width

The *ratio of hoof wall thickness to hoof wall width* is obtained by measuring the hoof width at its widest part, and the hoof wall thickness at that point (◆ fig 4.4). These measurements can be obtained with calipers. To keep measurements constant, the hoof wall thickness is measured from the outer hoof wall to the beginning of the white line. Measurement should be taken immediately following hoof trimming in order to minimize the effect of contraction due to moisture loss.

The ratio obtained from the two measurements provides a value that can be used for comparison between horses. The ratio of body weight to hoof size may be added to the comparison.

THE HOOF LEVER ARM

THE *hoof lever arm* (HLA) IS A FULCRUM that is measured from the center of rotation of the DIP joint to the tip of the toe wall (◆ fig. 4.5). The *center of rotation* (COR) of a joint is the pivot point of the joint. The COR of the DIP joint is located at the distal 1/3 of the second phalanx; this point is measured by extending the joint arc into a circle and finding the center of the circle (Craig et al., 2001). As can be seen, the length of the HLA is affected by hoof growth, trimming and shoeing.

The HLA has significant affect on locomotion. During motion, the DDFT flexes the digit and the hoof begins to cut into the

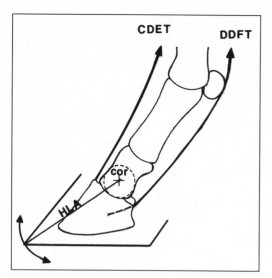

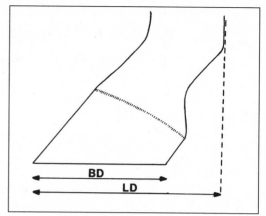

◆ Fig. 4.5. The hoof lever arm. The DDFT and CDET oppose each other around the fulcrum created by the HLA.

HLA= hoof lever arm, COR= center of rotation of the DIP joint, DDFT= deep digital flexor tendon, CDET= common digital extensor tendon.

◆ Fig. 4.6. Support dimensions of the foot, lateral view. (Reprinted with permission from Snow, V.E. and Birdsall, P.D. 1990, fig. 5. Illustration modified to text.

BD=Base distance, LD= Load distance.

ground prior to breakover; any increase in the length of the HLA requires more force to rotate the foot, hence more tension is placed on the DDFT. Another factor that is involved is *ground resistance,* which depends on the type of soil the horse is moving on. Soft ground has relatively low resistance and the foot can rotate into the ground easily, thus the effective length of HLA is diminished (see ◆ fig. 8.4). Hard ground resists the rotation of the foot and the DDFT has to function against the full fulcrum of the HLA in order to lift the limb. Therefore, an increase in the hoof lever arm and ground resistance predisposes the horse to stay apparatus injuries. A common predisposing factor for this type of injury is long-toe low-heel hoof conformation.

 SUPPORT DIMENSIONS OF THE FOOT

THE *support dimensions of the foot* DESCRIBE two parameters of foot balance. These parameters are the base distance and the load distance of the foot (Snow and Birdsall, 1990). The *base distance* (BD) is the distance from toe to heel, or the hoof length, viewed from the side. The *load distance* (LD) is the distance from the toe to a point where a perpendicular line is dropped from the palmar/plantar aspect of the fetlock to the ground (◆ fig. 4.6). Snow and Birdsall (1990) indicated that the base distance should be at least 60 percent of the load distance; at this point, the heels are typically positioned directly beneath the center of the cannon bone (see below). Actual measurements of the support dimensions of the foot are not taken, but established intuitively as the farrier balances the foot.

Several factors affect the ratio between the support dimensions, including hoof growth, foot balance, abnormal foot conformation, horseshoes and horseshoe adjuncts. The base distance is determined primarily by hoof wear, horseshoes and horseshoe adjuncts, whereas the load distance is determined primarily by hoof growth and limb conformation. As the hoof grows in a dorsal-distal direction, the position of the base distance is shifted forward. If wear is even, the length of the base distance remains constant while the length of the load distance increases. Thus, the ratio between the two parame-

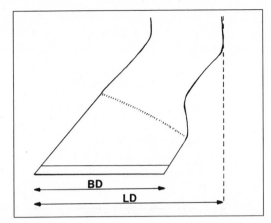

◆ **Fig. 4.7.** The effect of hoof growth on the support dimensions of the foot with the same growth at the bearing surface, note that the base distance remains constant and the load distance increases in length.

BD=Base distance, LD= Load distance.

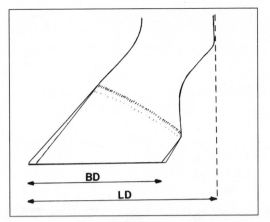

◆ **Fig. 4.8.** The effect of hoof growth on the support dimensions of the foot when hoof growth is accompanied by wear at the quarters and heels. Both the base distance and the load distance increases in length.

BD=Base distance, LD= Load distance.

ters changes and the base distance become relatively smaller (◆ fig. 4.7). More commonly, hoof growth is accompanied by excessive wear at the bearing surface of the quarters and heel resulting in acute hoof angle; in this case, both the base distance and load distance are increased and the ratio between the two parameters may not change as in the first example (◆ fig. 4.8). However, the long toe that develops increases the hoof lever arm and the risk for suspensory apparatus failure.

Other factors that alter the support dimension of the foot include abnormal foot conformation such as clubfoot and under-run heels (◆ fig. 4.9). An increase in the load distance can be observed in sloping pasterns, and a decrease in base distance results from application of beveled horseshoes. In some cases, the proportions between the support dimensions of the foot can be improved with therapeutic horseshoes. Factors that alter the HLA and the support dimensions of the foot may affect the palmar/plantar support of the digit (see chapter 9).

Heels Position

Ideally, the *position of the heels* should be at a point where a perpendicular line that bisects

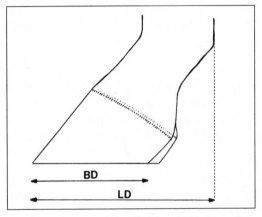

◆ **Fig. 4.9.** The effect of under-run heels on the support dimensions of the foot.

BD=Base distance, LD= Load distance.

the cannon bone reaches the points of the heels when viewed from the side (Balch, 1991a); note that this line is more dorsal than a line that transects the limb. Normal conformational variations among horses may affect heels position.

BODY SIZE TO HOOF RATIO

THE *body size to hoof ratio* DESCRIBES THE proportion of the horse's weight to its feet. The weight may be compared to the *solar surface area*, which includes the area occupied by the hoof wall outline and a line made between the corners of the heels (Kane et al., 1999). During motion, loads are being transmitted to the ground through the solar surface area (Bertram and Gosline, 1986). Horses with small feet have poor ability to absorb shock, and become predisposed to concussion related lameness. Turner (1988) indicated small feet are more common in horses afflicted with navicular disease.

Based on the proportions between the upper limb-bones relative to the lower limb-bones, fossil researchers in the early 1900s concluded that the horse has reached the limit where large body size provides speed, and that any further increase in size will result in slower speed or increased injuries (Simpson, 1951). Domestication of the horse resulted in increased in body size, aimed at producing stronger draft horses, faster racehorses and more impressive show horses. Consequently, many horse breeds have developed smaller feet relative to body size, accompanied by myriad of foot disorders.

Since small feet are a very common hoof conformation, calculating the body size to hoof ratio for comparison between horses can be an important tool in selecting horses. Small feet have been defined as a weight to hoof ratio of greater than 78 pounds per square inch (Turner, 1992). In a different study, a ratio of 83 pounds per square inch was applied (Turner, 1986). This ratio can be calculated for the forelimb using the following formula:

12.56 x wt /C²

The horse's weight **(wt)** in pounds is multiply by 12.56, and than divided by the hoof wall circumference **(C)** squared. The hoof circumference is measured in inches immediately below the coronary band and around the foot (Turner, 1992). The approximate weight of the horse can be obtained by measuring its girth with a weight tape (Lewis, 1982).

Kaneps et al. (1998) calculated the approximate bearing surface area in young foals by using the calculation for ellipse:

π/4 x hoof length x hoof width

Estimation of hoof size can be made by comparing horses, but the hoof length, age of the horse, and breed variations have to be considered. Overgrown hooves and flat feet may give the impression of oversize. The body size to hoof ratio of obese horses can be improved by exercising the horse and correcting its diet.

LAMINAR SURFACE AREA

THE SUSPENSION OF THE THIRD PHALANX WITHIN the foot is maintained by the bond between the dermal and epidermal laminae. The direct area of contact between these two structures is about 25 square inches (Kilby, 1982), whereas the dovetail arrangement between the laminae increase this *laminar surface area* to an area of eight to nine square feet (Smithcors, 1961c, Butzow, 1961). The large surface area reduces the distribution of the horse's weight per unit area (Smithcors, 1961c) and makes the suspension of the third phalanx possible.

The laminar surface area appears to be proportional to hoof size and hoof wall thickness. If this is the case, horses with good body weight to hoof ratio should have a strong bond between the dermal and epidermal laminae. A strong bond implies better attachment of the suspended third phalanx and better dissipation of shock by the laminae. Hooves with a stronger bond between the dermal and epidermal laminae may resist laminitis better and recover better from the disease. Cripps and Eustace (1999) indicated that horses with wide, flat feet with poorly developed heels, and thin walls and sole are more sensitive to laminitis compared to horses with more upright foot and stronger horn. If the laminar surface area is positively correlated with better tolerance to disease, it can be used as a tool for selection of horses with better feet.

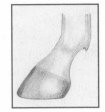

Chapter 5

The Hoof Capsule

 HORN PRODUCTION

THE PROCESS OF HORN PRODUCTION IS TERMED *cornification*. Cornification begins with the synthesis of *hard keratin* by epidermal cells termed *keratinocytes* (◆ fig. 5.1). The keratin that is being produced becomes incorporated into the internal skeleton of the keratinocyte cells. Production continues with the synthesis of sulfur-rich proteins that form the cell envelope (Grosenbaugh and Hood, 1993); the stability of the keratin is enhanced by *disulfide cross links* within its molecular structure (Bertram and Gosline, 1986). Protein production is followed by secretion of lipids that bond adjacent keratinocytes together. The proliferating keratinocytes are pushed downward during the process of horn production, and begin to die from lack of nutrient supply. The horn that is formed is "tough enough to endure enormous forces and flexible enough to resist permanent deformation" (Grosenbaugh and Hood, 1993). The perioplic keratinocytes produce soft keratin similarly to skin.

The keratinocytes responsible for the production of the hoof wall cover the coronary dermis. Keratinocytes that cover the dermal

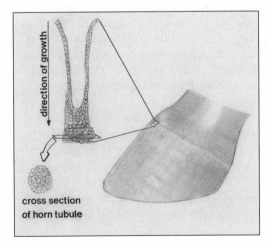

◆ **Fig. 5.1.** Hoof wall production, schematic illustration. A single papilla is shown; the keratinocytes that cover the papilla give rise to a single horn tubule. (Adapted from Grosenbaugh D.A. and Hood D.M. 1993, fig. 1, and from Banks J.W. 1986, fig 20.33 A and B).

papillae give rise to horn tubules (see page 15). Each horn tubule is produced by a single papilla and is formed by concentric layers of epithelial cells. The keratinocytes that are located between the dermal papillae produce the less organized intertubular horn (Banks, 1986). The keratinocytes that cover the laminar dermis give rise to the epidermal laminae. Some texts describe the hoof wall horn as tubular horn, and its laminae as laminar horn.

Abnormal Horn Production

Abnormal horn production may result from coronitis, systemic diseases that affect the feet, and other ill-defined causes. One possible complication of coronitis include the production of soft, rubbery horn with chalky surface (one case observed by the author). Chronic coronitis may result in development of rough and porous hoof described as *pumiced hoof* (as seen in some horses with chronic laminitis). Menzies-Gow et al. (2002) described a rare disease of the foot termed *coronary band dystrophy*. The coronary band and surrounding skin are scaled and crusted, the hoof wall is poorly keratinized and growth is accompanied by scaling and rings. The cause of this disease is unknown, and affected horses are not lame. Goubaux and Barrier (1892) described a hoof disorder termed *crapaudine*, which affects primarily donkeys. This disorder is characterized by longitudinal and transverse ridges on the hoof wall.

Several systemic diseases can effect keratin production and cause malformed hoof wall growth. One of these is *pemphigus foliaceous* (Knottenbelt, 2006), an immunological disease that is rare in horses. Another cause include excessive intake of selenium (see chronic selenosis, page 200).

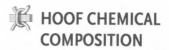

HOOF CHEMICAL COMPOSITION

STUDIES ON THE CHEMICAL COMPOSITION OF THE horse's hoof are scarce. Ley et al. (1998) reported that the season of the year and diet management had significant effect on *hoof mineral composition*. The study included measurements of phosphorus, potassium, calcium, magnesium, sulfur, zinc, manganese, copper and iron. An earlier study (Weiser et al., 1965) provided data on the mineral concentrations of sodium, potassium, magnesium, calcium, phosphorus, zinc and copper measured from horn samples taken from various regions of the hoof capsule. Butler and Hintz (1977b) studied the hoof wall content of iron, zinc and nitrogen. Jackson (1996) pointed out that the protein concentration of the hoof wall is about 93 percent. Weiss et al. (1984) suggested that examination of the hoof keratins and their associated proteins might be applied as a tool for investigating pathologic conditions of the hoof.

Future studies on hoof chemical composition should reveal why some horses have excellent quality hoof horn while others do not. If such correlation is found, a much-needed objective test for determining hoof quality can be developed. The use of hoof clippings for analysis of chemical composition may provide erroneous results due to aging of horn and environmental effects. Singh et al. (1993) described a simple method for obtaining hoof biopsy samples from cattle hooves.

 ## HOOF PIGMENTATION

THE COLOR OF THE HOOF MAY BE BLACK, WHITE or striped. A striped hoof is a combination of black and white and is common in the Appaloosa breed and horses related to it (Gower, 2000) (see ◆ fig. 6.3). Pigmentation (black coloration) of the hoof keratin takes place at the coronary band. In some foals born with white hooves, a change into black may

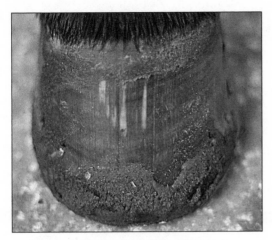

◆ **Fig. 5.2.** Hoof pigmentation. White stripes on the surface of a dark hoof. (Photo by author.)

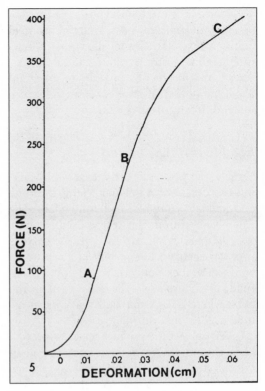

◆ **Fig. 5.3.** Force-deformation curve. The loads in Newtons (N) are plotted against the change in length of the horn sample (deformation); the yield point is calculated from the upper portion of the curve (c) where sample failure takes place. (Reprinted with permission from Leach, D.H. and Zoerb, G.C.1983, fig. 5.)

begin at few weeks of age; this change can be observed as a dark band of horn growth from the coronary band downward (Gower, 2000). Occasionally, light stripes of horn develop on the surface of dark hooves. These stripes result from interruption of normal horn pigmentation caused by an injury to the coronary band (◆ fig. 5.2).

Anecdotally, the common belief was that dark hooves are stronger than light hooves. Contrary to that belief, poor and excellent quality hooves can be observed in horses with black or white hooves or striped ones. Results of different studies on pigmented and non-pigmented keratin show no significant difference in hoof hardness (Benedetti, 1948; Dinger et al., 1973; Landeau et al, 1983; Douglas et al., 1996), chemical composition (Weiser et al., 1965), moisture content (Miyaki et al., 1974; Ley et al., 1998), relative elasticity, tensile strength, mineral content (Ley et al., 1998) and fracture toughness (Bertram and Gosline, 1986). Runciman et al. (2004) measured the strength of horseshoe nail fixation of light and dark hooves and found no significant differences between the two types of hooves when the mean forces were compared.

MECHANICAL PROPERTIES OF THE HOOF WALL

THE FORCES THAT ACT ON THE HOOF WALL RESULT in compressive, tensile and deformation stress (Leach, 1980). Compressive forces develop by the hoof pressing against earth. Tensional forces develop by the tendency of the third phalanx to separate from its laminar hold, and deformational forces develop from changes in the hoof shape as it yields to the forces applied to it. The mechanical ability of the hoof horn to resist these forces is determined by factors such as genetics, moisture content and nutrition.

Data on the mechanical properties of hoof keratin is obtained by measuring rigidity, yield point, relative elasticity, tensile strength, fracture toughness, strain patterns and hardness. These measurements provide information about the quality of the hoof horn substance under different stress conditions.

Rigidity and Yield Point

Rigidity and yield point are measured by placing a section of hoof wall in a testing machine and gradually compressing it until it fails. The data obtained from this test is used to plot a *force-deformation curve* (◆ fig. 5.3). The curve is used to calculate the *rigidity* of the sample which describes how elastic (or how stiff or rigid) the sample is. The *yield point* is the point where the sample fails and it is measured in Newtons/mm² (N/ mm²).

Vertical compression tests of hoof wall horn, compressed from top to bottom, had an average yield point of 177.1 N/mm² for sections taken from the outer hoof wall (Leach and Zoerb, 1983c). Similar samples that were compressed from side to side had an average yield point of 220N/mm². The results of the last test indicate that other forces beside simple compressive forces may be acting on the hoof. Butler and Hintz (1977b) measured an average yield point of 146N/mm² taken from moist samples. Konig and Budras (2003) showed that horn hardness decreases toward the distal portion of the hoof wall; they proposed that this change is the result of the aging process of the horn.

Tensile Strength

The *tensile strength* of the hoof horn is measured by placing a prepared horn sample in a device and gradually stretching it until it fails. The tensile strength is calculated from the maximum load applied and the cross-sectional area of the sample; the results are expressed in N\mm². Zenker et al. (1995) indicated that tensile strength values of less than 50 N/mm² in samples from the proximal part of the hoof wall are abnormal. Küng

(1991) measured a mean tensile strength of 52 N/mm² in the bearing border of hooves of ten Warmblood horses. Values for the middle and outer zones of the proximal hoof wall were 68.7 N/mm² and 58.9 N/mm² respectively.

Results of tensile strength measurements on hooves of 48 mature Thoroughbred mares showed that both season and nutritional plan affected the hoof mineral composition and hoof wall strength. The tensile strength of the keratin was positively associated with its sulfur content (Ley et al., 1998). In a different study (Monhart, 2002), the tensile strength of hoof horn from ten horses varied significantly between individuals.

Fracture Toughness

The *fracture toughness* of the hoof wall provides an indication of the ability of the hoof wall to resist vertical cracks. Bertram and Gosline (1986) indicated that fracture toughness is higher in the direction of the horn tubules. Their study and a study by Kasapi and Gosline (1997) showed that the intertubular horn has a *crack diversion mechanism* that prevents proximal progression of cracks by diverging them into a horizontal direction (◆ fig. 5.4). Bertram and Gosline (1986) found that the fracture toughness of the most distal

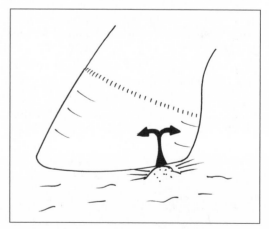

◆ **Fig. 5.4.** Crack diversion mechanism, schematic illustration. The forces that develop in the hoof wall following stepping on a stone are being diverted from a vertical into horizontal direction.

hoof wall was significantly lower compared to that in locations that are more proximal. They proposed that this difference was due to fatigue damage of the older, more distal horn.

Strain Patterns

In a study on hoof capsule *strain patterns* under weight bearing, two strain field epicenters developed on each side of the hoof. Each epicenter was located between the middle and distal third of the hoof wall, along a line that anatomically corresponds to the free edge of the third phalanx (Dejardin et al., 2001). Interestingly, the position of the palmar epicenter seems to correspond to the region of quarter cracks and corn development.

 HEALING OF FOOT WOUNDS

ALTHOUGH THE HOOF CAPSULE IS A RIGID structure, it has healing capacity. Healing of foot injuries, with some exceptions, is similar to that of skin. The main differences are due to the rigid hoof capsule structure that prevents swelling of tissue and drainage of exudates from the wound (Parks, 1999).

The healing process of foot wounds depends on the extent of the injury. Superficial wounds begin to heal by the process of *keratinization* (Steckel, 1987). This process involves direct keratin production by *germinal cells* that remain attached to the dermis following an injury. Production of new horn or cornification takes about 10 days (Fessler, 1989). Deep wounds accompanied by destruction of germinal cells begin to heal by formation of *granulation tissue* (see plate 3). Healthy granulation tissue is essential for healing to proceed (Steckel and Fessler, 1983). The granulation tissue fills the wound space, than, the outer layer gradually becomes covered with *keratogenic tissue* (Fessler, 1971b). This tissue is formed by new epithelial cells that migrate from the margins of the wound over the surface of the granulation tissue (Park, 1999). The new epithelium is very thin and disrupts easily.

The laminar dermis has limited proliferation capability, thus healing of deep wounds that involve the hoof wall depends on new hoof wall growth from the coronary band toward the weight-bearing surface (Fessler, 1989; Park, 1999). Until then, new horn made through the process of cornification covers the damaged laminar dermis (Stashak, 1987; Park, 1999; Fessler, 1989) (see plate 20). Pollitt and Daradka (2004) showed that following wall stripping in the normal hoof, most of the laminar *basement membrane,* which is a supporting layer that underlies the epidermis, remains in the dermis. The basement membrane forms a template over which migrating keratinocytes can reconstruct the laminae. Their study showed that the resulting new laminae had near normal anatomy.

Factors that Interfere with Wound Healing

Hoof wound healing may be interrupted by several factors that include low ambient temperature (Silver, 1973), exposure to soil and manure, edema of the lower limb (Allen et al.,1988; Robinson et al., 1975), motion of the injured part, strong astringents, infection, and trauma (Fessler, 1989). Delay between injury and initial treatment favors infection, and should be considered the greatest limitation to healing (Fessler, 1989). Neglected wounds may result in development of excessive granulation tissue or *proud flesh* that is difficult to treat (Fessler, 1971a). Immobilization of the foot aids in epithelial migration in wounds situated in areas of motion (Hackett, 1982; Peacock and Van Winkle, 1976). The foot may be immobilized with a lower limb splint or a distal limb cast. Healing of foot injuries depends not only on the healing capacity of the foot but also on the use of aseptic procedures, antibiotics, and application of acrylics (Fessler, 1971a). Foot injuries involving elastic structures such as the digital cushion, lateral cartilages and heel bulbs, heal by collagen fiber replacement that results in *scar tissue*. The scar tissue has reduced tensile strength and elasticity that may compromise the shock absorption function of these structures (Fessler, 1989). Scar tissue that develops following laceration injuries to the coronary band might cause permanent hoof wall cracks. Migration of epithelial cells to the margin of the coronary band and developments of a *horn spur* may complicate healing (Park, 1999; Fessler 1971a) (see fig. 16.61).

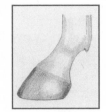

Chapter 6

Hoof Quality

Hoof quality REFERS TO HOOF CONFORMATION and hoof substance. Genetic, environmental and nutritional factors determine these qualities. Observations show that the degree of hoof quality among horses is quite variable. Few horses have exceptionally good quality hooves that permit them to work barefoot on rigid terrain for a prolonged time. Horses that work barefoot extensively, such as the Peruvian Paso horses, have some individuals with excellent hoof quality. Good quality hooves include hooves with good proportion to body size, thick hoof wall, hard, dry hoof capsule and concaved sole. Kempson and Campbell (1998) described the quality of the hoof horn as "good" in well-shaped feet with shiny, even, normal horn, minimal growth ridges and no cracks or defects. Mackay-Smith (in Sellnow, 2004) described the desirable feet qualities for a distance horse as having thick, tough, "flinty" walls, moderate slope, deep open heels, an "oversized" look, and matching hooves left and right. In a description of hoof criteria set by the Arabian Horse Club of America, the desired character-istics of the hoof include hard hoof, large, round and wide, and low at the heel (Lawrence and Huddleston, 1951). Unfortunately, most horses have hoof quality that can be classified as poor to average.

POOR HOOF CONFORMATION AND SUBSTANCE

Poor hoof conformation and substance IS A common condition among horses. Descriptions of poor hoof quality from various sources include hooves that are dull, cracked with damaged horn (Kempson and Campbell, 1998), brittle, chipped hoof wall, thin quarters and softness of the white line (Josseck et al.,1995), crumbling lower parts, thin sole, small split frog, low heels, weak quarters that break away around the horseshoe nails, dished walls, horizontal ridging, vertical ridging, rough hoof wall surface and lack of periople (Comben et al., 1984), tender feet (Comben et al., 1984; Jossek et al., 1995) and

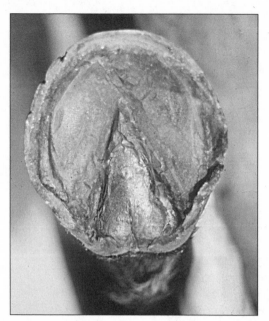

◆ **Fig. 6.1.** Poor hoof quality. Note the weak hoof wall, separation at the white line and lack of bars. (Photo by author.)

flat sole (◆ fig. 6.1). Horses with poor hoof quality may have one or more of the above conditions.

One of the protective functions of the hoof capsule is its low permeability to water-soluble substances. This barrier becomes compromised in horses with poor quality hoof horn that is damaged (Kempson and Campbell, 1998). Zenker et al. (1995) investigated the hoof wall microscopic features in a group of Lipizzaner horses with poor hoof quality. Most of the horses in this study had hoof wall micro-cracks, damaged connection between the terminal horn and horn leaflets (the white line) and damaged horn tubules. In some cases, the micro-cracks caused the formation of visible clefts. Kempson (1987) found complete loss of tubular structure in the middle and inner zones of the hoof wall in 32 out of 35 horses of different breeds that had crumbly bearing horn. She proposed that this change might relate to production of inferior horn. Zenker et al. (1995) indicated that one of the characteristics of poor horn quality is reduced tensile strength. Their study showed

mean tensile strength values of 36 N/mm² measured at the lateral and medial hoof wall and 46 N/mm² for measurements at the dorsal wall. Poor hoof quality may develop from slow growth rate which may be affected by season of the year, level of nutrition, the age of the horse, and diseases. Several authors (Keller et al., 2000; Kuwano et al., 1996; Kuwano et al., 1998) investigated the rule of fungi in horses with poor horn quality; a positive correlation between poor hoof quality and presence of keratinopathogenic (horn destroying) fungi were found (Keller et al., 2000) but the rule of the fungi is still not clear (see onychomycosis, page 199).

Poor hoof substance is commonly accompanied with small feet conformation. In some horses, the feet have normal proportion to body weight but the hoof walls are too thin. The quality of the hooves may be so poor that they require regular protection in the form of horseshoes. Paradoxically, driving horseshoe nails through these hooves weakens them further. Application of glue-on shoes to horses with poor hoof quality may solve this problem, although the genetic factors that cause the problem will remain.

FOOT GRADING

EXAMINATION OF THE FOOT PROVIDES important information on the ability of the hoof to function properly. This includes the ability of the hoof to endure concussion, the "match" between the foot and suspensory apparatus, and the ability to work barefoot or "tolerate" horseshoes. The examination may provide clues to possible conformation faults above the foot that could alter the conformation of the hoof. Evaluation of the foot should include a thorough examination of the conformation of the digit and limb in relation to the foot and to general body conformation. The *intended athletic activity* of the horse has to be considered as well. The data obtained from such examinations can give the horse owner an idea as to how suitable the horse is for different working conditions.

TABLE 6.1 ◆ Example of foot grading records

Age	Breed	Gender	Environment Type	Foot Care	Type /Amount of Work	Comments	Foot Grade
8 yr	QH	Gelding	Dry pasture	Trim every 3 months	Walk	Crumbling horn, dry hooves, vertical cracks, small feet, frequent shoe loss	2
6 yr	Mixed	Gelding	Stable, clean	Trim and front shoes every 8 weeks	None	White line disease, foot grade was 3	1
13 yr	TB	Mare	Dry gravel paddock	4 shoes every 2 months	Walk	Laminitis, very thin sole, can't walk barefoot	1
5 yr	MST	Stallion	Dry pasture	None	Self exercised	Has a potential for grade 5	4

QH=Quarter Horse, TB=Thoroughbred, MST=Mustang.

Foot grading can be used as a tool in the evaluation of hoof quality; this system can be useful in prepurchase examination, selection of breeding stock and for communication between horse owners, farriers and veterinarians. The proposed grading system is based on subjective evaluation of the foot based on five grades. The addition of objective tests in the future should increase the accuracy of hoof evaluation. Examples of hoof grading are given in ◆ Table 6.1.

Grade Groups

The proposed foot grading system includes the following groups:

Grade 1. Chronic foot disease. This category includes horses with chronic foot conditions that permanently limit their use. Examples: clubfoot, navicular disease, chronic laminitis, and weak suspensory apparatus. Horses within this group with non-heritable disorders (i.e. laminitis) may be used for breeding.

Grade 2. Poor hoof quality. This group includes horses with hoof conformation and substance that significantly limits their use.

Examples: thin hoof wall, small feet, crumbling horn, flat sole, sheared heels, underrun heels, offset pasterns and poor limb conformation with pronounced uneven wear at the hoof-bearing surface. Horses in this group should not be used for breeding (see ◆ fig. 6.1).

Grade 3. Average hoof quality. This group includes horses with hoof conformation and substance that requires protection for most types of activities. These horses are able to work barefoot on soft terrain. Examples: average hoof size, average wall thickness, mule foot, splitting at the hoof margins, soft horn, and moderate toeing-out with some uneven wear at the bearing surface. Horses in this group should not be used for breeding.

Grade 4. Good hoof quality. This group includes horses with hoof conformation and substance that permits them to work barefooted on most types of terrain. Examples: thick hoof wall, good hoof to body-size ratio, hard and resilient hooves, concave sole, even wear at the bearing surface, good limb conformation. Horses in this group can be used for breeding (see ◆ fig. 6.3).

Grade 5. Excellent hoof quality. This group includes horses with excellent hoof conformation and substance. These horses can be worked barefoot on all types of terrain. Horses in this group are very rare. Examples: dry, hard and resilient hooves, "oversized" hooves, very thick hoof wall, concave sole, strong bars, good limb and body conformation. Horses in this group should be tested further as candidates for hoof improvement breeding programs. Tests may include endurance riding, genetic profiling, and mechanical tests of the hoof horn.

Tests for Hoof Quality

Evaluation of hoof quality is commonly done by subjective evaluation. The results of such evaluation may vary according to the observer's opinion and experience. Since there are significant differences in hoof quality among horses, an objective method for evaluating hoof quality would be practical. Currently there are no objective tests for evaluating hoof quality and more research is required in order to develop these tests. Hoof quality tests could include testing the genetic makeup, chemical composition and mechanical properties of the hoof.

Evaluation and examination of hoof quality through endurance testing is another possibility. These tests could be conducted on barefooted horses by applying data from endurance riding clubs. Current tests for hoof conformation include measuring the ratio of body weight to foot size, and hoof wall width and thickness. These measurements are best don by comparing horses.

 HEREDITY AND HOOF QUALITY

THE *inbreeding and line-breeding* PRACTICED in the establishment of the various modern horse breeds has had a major influence on the development of horses with poor hoof quality. The condition is common in different breeds, family lines, and individual horses. Unfortunately, studies on the effect of heredi-

ty on hoof quality are rare and most of the data is observational.

Certain Thoroughbred sire lines have a dominant effect on hoof conformation; some stallion lines produce narrow, almost donkey-shaped feet, others produce a flat, shallow heeled hoof (Ellis, 1998). Cannon (1979) described various hoof characteristics observed in some Thoroughbred breeding lines as having thin-wall, brittle hooves, white hooves, contracted heels and flat soles. Turner (1988) indicated that in some horses, small feet might be an inheritable trait that is difficult to modify. Rich (1907) noted that many Hambletonian trotters have thin hoof wall (Hambletonian was a leading Standardbred sire). Large numbers of disproportionably small feet can be observed in Quarter Horses. A relationship between heredity and poor hoof quality in a herd of Lipizzaner horses has been described by Josseck (1991) and Josseck et al. (1995); the usage of these horses was affected by the hoof quality (Josseck et al., 1995). Schmitt (1998) found significant variability in hoof quality among young Lipizzaner stallions; some with very poor hoof quality and others who had superior hoof horn quality. He concluded that the effects of genetics on horn quality are considerable and should not be underestimated. In a study on the hoof quality of 116 Lipizzaner stallions, Munzinger (2005) observed that hoof quality began to deteriorate in many horses at the age of four to five years.

Young (1993) indicated that some horses affected by white line disease might have hereditary vulnerability for the disease. In Japan, under-run heels among Thoroughbred horses are considered a genetic problem (Oikawa and Kasashima, 2002). Budras and Schiel (1996) concluded that the Przewalski's horse has a better barrier against bacterial decomposition of the white line compared to the domesticated horse. Unfortunately, as the last true wild horses gradually disappear, the chances of preserving these genetic qualities are diminished.

Abnormal hoof conformation may develop secondary to conformation faults above the foot. These conformational faults, which are mostly heritable, alter the weight distribution on the foot, thus causing uneven hoof wear. Examples of this type of conformational fault include toeing-in, toeing-out, offset pasterns, and club foot. Clubfoot is not uncommon in certain family lines of Arabian horses and Quarter Horses.

🐾 ENVIRONMENTAL EFFECT ON HOOVES

Environmental factors THAT AFFECT HOOF quality include the stable, pasture, and the working area, as well as the hoof care management practiced on each horse. The hoof horn may become exposed to a variety of environmental conditions ranging from acidic bog water to dry deserts (Kempson and Campbell, 1998). Lack of exercise, prolonged stabling in dry stalls, hoof dressings, sand, manure, urine and wood shavings tend to dry the hoof. This predispose the hoof to development of contracted heels, dry and cracked hooves, and shriveled frogs (Dickson and O'Malley, 1987). Josseck et al. (1995) indicated that Lipizzaner horses that are kept mainly on hard, and often stony ground, had better quality hooves compared to horses of the same breed that were kept on pastures and bedded stables. The former group had white line that was better connected and drier, hoof wall with fewer cracks and sole that was drier and harder. They proposed that defects in horn formation might result in inferior quality horn that cannot resist stable environments such as manure and urine. Moyer (in Sellnow 2002) indicated that feral horses that travel over hard surfaces wear their hooves down in a balanced fashion; this wear and natural selection resulted in horses with strong hooves. He indicated that hoof strength depends on environmental challenges such as motion and stress. Placement of horses in artificial environments such as soft ground results in reduced hoof strength. According to Smyth and Goody (1972) native Welsh ponies, developed hard hooves suited to the outdoor environment whereas Moorland ponies that kept

indoors tend to develop laminitis; the former group commonly live on a meager diet whereas the later group commonly being overfed on corn.

Dry paddocks covered with fine gravel appeared to have beneficial effect on the hooves when stocked at 400 square meters per horse. Under these conditions, the hooves remained clean and at proper length (see ◆ fig. 12.1.)

Sweeny et al. (2000) concluded that the application of sodium bisulfate to the horse stall may be safe for hooves at recommended amounts. Sodium bisulfate is used to reduce ammonia concentration in stables in order to decrease fly population. Suchorski-Tremblay et al. (2001) listed ammonia among many other possible causes (variables) for hoof crack formation. Küng (1991) showed that manure and urine reduce the tensile strength of horn.

Monhart (2002) tested the effect of different organic environments on the hoof horn. The organic media that contained urine, and one of the hoof conditioners tested, tended to reduce the hoof horn tensile strength. She concluded that good quality horn seemed to be less sensitive to damage by environmental factors. Kempson (2004) indicated that regular application of disinfectant to hooves of horses with persistent hoof horn defects could improve horn quality.

The external appearance of the hoof may change by the effect of environmental moisture. The periople is polished and glistening in dry hooves, but whitish, swollen, and fibrous when moist (Bradley and Grahame, 1946). Excessive moisture can be harmful to hooves; horses raised in low, marshy areas lose the spring action of the foot from too much moisture (Lambert, 1966). In temperate climates, exposure of the horn to excessive moisture weakens the horn and causes more wear at the heels (Östblom, 1984b). Placement of horses for prolonged periods in wet bedding leads to deterioration of the hooves, whereas prolonged foot soaking softens the hoof and predisposes the white line to penetrating microorganisms (O'Grady, 1996). Josseck et al. (1995) indicated that increased moisture content of the hoof was associated with more severe changes in the white line quality in a group of Lipizzaner horses. Kempson and Campbell (1998) indicated that in winter, some horses spend the day in wet mud and the night in absorbent material with no ill effect.

The Effect of Hoof Dressings on Hoof Quality

The horse market offers a large number of hoof care products, including hoof dressings aimed at improving hoof quality. Some of the label claims on these products include moisture preservation and increased hoof wall growth and strength. Few of these claims are supported by scientific studies and the efficacy of many of these products is questionable (Butler, 1977; Butler 1978). Some products may even be damaging to the hoof (Kempson in King, 2002; Geyer, 2005). One product that has been tested and showed a positive effect on the hoof is pine tar (Robertson and Hood, 1996).

Products that are made for hoof wall moisture preservation are based on various oils, pine tar, petroleum, lanolin, glycerin and on drying agents such as formalin. Wagner (in King, 2002) indicated that over-moisturizing the hoof with dressings weakens the hoof wall. Kempson (in King 2002) indicated that tar-based products can damage hooves with poor-quality horn. She also indicated that formalin causes the horn to lose its elasticity and this leads to development of brittle horn that is more liable to crack. One case report (Dart and Pascoe, 1988) pointed to a possible link between prolonged topical application of formalin for treatment of a foot wound and development of laminitis. In addition, formalin is hazardous substance to humans. Covering the hoof with an impervious dressing may result in a sodden hoof by preventing normal loss of water by evaporation (Smithcors, 1961c). Budras et al. (1998) indicted that greasing the solar area softens the horn further and predisposes it to bacterial decay. Kempson (in King, 2002) indicated

that good quality horn has a permeability barrier that resists the deleterious effects of external factors such urine and manure without the need of hoof dressings. Good quality hooves that appear dry reflect an adaptation to arid areas and do not require any addition of hoof dressings (Wagner in King, 2002).

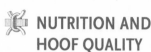 ## NUTRITION AND HOOF QUALITY

HORSES FED A BALANCED RATIO SHOULD HAVE adequate amount of nutrients necessary for normal hoof growth. A deficiency or an excess of nutrients may affect hoof substance. Grosenbaugh and Hood (1993) indicated that a deficiency in a substance essential for horn production, or a circulatory problem that prevents the substance from being provided, could compromise the quality of the hoof. Some horses that receive adequate nutrition may still have poor quality hooves due to their genetic makeup. Some horses may have higher individual requirements for certain elements in their diet. Jackson (1996) indicated that the addition of a *feed supplement* to traditional diets can result in significant improvement of hoof quality. Butler (1977a) indicated that the market offers a large selection of feed additives for horses, but they have not been shown to have any effect on hoof quality. Cuddeford (1994) indicated that alfalfa contains crude protein, sulfur-containing amino acids and certain minerals that can improve hoof horn quality.

Excessive amounts of certain nutrients may be detrimental to the health of the hoof horn (Kempson, 1996). Some elements may interfere with the absorption and utilization of others. Nutrients that have been found under controlled studies to affect the hoof include vitamin A (deficiency), biotin (supplement), and selenium (toxicity).

Horse owners and breeders should check their feeding program periodically with an animal nutritionist in order to detect and correct deficient or excessive nutrients in the diet. Additional source include the National

Research Council (NRC) publications on nutritional requirements of horses. Deficient diet should be corrected by providing the deficient nutrient(s) rather than by supplementation that contain unnecessary ingredients.

Nutrients

The following list includes *nutrients* that may affect hoof growth and substance.

vitamin A. *Vitamin A* (Donoghue and Kronfeld, 1980) is involved in the maintenance of epithelial integrity and may have an important role in the health of the hoof (Jackson, 1996). Experimentally, Vitamin A deficiency resulted in development of a band of rough, scaly hoof below the coronet; however, normal growth resumed after correction of the deficiency (Madsen, 1942) (◆ fig. 6.2). This condition is probably rare due to current feeding practices; it may be more common in countries with poor animal husbandry practices.

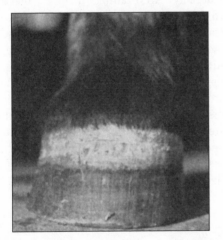

◆ **Fig. 6.2.** Vitamin A deficiency. The appearance of the foot of a yearling Belgian filly following a period of vitamin A deficiency. (Reprinted from Madsen, L.L. 1942, fig. 5A.)

biotin. *Biotin* (vitamin H) is a water-soluble B-group vitamin essential for growth (Whitehead, 1981) and maintenance of epidermal tissue (Geyer and Schultz, 1994). Biotin

deficiency may affect hoof horn quality in horses (Josseck et al., 1995). Studies in cattle show that biotin is required for production of keratin proteins (Sarasin, 1994). Significant improvement in growth rate, hardness (Buffa et al., 1992) and elasticity (Wintzer, 1986) of hooves was measured in a group of horses that received biotin supplement for 10 months. Horses with weak, crumbly hooves, ridging of the hoof wall and soreness may benefit from daily biotin supplementation. A dosage of 10 to 30 mg biotin/day for horses and 5 to 10 mg/day for donkeys and ponies has been recommended; supplementation should continue for six to nine months (Comben et al., 1984). Josseck et al. (1995) found a significant improvement in white line quality and hoof wall quality in Lipizzaner horses supplemented with a daily dosage of 20 mg biotin for nine months or longer. The same group of horses had slight improvement in hoof wall microscopic features (Zenker et al., 1995). Schmitt (1998) observed a significant decrease in hoof horn strength developing one and one-half years following withdrawal of biotin supplementation in a group of horses with initially poor hoof quality. He recommended continuous supplementation of biotin to horses with hoof horn problems.

Sources of biotin include young green grasses, growing green cereals and legumes (Naylor and Raltson, 1991). Since hoof horn production is a continuous process, it is important to maintain a constant level of biotin supplementation when required.

calcium. *Calcium* is an important element in the formation of cell-to-cell attachments in the hoof horn (Kempson, 1987).

methionine. *Methionine* is a sulfur-containing essential amino acid necessary for the production of *cystine*, an amino acid found in keratin. Colles and Jeffcott (1977) recommended the addition of methionine as a feed additive to increase hoof growth and strength in cases of chronic laminitis.

pyridoxine. *Pyridoxine* (vitamin B6) is a key factor in the process of the conversion of methionine to cystine.

selenium. Excessive *selenium* fed to horses and cattle results in abnormal hoof growth caused by *chronic selenosis* (O'Toole and Raisbeck, 1995; Witte et al., 1993) (page 200). The source of selenium may be from eating selenium-accumulating plants, or from salt blocks containing selenium made for cattle. Valberg (in Corum, 2004) recommended the supplement of *vitamin E* and selenium to horses kept in areas of low soil selenium. Recommended daily amounts of selenium can be found in the National Research Council (1989).

sulfur. Data from Ley et al. (1998) shows that *sulfur* is the most abundant mineral element in hoof keratin. Sulfur is found in the *sulfur-containing amino acids*: methionine, cystein and cystine (Reeves et al., 1989). Sulfur forms *disulfide bonds* that increases the strength of the keratin structure (Bertram and Gosline, 1986; Ley et al., 1998).

zinc. *Zinc* is a trace element important for tissue growth and repair. Zinc deficiency results in depressed amino acids and sulfur utilization; therefore, it is essential for hoof growth. Proper zinc to copper ratio is important for optimal absorption of both minerals. Zinc deficiency may be caused by excess calcium. Horses may respond better to zinc supplementation in the form of *zinc methionine* (Jackson, 1996), which is an organic form of zinc.

⚒ IMPROVEMENT OF HOOF QUALITY

HORSES HAVE MANY FOOT DISORDERS DUE TO inbreeding, line-breeding, lack of genetic variation, and banning the introduction of outside breeding stock to existing breeds. The end result is a large number of horses with poor hoof quality, including small feet and weak keratin. Some horse breeds have higher incidence of navicular disease, under-run heels, and contracted tendons in foals.

Many foot problems can be prevented by careful selection of horses with *good quality hooves*. Unfortunately, little attempt is made by horse breeders to improve hoof quality through selective breeding. Most horse-breed associations provide a vague description of the desired hoof traits for their horses; none of them limits the registration of horses with poor quality hooves (Lawrence and Huddleston, 1951).

In most cases, the hoof problems are treated with some form of farriery. Horses with small feet that cannot be shod with iron horseshoes are fitted with glue-on shoes. These horses are bred and the result is propagation of similar horses.

There are ways to improve hoof quality without complicated research. Selective breeding for horses with good quality hooves is practiced in many places, sometimes unintentionally. An example includes breeding two different populations of horses, such as Quarter Horses and mixed Arabian horses, a practice done in Israel that results in significant improvement of the hoof quality of the offspring compared to their Quarter Horse parents. Another example includes raising horses in rough terrain and keeping them barefoot during work. This practice, which is done in Peru, produces horses with good and excellent quality hooves through natural selection. Indigenous ponies such as Welsh ponies that live in their natural habitat have superior quality hooves (Smyth and Goody, 1972).

Any *hoof improvement-breeding program* should start by identifying and preserving horses with superior hoof quality. These horses can be found in the Mustang herds in North America, the Barb horses in North Africa, and the Peruvian horses in Peru. In addition, many Arabian horses that have not been subjected to inbreeding have good quality hooves (◆ fig. 6.3). Unfortunately, many horses with good quality hooves are unintentionally gelded.

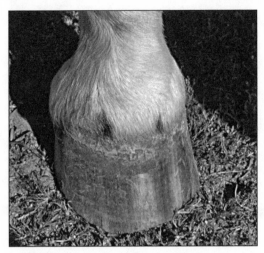

◆ **Fig. 6.3.** Good hoof quality in a mustang horse. (Photo by author.)

Not all feral horses have good quality hooves, and in fact, many have average hoof quality. This may be due to ongoing affect of past domestication, or from lack of selective pressure, or both. Since poor hoof quality is not a new problem, as data from the last 100-200 years show, it may influenced these feral horses as well. In one herd, managed by the Bureau of Land Management (BLM) in Nevada, a serious problem of gravel appears to be prevalent in mustang foals (Hartgrove in West, 2004). It is not clear whether the problem resulted from poor quality hooves or as a secondary complication of other conditions.

Veterinarians and farriers should advise horse owners to avoid breeding horses with inferior hooves. Horse breeding association should encourage the introduction of horses with superior hoof quality into their breeding programs. Horse breeders that produce horses with excellent hoof quality should receive premium prices for their weanlings, and buyers should be able to enjoy their horses under any working conditions.

Chapter 7

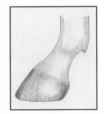

Hoof Physiology

 HOOF GROWTH RATE

Hoof growth rate IS THE TOTAL HOOF GROWTH IN a given time (Josseck et al., 1995). Hoof growth is measured by marking a groove at the proximal toe wall, at a predetermined distance from the coronary rim or hairline. The change in the location of the groove over a specific period is measured in order to calculate growth rate. The hoof length is maintained by hoof growth and hoof wear. In feral horses, hoof growth and wear are maintained at the same rate, while in domestic horses horseshoes and other environmental factors affect this process.

Hoof growth rate is affected by age, season and nutrition. The monthly hoof growth rate is approximately 15.5 mm in nursing foals, 11.5 mm in weanlings and 8.5 mm in mature horses (Butler, 1977). Fessler (1989) indicated that it takes 9 to 12 months for the toe at the dorsal hoof wall to grow out. Josseck (1991) reported that the renewal rate of hoof horn lies between 301-378 days. The hind

hooves grow approximately 12 percent faster than the fore hooves in foals and 7 percent faster in weanlings (Butler, 1977). Hoof growth decreases with age and is slowed by cold and dry environments (Fessler, 1989). The rate of horn growth is greater in regions with warm climate, or in the summer, as compared with winter (Smithcors, 1961c; Dinger, 1976). Hoof growth rate peaks in the spring (Butler, 1977). Slow horn growth during cold seasons may represent an adaptation to reduced ground friction. Due to their lower metabolic rate, hoof growth rate in draft horses is slower, compared to that of light horses.

Factors Affecting Hoof Growth

Hoof growth rate may increase by injuries to sensitive structures of the foot, and by counter-irritants, blistering and massage applied to the coronary band region (Butler, 1977). Lockard and Reinertson (1986) demonstrated an increase in growth rate of hooves after application of counter-irritants to the coronary band region.

Butler and Hintz (1977) compared the hoof growth rate of two groups of eight-month-old ponies. One group received a limited diet and the other group received an unlimited diet. The hoof growth rate was 50 percent greater in the second group; this group also had a larger solar surface area. The sex of the animals did not affect hoof growth rate. Reilly et al. (1998b) reported a 15 percent higher growth rate in ponies supplemented with biotin.

Dinger (1976) reported that the medial hoof wall in horses that toe-out grows at a slower rate compared to the lateral side. He proposed that this difference might be caused by higher ground pressure exerted on the medial hoof wall. Glade and Salzman (1985) reported that hoof growth was significantly slower in forelimb hooves trimmed with short toe compared to hooves with long toe. The underlying cause for this difference was not clear.

Some hooves have hoof wall rings or *keratin rings* on the outer surface of the wall. These rings represent a period of active hoof wall growth alternating with slower growth rate (see hoof wall rings, page 225).

A common disease that affects hoof growth is laminitis. No information was found on hoof growth rate in horses with Cushing's disease.

Factors Affecting Hoof Wear

Factors that affect hoof wear include the type of ground, distance of travel, hoof substance, habits, and horseshoes. Ground type depends on geographical location and may include rocky basalt, abrasive gravel, soft sand and heavy mud. Some individual horses of the Peruvian breed are able to travel thousands of miles on rigid terrain without protective horseshoes. On the other hand, some horses grow their hooves at a very slow rate and have to be shod regularly, even when kept in pasture and not worked. Application of horseshoes prevents wear, but in working horses

the quarters and heels continue to wear against the horseshoe, consequently a lower hoof angle develops toward the end of the shoeing interval.

 ## HOOF MOISTURE CONTENT

THE KERATINIZED PARTS OF THE FOOT CONTAIN water, which maintains the elasticity of the hoof horn. Lack of moisture results in reduced elasticity that affects the shock absorption properties of the hoof (Fraser et al., 1972; Butzow, 1961; Emery et al., 1977). The hoof moisture content is supplied by blood circulation (Butler, 1977) and by water absorption from the environment (Butler, 1977; Wagner and Hood, 2002). Dynamic movement of the hoof during exercise increases the circulation within the foot and maintains the moisture level of the keratin (Butzow, 1961).

Smithcors (1961c) indicated that the periople protects the wall from excessive drying, but it scales off more distally and it may be entirely lacking at the toe. Butler (1977) indicated that the periople has a minor role in moisture retention within the hoof.

The percentage of relative moisture content in the keratinized parts of the hoof varies considerably (Miyaki et al. 1974). The hoof moisture content is approximately 25 percent in the hoof wall, 33 percent in the sole and 50 percent in the frog (Butzow, 1961). These areas vary in their elasticity; the sole is less rigid than the wall, and the frog is soft and pliable (Bradley and Grahame, 1946). The average mid-toe hoof wall moisture level in pony yearlings were 27.8 percent (Butler and Hintz, 1977b). In a different study, the average moisture content of dorsal outer wall and dorsal inner wall were 27.9 percent and 35.5 percent respectively (Douglas et al., 1996). The moisture content of the hind hooves is slightly higher than that of the fore hooves (Butler, 1977).

The pliability of the hoof wall increases toward the coronary border (Bradley and

Grahame, 1946). Since younger horn contains more moisture, there is a moisture gradient from toe to heel, with higher moisture content at the palmar/plantar aspect of the hoof (Kainer, 1989). The higher moisture level at the back of the hoof, combined with the gradual thinning of the hoof wall toward the quarters and heels, forms a flexible structure that can expand during weight bearing.

Bertram and Gosline (1987) indicated that keratin stiffness is reduced at higher moisture levels and the hydrated horn is more prone to crack propagation. Douglas et al. (1996) indicated that the differences in stiffness between the outer and inner wall is inversed to their moisture content. Measurements of rigidity and yield points showed that the behavior of hoof samples is affected by the level of its moisture content. Moist samples or samples from the inner wall are less rigid and have a lower yield point compared to dry samples (Leach, 1983c; Butler and Hintz, 1977).

Evidence on hoof wall moisture loss and its effect on keratin can be observed following hoof trimming. The exposure of the fresh hoof cut to the environment causes it to contract and shrink; after a while, hands can break the hoof cut easily. Another evidence for moisture loss is seen as a damp print of the hoof outline on the floor mat following trimming. Following moisture lost from the keratin, the hoof wall begun to contract similarly to a fresh horn cut, but to a lesser degree. The degree of contraction may be sufficient to cause slight bulging of the sole above the level of the wall-bearing surface. This bulge has to be trimmed prior to application of horseshoes in order to prevent sole pressure. No data was found on the degree of hoof contraction following water loss from the hoof.

Under excessively dry conditions, the horn becomes hard and brittle and may crack or chip off (Smithcors, 1961c; Dickson and O'Malley, 1987). Dry hooves may develop as a result of interference to the blood circulation of the foot (Smithcors, 1961c).

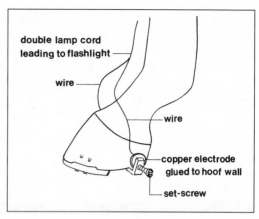

♦ **Fig. 7.1.** Lambert's experiment. The instrumented horseshoe was nailed to the hoof and the setscrews were adjusted until they made contact with electrodes that were glued to the hoof, completing a circuit and causing the light of the flashlight to show. Following contraction of the heels, the light turned off. The light returned when the hoof was placed in water and the heels expanded. (Reprinted by permission from Lambert, F. 1968, fig. 3.)

Lambert's Experiment

Lambert (1968) conducted an experiment that tested the effect of moisture loss from the hoof following trimming. In this experiment, horses were trimmed and fitted with an instrumented horseshoe equipped with an electrical circuit and a flashlight (♦ fig. 7.1). Hoof contraction caused the flashlight to be turned off while expansion caused it to turn on. Hoof contraction at the heels was detected within a few minutes following trimming; once the trimmed hoof was placed in water, the heels expanded back rapidly (♦ table 7.1). These findings demonstrate the importance of the solar area in retention of moisture within the hoof. Moisture loss may be prevented by sole flakes, abrasion that smooth down the solar surface, and by accumulation of dirt under the sole and frog. The experiment also shows that moisture can be supplemented from external sources as well.

Table 7.1 ◆ Time measurements for heel contraction and expansion obtained with instrumented horseshoe.

Experiment No.	Foot	Time of preparation[1]	Time from "ready" until light went out[2]	Time until light came on after hoof was placed in water[3]
1	LF	4 min, 49 sec	3 min, 24 sec	15 sec
2	RF	4 min, 21 sec.	4 min, 27 sec	Instantly
3	LF	6 min, 47 sec.*	1 min, 37 sec	5 sec

LF=left front, RF=right front

1. Time of preparation began when the old horseshoe was removed.
2. "Ready" was recorded when the horse was standing on the experimental horseshoe with the set-screws adjusted and making contact with the electrodes.
3. An interval existed between "light out" and putting the foot into a pan of water. The experiment would be more conclusive if the entire procedure was carried out in a dry pan, with water being added when the light went out.

* Delay in fastening one electrode to foot.

Reprinted with permission from Lambert, F. 1968, table 1.

Part 2 Locomotion

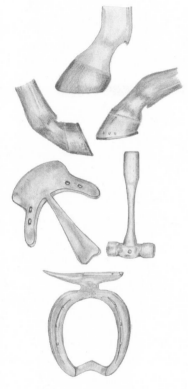

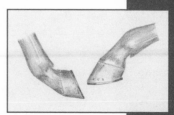

Chapter 8

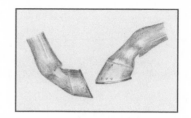

Foot Locomotion

 ## LOCOMOTION TERMINOLOGY

THE FOLLOWING LIST INCLUDES locomotion terms that appear in the text:

breakover. The last portion of the support phase, between heel off and toe off (Clayton et al. 1990) (◆ fig. 8.1).

breakover point. The last point of contact between the hoof and ground before suspension.

breakover time. The time between heel off and toe off (Clayton et al. 1990) (◆ fig. 8.1).

force vector. A physical quantity, commonly given in Newtons, that describes the magnitude and direction of a force, represented by a line and arrow. See also, resultant force.

gait. A sequence of limb movements within each stride.

ground reaction force (GRF). The force developed between the limb and ground; this force changes its magnitude and direction during the support phase. See also, point of force application.

hoof flight pattern. The trace made by the toe of the foot during suspension as viewed from the side.

mid-support. The point during the support phase where the limb is perpendicular to the horse's body.

newton (N). A unit of force commonly used in equine biomechanics. One newton is equal to the force that causes a mass of 1 kilogram (2.2 pounds) to accelerate 1 meter per second per second.

point of force application. A point that represent the position of the GRF on the solar area at certain time during hoof and ground interaction.

resultant force (R). A single force with an effect equal to that of two or more forces acting together (see ◆ fig. 8.8).

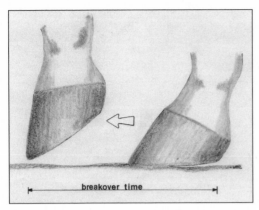

◆ Fig. 8.1. Breakover, schematic illustration. Break over time begins at heel-off and ends at toe-off.

step. The act of one of the limbs during progressive motion (Muybridge, 1957).

stride. A complete cycle of limb movement in a particular gait (Muybridge, 1957; Clayton, 1989).

stride length. The distance between successive limb placements.

support phase. The part of the stride where the limb is in contact with the ground, also called stance phase.

suspension phase. The part of the stride where the limb is off the ground, also called swing phase.

HOOF STRIDE KINEMATICS

Hoof stride kinematics IS THE STUDY OF THE hoof in motion during support and suspension phases. This study involves the measurements of various parameters including the hoof flight pattern or the shape, length and height of the moving hoof, duration of the stride, the degree of limb protraction, landing patterns, breakover time and more. Although measurements of the hoof in motion (kine-

matics) and the energies (kinetics) involved are done mostly under laboratory conditions, these studies provide valuable data on the distribution of forces within the foot, the effect of horseshoes and horseshoe adjuncts, and gait alterations in lame horses. The function of the foot may be affected by lameness, fatigue, track type, horseshoe design and conformation.

The hoof stride may be divided artificially into a suspension phase where the foot is airborne (forming a flight pattern), and a stance phase where the foot interacts with the ground.

Suspension Phase

Historically, the *hoof flight pattern* or the trace of the hoof traveling in air was described as a single-humped parabolic arc. The arc was at its highest point when the foot passed the opposite limb (Adams, 1974). The held theory was that the shape of the flight arc can be affected by changing the hoof angle. Lowering the hoof angle was aimed at shifting the highest point of the arc backward, whereas increasing the hoof angle was aimed at shifting the highest point of the arc forward (Adams, 1974). Based on this theory, the hoof angle was modified in order to correct accidental limbs contact.

Later studies showed that the shape of the hoof flight tracing is quite different. The shape of the hoof flight pattern in normal trotting horses has a double-hump shape (Ratzlaff and Grant, 1986; Clayton, 1990a; Ratzlaff, 1988; Balch et al., 1994) with the highest part of the trace occurring soon after breakover, followed by gradual reduction in the height of the arc (◆ fig. 8.2). Toward the end of suspension, a second moderate elevation of the trace appears; this trace represents the preparation of the foot for impact (Clayton, 1990).

Changing the hoof angle did not affect the shape of the double-bumped flight arc pattern (Ratzlaff, 1988; Clayton, 1990a; Clayton, 1987). Clayton (1987) found no significant

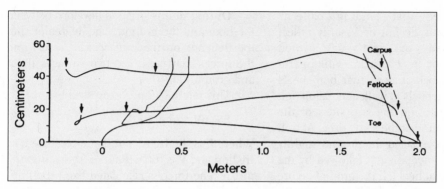

◆ **Fig. 8.2.** Hoof flight pattern of the right forelimb recorded at a trot. The flight pattern has a double-humped trace. (Reprinted by permission from Ratzlaff, M.H. 1988, fig. 2.)

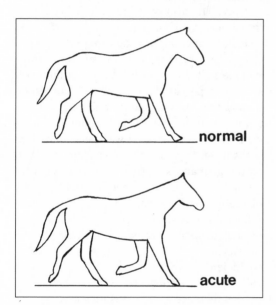

◆ **Fig. 8.3.** Tracing of a horse during motion in a horse with normal hoof angles and acute hoof angles. Acute angle causes the horse to land toe first. (Reprinted by permission from Clayton, H.M. 1990a, fig. 1)

differences in stride height, shape and length between normal and broken-backed hoof angles with a difference of 10 degrees. However, low hoof angle was associated with a significantly slow breakover time in the fore and hind limbs (Clayton, 1990) (see page 53). Moyer (1988a) indicated that horses with acute hoof angle have a greater tendency to land toe first. Clayton (1990) showed that lowering the hoof angle by 10 degrees causes a significant shift toward toe-first impact, particularly in the forelimbs (◆ fig. 8.3). Clayton (1987) indicated that these changes may cause stumbling and may create abnormal loading patterns in the early part of the support phase.

Foot and Ground Interaction

Although the *support phase* of the stride is a single event, it may be divided for convenience into the following components:

hoof impact ➤ sliding ➤ rotation ➤ breakover

HOOF IMPACT

During motion, the natural unshod hoof lands heel-first or flat-footed. In racing Thoroughbreds and Standardbreds, the impact of the hoof with the ground is usually heel-first (Rooney et al., 1978b; Fredrickson et al., 1975). In a study on trotting horses with normal hoof angle, the frequencies of landing heel first were lower than landing flat-footed. None of the horses landed toe first (Clayton, 1990). Toe-first landing was observed in lame horses (Clayton, 1986) and in horses with acute hoof angle (Clayton, 1987). Balch et al.

(1994) indicated that landing patterns observed at a walk do not necessarily reflect those observed at trot or canter. Measurements of hoof contact with instrumented horseshoes showed that both heels landed simultaneously at walk and gallop, followed by the toe, and the two sides of the heels left the ground at the same time. At trot, the lateral heel contacted the ground slightly earlier than the medial side, followed by the toe, and the lateral heel left the ground before the medial heel (Ratzlaff, 1988). Under natural conditions, these contact patterns may vary according to the position of the horse's body in relation to the ground, the type of gait and the contour of the terrain.

Causes that lead to abnormal landing patterns include conformational deviation, unbalanced feet, horseshoe adjuncts, track type, fatigue and lameness. Uneven landing predisposes the horse to concussion related lameness, including DIP joint disease, ringbone, sheared heels, side bone and navicular disease (Anderson, 1992). Two common foot diseases characterized by modification of the landing patterns include laminitis and navicular disease. In laminitis, the horse places the limb forward and lands heels first in order to avoid loading the painful toe. In navicular disease, the horse lands toe first in order to avoid loading the painful palmar region.

SLIDING

The natural unshod hoof contacts the ground and begins to slide forward from the point of impact until near mid-support (Smithcors, 1961c; Sparks, 1970; Rooney, 1977b). Pardoe et al. (2001) determined that the slipping of shod horses occurs in the first 10 percent of the stance phase (tested at a trot on concrete); this slippage takes about 20-30 milliseconds. Hoof sliding attenuates the kinetic energy of the foot after impact (Pardoe et al., 2001) and reduces strain from the musculoskeletal system (Back et al., 1995). Pardoe et al. (2001) indicated that sliding over soft yielding surfaces is more pronounced at slow speeds, whereas at high speeds the feet tend to interdigitate with the ground.

During sliding, friction develops between the hoof and the ground. The degree of sliding depends on the *coefficient of friction* and the forces that press the two surfaces (hoof and ground) together.

This relationship is expressed by:

$$F = \mu V \text{ and } \mu = F/V$$

Where **F** is the friction, **μ** is the coefficient of friction and **V** is force (Rooney, 1981a; Rooney, 1999). The force is calculated from the horizontal and vertical components of the *ground reaction forces* (GRF) that act on the limb (Pardoe et al. 2001).

The friction between the hoof (or with the horseshoe) and ground determines the *slide distance*. The average slide distance of a trotting horse wearing regular iron horseshoes, tested on concrete, was 15.2 mm (Pardoe et al., 2001). Factors that alter the frictional force include gait, fore and hind limb differences, surface type, angle of surface, horseshoe material and design, horseshoe adjuncts and animal compensation. The *dynamic* coefficient of friction for sand was calculated to be 0.585 (Clanton et al. 1991). In a study that tested the grip and slippage of the hoof on various surfaces, a dynamic coefficient of friction of 0.281, 0.638, 0.710, 0.821 and 0.846 was calculated for steel, asphalt, concrete, patterned rubber and smooth rubber respectively (McClinchey et al., 2004). A low dynamic coefficient of friction implies that the hoof will slip longer, consequently the deceleration (brake) distance and time is increased.

CUTTING INTO THE GROUND

Following sliding, the hoof begins to rotate forward (Smithcors, 1961c; Sparks, 1970; Rooney, 1977b) and push against earth (Rooney, 1977b). Forward (downward) rotation or *cutting into the ground* provides sideways stability to the hoof and reduces energy expenditure. As the hoof rotates, the effective length of the limb decreases and the horse invests less energy to lift its weight over the foot (Rooney, 1977b). In essence, the effective length of the hoof lever arm is decreased (◆ fig. 8.4A).

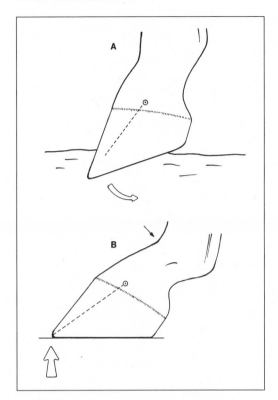

◆ **Fig. 8.4.** Cutting into the ground. A. Forward rotation of the hoof in soft ground (curved arrow). In this case, the effective length of the hoof lever is shorter than the actual length. B. Interference with forward rotation of the hoof by hard ground (large arrow) leads to excessive fetlock dorsiflextion (small arrow).

The ability of the hoof to cut into the ground may be disrupted by horseshoes and hard ground (Sparks, 1970; Rooney, 1977b). This disruption places excessive strain on the stay apparatus. In addition, there is a loss of sideways stability and increased concentration of pressure on the toe wall that may lead to development of toe cracks. Interference with cutting into the ground forces the horse to invest energy in order to lift its weight over the foot, which results in delay in breakover and consequently in excessive fetlock dorsiflexion (Rooney, 1974a) (◆ fig. 8.4B). Sparks (1970) indicated that at 90° fetlock dorsiflexion, the tension on the digital flexor tendons increases by 90 percent, and that normal maximum fetlock dorsiflexion is at or near

95°. At high speeds, this upper limit may be exceeded. Excessive fetlock dorsiflextion predisposes the horse to suspensory ligament and digital flexor tendons injuries, as well as third phalanx and sesamoidean bones fractures (Rooney, 1974b).

BREAKOVER

The last component of the support phase before the foot leaves the ground is *breakover*. Breakover is the period between heel lift and toe lifting (◆ see fig. 8.1). This stage is accompanied by the release of elastic energy stored in the suspensory apparatus. In practice, breakover reflects the ease by which the foot leaves the ground. An increase in breakover time predisposes the horse to lameness.

Breakover may be affected by horseshoes, horseshoe adjuncts, ground type and foot conformation. Balch et al. (1994) showed that low or high hoof angle did not affect stride length, but low hoof angle increased the breakover time, and high hoof angle reduced the breakover time; similar results were obtained when 4° wedges were used to elevate and lower the hoof angle (Balch et al., 1991b). A relationship between increased breakover time and low hoof angle was shown by Clayton (1990). Application of weighted horseshoes fitted with thick pads resulted in increased breakover time (Balch et al., 1996).

The increase in breakover time associated with acute hoof angle is caused by the long lever arm created by the long toe. This increased leverage requires more force to rotate the heel around the toe (Clayton, 1987) (◆ fig. 8.5). The greater effort required to rotate the hoof is associated with increased tensile stress in the DDFT and with greater compressive force on the navicular bone (Schryver et al., 1978). Furthermore, the delay in breakover causes the horse's body to move forward relative to the limb (Balch et al., 1991a), thus predisposing the horse to lameness by increasing the tension in the DDFT and the navicular ligaments that are maximally stretched at the start of breakover (Leach, 1983a). Prolongation of breakover caused by

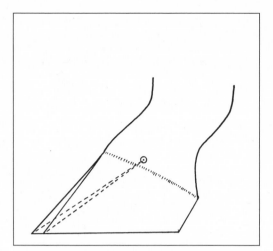

◆ **Fig. 8.5.** The effect of long-toe low-heels conformation on the hoof lever arm as compared to a normal hoof.

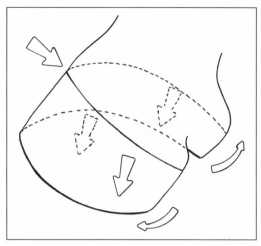

◆ **Fig. 8.6.** Hoof deformation during impact. The arrows indicate hoof wall expansion (curved arrows), decreased hoof wall height, sole flattening, and inward motion at the coronary band (large arrows). (Data from Lungwitz A. 1891.)

acute hoof angulations may limit the horse's ability to increase stride frequency (Leach, 1986b).

 HOOF DEFORMATION

DURING NORMAL WEIGHT BEARING, THE HOOF capsule deforms in a consistent pattern (Douglas et al., 1996), yielding under the pressure of impact and dissipate concussive forces (Sack and Habel, 1977). Lungwitz (1891) investigated the changes in hoof form during loading by using an instrumented horseshoe connected to an electrical apparatus. He was able to detect concurrent expansion of the heels, flattening of the sole, diminution of the height of the hoof capsule with sinking of the bulb of the heel, and inward movement of the dorsal aspect of the hoof wall at the height of the coronary band (◆ fig. 8.6). He also observed that heel expansion in horses with contracted hooves was minimal. Reduced heel expansion in contracted heels cases may result from the steeper hoof wall, dry hoof capsule or chronic heel pain that commonly

accompanied the condition. Dejardin et al. (1999) showed that the lower margin of the hoof wall, distal to the free edge of the third phalanx, tends to spread farther than its proximal surface.

The most pronounced change in the hoof shape during foot impact includes the expansion of the quarters and heels. This expansion can be readily observed by development of grooves over the hoof surface at the branches of metal horseshoes. These grooves are caused by constant friction between the hoof wall and the horseshoe. Historically, expansion of the heels during motion was explained by the frog pressure theory. Later works suggest that the role of frog pressure in heel expansion is small (Colles, 1989a), although Roepstorff et al. (2001) showed that increased pressure on the frog and sole resulted in higher expansion, compared to pressing the hoof wall only. Interestingly, they also detected slight contraction of the heel prior to breakover. Another explanation for hoof expansion during foot loading was that the second phalanx compresses the digital cushion, which in return expands the quarters and heels. A study by Taylor et al. (2005) showed that hoof wall expansion is not affected by the digital cushion. The degree of expansion at the quarters and heels is also influenced by the degree of friction between the hoof and surface (McClinchey et al. 2004). Roepstorff et al. (2001) determined that maximum heel expansion occurs at 20 percent and 33 percent of the stance phase in walk and trot respectively.

The expansion of the quarters and heels is made possible by the frog, digital cushion, lateral cartilages and the bulbs of the heels. At the same time, the bars stabilize the hoof without decreasing its ability to expand (Smithcors, 1961c). The horn moisture content also has a rule in hoof deformation. The distal hoof wall at the heel has shorter growth distance, therefore it is made of younger horn which contains more moisture; therefore, it is more yielding and deformable under pressure (Kainer, 1989). The to-and-fro movement of the heels may be explained by the presence of the flexible lateral cartilages at the palmar/plantar regions of the foot (Sisson and Grossman, 1953). The white line may play a role in hoof yielding during motion by forming a flexible zone between the rigid hoof wall and the moderately soft sole (Budras et al., 1998).

Proper function of the foot can be described by the following association:

circulation ➤ **moisture** ➤ **elasticity** ➤ **deformation** ➤ **shock absorption**

Hoof deformation during locomotion depends on hoof horn elasticity. The optimal elasticity of the horn depends on its moisture content, and the moisture level is maintained primarily by the foot circulation; circulation is optimal when hoof deformation is normal (Lungwitz, 1891). Therefore, any interference with these events may affect the shock absorption capability of the foot. Factors that may interfere with proper hoof function include lameness, imbalance, horseshoes and their adjuncts, lack of exercise, and the physical environment.

SHOCK ABSORPTION

Sack and Habel (1977) and Dyhre-Poulson et al. (1994) indicated that the hoof is remarkably adaptable to accommodate concussion produced by contact with the ground. During locomotion, the hoof strikes the ground with great force and frequency; in the galloping horse, the vertical concussive force may reach 9000 N (Quddus et al., 1978; Geary, 1975) which is equivalent to twice the bodyweight of the animal (Newlyn et al. 1998). This force is being transmitted to the bearing surface of the hoof wall over a total area of ~20 cm² (Bertram and Gosline, 1986). Therefore, the relatively small foot has to adapt to distributing the horse's weight and reducing concussion (Smithcors, 1961c). Although the full mechanism of shock absorption in the foot has yet to be explored, it most likely involves several structures including the hoof capsule (Sack and Habel, 1977; Lambert, 1971), frog and bars (Lambert, 1971), laminae (Lanovaz et al., 1998), lateral cartilages and digital cushion (Stump, 1967; Bowker et al., 1998) and the hoof venous system (Stump, 1967; Ratzlaff et al., 1985; Bowker et al., 1998).

Wright and Douglas (1993a) indicated that foot expansion reduces vertical impact forces. During impact, the horse's weight causes an outward expansion of the hoof at the quarters and heels; this response can be compared to the function of a loaded spring, with deformation resulting in absorption of some of the impact forces. The expansion of the quarters and heels is permitted by the frog, the open palmar/plantar area of the foot, the slope of the hoof wall and by the lateral cartilages. During hoof deformation, the bars function as supporters that prevent excessive expansion. Once the foot is lifted, the bars assist in the return of the quarters and heels to preload position (◆ fig. 8.7). At the same time, the frog functions as a hinge that permits outward expansion of the hoof while protecting sensitive structures within the foot (Avisar, 1995). This hypothesis can be tested by designing an experimental horseshoe or a

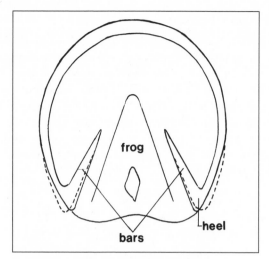

◆ **Fig. 8.7.** Proposed shock absorption mechanism of the foot, schematic illustration. During impact, the hoof expands like a spring, absorbing forces of impact. Once the foot is lifted, the hoof returns to preload position. The dashed line represents the position of the hoof wall during impact.

device that prevents sideway expansion of the hoof wall during motion. Once the device is fitted, the forces transmitted in the hoof wall can be measured and compared to these in hooves without restricted movement.

The laminae, although its primary role is the suspension of the third phalanx, may be involved in dissipation of shock through its large surface area formed between the epidermal and dermal laminae. Lanovaz et al, (1998) proposed that the distal hoof wall and its laminar dermis absorb and transmit the impact to the bones of the limbs. They proposed that the digital bones and joints might play a larger role in attenuation of shock than the hoof wall and digital soft tissue.

Ratzlaff et al. (1985) demonstrated rapid increase in digital venous pressure at the onset of the stance phase in walking and trotting horses. They proposed that the hydraulic components of the hoof venous system absorb some of the initial impact during locomotion. Bowker et al. (1998) proposed that during impact, energy is dissipated by blood that is being forced into the venous system of the lateral cartilages. This process is followed

by build-up of negative pressure within the digital cushion (Dyhre-Poulsen et al., 1994) that enhances the refilling of the veins within the lateral cartilages (Bowker et al., 1998). Being a large and enclosed pad by itself, the digital cushion that occupies most of the palmar/plantar area of the foot may have an important role in shock absorption.

The shock absorption mechanism of the foot may be disrupted by abnormal foot conformation such as thin hoof wall, contracted heels, small feet, mule feet, sheared heels and imbalanced feet. In addition, horseshoes, dry hooves and excessive moisture may interrupt the outward expansion of the hoof. Therefore, any condition that interferes with normal hoof deformation can eventually lead to lameness. Studies on the relationship between shock absorption, abnormal foot conformation and lameness are lacking.

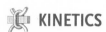 KINETICS

Kinetics IS THE STUDY OF FORCES INVOLVED IN the interaction between the limb and the ground during motion (kinematics). These forces continuously change their magnitude and direction during impact, sliding, cutting into the ground, and breakover. The magnitude and direction of these forces are described by pairs of *vertical* and *horizontal force vectors*. Each pair of these forces has a *resultant force* that is equal to the effect of the vertical and horizontal forces acting together (◆ fig. 8.8).

From the initial contact of the limb until mid-support, the horizontal force is dominated by *braking force*. At mid-support, the hoof begins to push back and the horizontal force is dominated by *propulsive force*. The vertical force results from the horse's weight pressing against earth; this force is the *supportive force*. Vertical forces increase in magnitude from impact until mid-support and then decrease (Rooney, 1977b; Hildebrand, 1982).

Force plate studies show that the vertical peak force exerted by the limbs during trot is approximately 1100 lbs and 1000 lbs for the

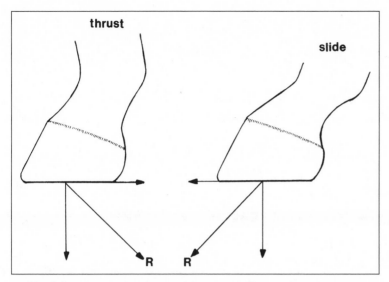

◆ **Fig. 8.8.** Horizontal and vertical forces and their resultant force (R) during slide and thrust. (Adapted from Rooney, J.R. 1977b, fig. 1, and Hildebrand, M. 1982, fig. 22.4F.)

fore and hind limb respectively (Ratzlaff, 1988). Schryver et al. (1978) indicates that the maximum vertical force exerted on the hoof is about 0.6 multiple by the body weight for the walk and about 0.9 multiple by the body weight for the trot. The average *ground reaction force* (GRF) or the force that developed by the interaction between the limb and ground in a group of Dutch Warmblood horses at normal trot was 11.59 N/kg and 10.21 N/kg for the fore limbs and hind limbs respectively (Merkens et al., 1993).

Foot Kinetics

Foot kinetics is the study of the force distribution within the foot during locomotion. As with the limb, these forces change their magnitude and direction during the support phase. To find the location of the force, a single force is calculated from a given number of force vectors. This force is the resultant force (Badoux, 1975). By knowing the normal location of the resultant force for each gait and at different phases of each gait, it becomes possible to study the effect of farriery manipula-

tions, gait alteration and ground type on these forces.

The location of the resultant force consistently changes as the horse's body passes over the hoof during the support phase, moving from palmar/plantar location toward the toe (Barrey, 1990; Balch et al., 1991b). The vertical component of the force is not distributed uniformly over the hoof surface (Barrey, 1990). Measurements of force distribution within the foot, with the use of instrumented horseshoes, showed that the vertical forces are higher on the medial heel compared to the lateral heel during walk, trot, and gallop; the vertical forces at the toe are lower than these measured at the heel. At breakover, a pronounced force spike developed at the toe (Ratzlaff, 1988).

Measurements of the horizontal and vertical forces exerted by the hoof showed that the location of a single vector representing all the forces applied to the digit was centered on the forward third of the frog at walk and trot (Schryver et al., 1978). Seeherman et al. (1987) and Barrey (1990) obtained similar results, but in some horses, the force was displaced away from the middle plane. Other studies

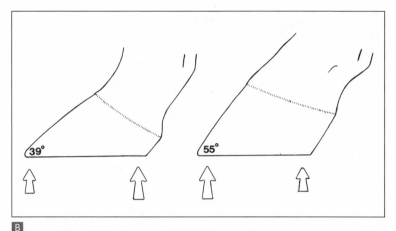

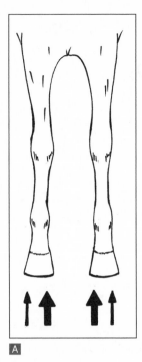

♦ **Fig. 8.9.** **Weight distribution.** A. Relative weight distribution between the medial and lateral sides of the limb in the normal standing horse, schematic illustration. Data from Colahan P. et al. 1993. B. Relative weight distribution between the toe and heels in a hoof with normal and acute hoof angles, measured at a walk. Data from Barrey, E. 1990.

showed that the location of the resultant force was medial to the center of the foot throughout the majority of the stance phase, in both the fore and hind feet (Williams, 1977a; Williams and Smith, 1977b). These studies show that force distribution in well-balanced hooves landing simultaneously on both heels or flat-footed is not even (Ratzlaff, 1988; Barrey, 1990; Balch et al., 1991b).

More evidence of unequal distribution of weight between the medial and lateral sides of the limb comes from examination of cross sections of the metacarpus. The medial side of the bone has a greater mass of supporting bone compared to the lateral side. This indicates that the medial side of the bone bears more weight (Nickel et al., 1986). Firth et al. (1988) showed that the medial surface of the metacarpal bone in young foals naturally receives more compressive strain than the lateral side. Mackay-Smith (1993) indicated that the asymmetry of the hoof itself causes the weight to be born eccentrically to the limb. Colahan et al. (1993) showed that the pressure in the hoof of standing horses is higher in the medial heel compared to the

lateral heel (♦ fig. 8.9A). Greater force placement on the medial side of the hoof may explain the higher incidence of quarter cracks and corns on that side.

From these studies it appear that unless there is a compensatory mechanism, the natural unshod hoof should wear faster at the medial side. Natural correction of this may be explained by the different angulations of the two sides of the hoof. At equal growth rate on both sides, the horn on the relatively acute, medial side, should reach the ground before the more obtuse lateral side. This compensatory mechanism may be enhanced by faster growth rate at the medial side.

The above studies and observations indicate that force distribution within the foot is an asymmetrical event. The force magnitude, direction and location continuously change during the support phase. Therefore, when the horse's foot is assumed to be balanced it does not imply an even distribution of forces over the solar surface, but an optimal distribution of forces that reduces the probability for lameness.

Effect of Farriery Manipulations on Foot Kinetics

Measurements of vertical force distribution taken at a walk from a horse with acute hoof angle (39°) and normal hoof angle (55°) showed greater force concentration at the heel region at low hoof angle and greater force concentration at the toe region at normal hoof angle (Barrey 1990) (◆ fig. 8.9B). No data was given on force distribution when the horse was standing. In a different study, the forces on the medial region of the heel increased when the angle of the hoof was either increased or decreased by 4.0 degrees (Balch et al., 1991b). Wilson et al. (1998) studied the effect of elevating the hoof sideways, and changing the hoof angle. They concluded that the resulting imbalance, accompanied by abnormal loads in the elevated regions of the hoof, could have a detrimental effect on hoof structure and horn growth.

These studies suggest that factors that interfere with normal distribution of weight predispose the horse to lameness; these factors include abnormal foot conformation, horseshoe adjuncts and foot imbalance.

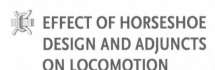

EFFECT OF GROUND TYPE ON LOCOMOTION

DOMESTICATION HAS LED TO THE USE OF THE horse on artificial ground that tends to alter the natural motion of the foot. In addition, horses are required to work at speeds and gaits that may not match their nature or the ground type. The ground type may alter the hoof flight pattern, foot and ground interaction, hoof deformation and distribution of forces. Studies on the effect of ground type on locomotion can provide information about surface suitability and horseshoe design.

Cheney et al. (1973) indicated that the maximal force of galloping on hard ground is approximately 900 kg and this force is reduced significantly over soft soil. According to Bartel et al. (1978) the loads from hard soil can be two and one-half times greater than

loads from soft surface. Kai et al. (1999) tested the effect of rough track surface on the vertical forces placed on the hoof in a group of cantering Thoroughbred horses. Their results showed a significant increase in vertical forces compared to a smooth surface.

Soil has higher resistance to hoof rotation and lower shock loading compared to sand (Zebarth and Sheard, 1985). Scheffer and Back (2001) indicated that a soft track allows natural forward rotation of the hoof, thus relieving pressure from the navicular area and decreasing fetlock dorsiflexion. Prolonged work on hard ground predisposes the horse to *road founder* caused by increased concussion and interference with forward hoof rotation (Rooney, 1978). A relationship between concussion and development of ringbone was described by Percivall (1865).

The type of ground should be considered when shoeing the horse. Horses that work on deep sand may walk easier with wide-web horseshoes, whereas horses that work on hard ground should be protected with a cushioned material. The addition of horseshoe adjuncts to the horseshoe in order to match the feet with the ground predisposes the horse to lameness (see below).

EFFECT OF HORSESHOE DESIGN AND ADJUNCTS ON LOCOMOTION

HORSESHOE DESIGN AND HORSESHOE ADJUNCTS may protect the foot and prevent lameness, or could interfere with normal hoof function and predispose the horse to injury. Horseshoes are commonly made from aluminum, steel or synthetic materials in various designs, dimensions and weights. In addition, the horseshoe may have adjuncts that aim at modifying foot function. The *horseshoe design* includes the horseshoe profile and the proportions between the horseshoe web and thickness. The *horseshoe profile* may be altered by rounding, rolling, squaring, tapering, seating and spooning the horseshoe. For example, rocker toe horseshoe provides rolling effect, which makes it suitable for horses that work on asphalt (Vanschepdael, 2006). The *horseshoe's dimensions* are related to the size of the hoof and intended type of activity. Historically, horseshoes were very thick and heavy and in many instances were fitted with odd adjuncts; with time, lighter horseshoes that places the foot closer to the ground replaced these horseshoes.

Horseshoe adjuncts are additions that modify the horseshoe. These may include traction devices such as toe grabs, trailers, stickers, mud nails, jar calks, heel calks and heel blocks. Other additions include pads and clips. With future advancement of glue-on shoes, horseshoe nails may be considered adjuncts too. Gross et al. (2004) pointed out that studies on the link between traction devices and lameness (non-catastrophic lameness) are lacking. They indicated that the type and number of devices applied to a horseshoe could affect the foot and ground interaction in different ways.

With the known data on the benefits and risks of horseshoes and their adjuncts, farriers, veterinarians and trainers can prevent many lameness cases. Hoof management should include proper balancing of the foot, leaving the horse barefoot whenever possible, fitting horseshoes with adequate palmar/plantar supports (see page 67) and avoiding using horseshoe adjuncts that predispose the horse to injuries.

The following sections provide examples on the effect of horseshoe design and adjuncts on the foot and stay apparatus.

Metal Horseshoes

Willemen et al. (1999) found a significant increase in the force placed on the navicular bone by the DDFT in horses with metal horseshoes compared to unshod horses (tested on a treadmill). Dyhre-Poulsen et al. (1994) and Benoit et al. (1993) showed that horseshoeing decreases the dampening action of the hoof and increases the impact shock. Marks et al. (1971) indicated that conventional horseshoeing greatly reduces the surface area of ground contact, which results in the spread of concus-

sive forces only to the wall. These findings deserve further investigation regarding the possible role of metal horseshoes as a risk factor for navicular disease in horses prone to the disease.

The low friction coefficient of iron can be a problem for horses working on hard surface (McClinchey et al. 2004). Sudden alteration in gait or direction may cause the horse to slip and could result in serious injury to the rider and horse. The horse's grip can be improved by welding borium to the ground surface of the horseshoe; but preventing hoof sliding strains the limb and predisposes the horse to lameness. Pardoe et al. (2001) indicated that on roadway surfaces, a compromise must be achieved between allowing foot slip and providing sufficient grip.

Slippage may be prevented by keeping horses barefoot when possible. Horses that work on paved surface, such as police horses, may be fitted with metal horseshoes with low profile, *spot borium*, welded to the ground surface of the horseshoes. Alternatively, the feet can be fitted with hoof boots that provide good traction. Trail horses ridden on slippery rocks may be fitted with *grooved horseshoes* made by making several parallel grooves across the horseshoe branches with a creaser; this result in ridges that increase traction with the ground (◆ fig. 8.10). The calks of ice horse-

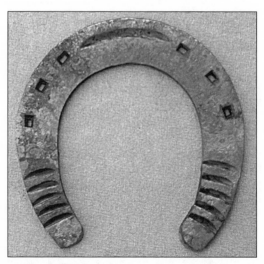

◆ **Fig. 8.10.** Grooved horseshoe. Additional grooves may be added as required. (Photo by author.)

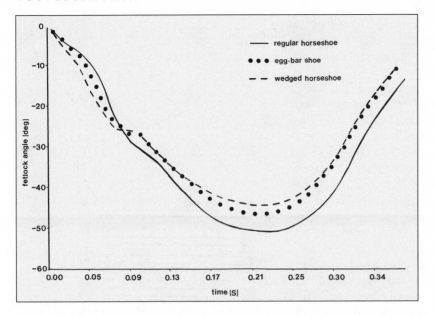

◆ **Fig. 8.11.** The effect of horseshoe type on fetlock dorsiflextion, tested at a trot on sand. Values that are more negative indicate increased fetlock dorsiflextion. (Reprinted by permission from Scheffer, C.J.W. and Back, W. 2001, fig. 3. Illustration modified to text.)

shoes should be filed smooth in order to reduce the risk of tread wounds. Wiseman (1968) recommended using screw-in-type calks and removing them when the horse is not working or using frost nails instead.

Horseshoe Design

Conventional horseshoes may interfere with forward rotation of the hoof by forcing the hoof to continue to slide forward and remain flat on the ground. The horse's momentum and the resistance caused by the "stubbing" of the toe against the dirt result in excessive fetlock dorsiflextion (Sparks, 1970). This effect becomes more pronounced when the horse is being worked on hard ground.

Scheffer and Back (2001) compared the effect of three types of horseshoes on limb kinematics at a walk and at trot. The tests were conducted on hard, semi-soft and soft ground. When trotted on sand, fetlock dorsiflextion was significantly smaller in horses fitted with a 5° wedged horseshoe compared to a regular horseshoe and an egg-bar shoe (◆ fig. 8.11).

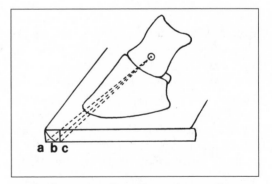

◆ **Fig. 8.12.** The effect of horseshoe profile on the hoof lever arm, schematic illustration. The examples include regular horseshoe (a), half-round horseshoe (b) and square-toed horseshoe (c).

The application of horseshoes that shorten the hoof lever arm (HLA) is a common practice aimed at reducing breakover time. Examples of this horseshoe type include half-round horseshoe, square-toe horseshoe, rolled-toe horseshoe and rocker-toe horseshoe (◆ fig. 8.12). Clayton et al. (1990b) showed that rolling, rockering, or squaring the toe does not hasten breakover in normal horses trotted on concrete. Similarly, horseshoes that were set back at the toe did not hasten breakover (Eliashar et al., 2002). In another experiment, van Heel et al. (2006) compared the affect of regular horseshoe and rolled toe horseshoe (the rolled toe horseshoes were very similar to worn out horseshoes). Their results show no significant difference in breakover time between the two horseshoes, but the rolled toe horseshoe improved ease of movement. In spite of these findings, horseshoes that shorten the HLA may allow greater natural forward rotation, and reduce strain from the stay apparatus in injured horses. For this reason, trainers attempt to reset worn horseshoes instead of fitting new horseshoes.

Horseshoes alter the support dimensions of the foot in several ways. Application of extended-heel horseshoes increases the base distance of the foot and increases palmar/plantar support. This practice is important for the prevention and treatment of stay apparatus injuries. Square-toe horseshoes decrease the base distance, but this effect may be offset by the reduced HLA obtained with these horseshoes, and by extending the heels in order to increase palmar/plantar support. Beveled horseshoes decrease the base distance of the foot and predispose the horse to stay apparatus injuries. Fitting the hoof with a short horseshoe has a similar effect; the horseshoe places abnormal stress at the palmar/plantar aspect of the foot (Wright and Douglas, 1993) by forming functionally under-run heels with a decreased palmar/plantar support (Anderson, 1992) (◆ fig. 8.13). Stanley (2004) indicated that bar shoes increase friction with the ground, and that could affect performance in Standardbred racehorses.

Effect of Horseshoe Nails

Data on the effect of horseshoe nails on hoof function varies. Miles (1846) indicated that normal heel movement during motion is restricted by excessive numbers of nails. Colles (1989b) used strain gauges applied to the hoof wall to measure changes in hoof shape during motion in shod and unshod

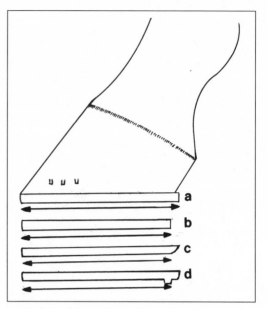

◆ **Fig. 8.13.** The effect of horseshoe dimensions, design and adjuncts on base distance. The examples include square-cut heels (a), short branches (b), beveled heels (c) and a horseshoe fitted with heel studs (d).

horses; the results indicated that the use of conventional nailed-on iron shoes had little effect on the degree of expansion of the heels. Hinterhofer et al. (2001) applied a model to test the effect of clips (see below) and horseshoe nails on hoof deformation and strain. The results show dominant stress areas in the bars, outer layers of the proximal dorsal wall and in hoof horn material surrounding nail fixations, particularly at the third nail. Moyer and Anderson (1975a) indicated that hoof expansion is limited with excessive number of nails and that the feet expand considerably following removal of horseshoes. Thomason (1998) reported that shoeing had little effect on hoof deformation compared to non-shoeing. Roepstorff et al. (2001) found significant differences between the average heel's expansion in barefoot and shod horses. The average heel expansion in the forelimb of five Standardbred trotters tested barefoot was 0.44 mm at a walk and 0.67 mm at a trot. When fitted with iron horseshoes, expansion decreased to 0.34 mm at a walk and 0.51 mm

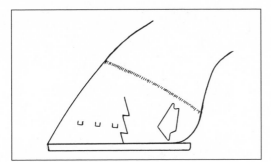

◆ **Fig. 8.14.** The effect of horseshoe nails on hoof expansion. Expansion (arrow) at the heel is restricted by the horseshoe nails. This results in stress areas at the hoof wall (zigzag line).

at a trot. McClinchey et al. (2004) indicated that although horseshoe nails may limit hoof expansion, the low coefficient of friction of iron horseshoes may result in greater expansion behind the nails compared to the rest of the wall; this can result in *bending stress* at the junction between the fixed wall and the free wall. This may explain the presence of hoof wall splits, chips, and cracks commonly observed at the quarters area (◆ fig. 8.14). Studies on possible effects of horseshoe nails in development of micro-fractures that may predispose the wall to cracks are lacking. No information was found on possible effects of horseshoe spreaders on the hoof.

Clips

Rich (1907) indicated that large toe clips can cause toe cracks; he recommended using low clips. Hinterhofer et al. (2001) measured stress areas in the hoof horn surrounding side clips; placement of toe clips and two side clips behind the third nail resulted in reduced deformation and stress values compared to regular horseshoes, toe clips and side clips, placed alone. No data was found on the effect of clips during motion.

Horseshoe Weight

Excessively heavy horseshoes can increase fatigue and lead to lameness. The weight of the horseshoe increases the inertia of the foot

and the energy invested during locomotion (Balch et al., 1995a). Balch et al. (1996) showed that application of weighted horseshoes (weight 724 to 869 grams) resulted in elevation of the flight path of the hoof and increased breakover time. Lengthening the hooves by 2.5 cm with the weighted horseshoes increased the height of the flight path further. Willemen (1994) found no effect of toe weights (weight 88 gm) on stride characteristics of the forelegs of Standardbred trotters tested on a treadmill. In a different study (Willemen et al., 1997), regular horseshoes (10 mm thick) with an average weight of 478 gm were fitted to the forelimbs of Dutch Warmblood horses. At trot, the horseshoes increased limb action and decreased limb extension during protraction. The height of the hoof above the ground increased (significantly) from an average of 10.0 cm in unshod horses to 17.4 cm in shod horses. In this study, fetlock dorsiflexion (extension) was not affected but fetlock flexion was significantly higher.

Toe Grabs

Fetlock over-dorsiflextion can occur when the foot cannot slide forward, as when wearing horseshoes with heel calks and toe grabs (Rooney, 1974b). Kane (1996b) reported an increased incidence of suspensory apparatus failure (SAF) in racehorses fitted with toe grabs. He indicated that the effect of the toe grabs was multiple. First, it elevated the toe and lowered the hoof angle; second, it increased the traction between the horseshoe and ground and interfered with normal hoof slide (◆ fig. 8.15). The risk of injury increased with taller toe grabs (Grubb and Kane, 1997; Kane et al., 1996a; Kane, 1996b); horses shod with taller toe grabs on the front shoes had odds 15 times greater for SAF compared with horses shod with regular toe grabs (Kane et al., 1996a). Toe grabs, which probably have a similar biomechanical effect to lowering the heels, may increase pressure on the navicular bone (Forssell, 1943) and concentrate impact forces at the toe (Moyer, 1988a). Gabel (1982) recom-

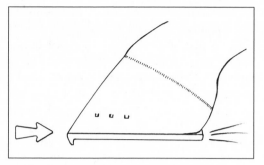

◆ **Fig. 8.15.** The effect of toe grabs on locomotion. The toe grab causes reduced sliding distance (arrow); this results in excessive stress on bones and joints as well as on the stay apparatus.

mended using horseshoe adjuncts that have minimal effect on traction in order to prevent tarsus injuries in Standardbred racehorses.

Heel Calks

Heel calks concentrate the energy of impact at the palmar/plantar portion of the foot (Moyer, 1988a). Rich (1907) pointed out that high calks are responsible for increased incidence of ring bone, curbs and spavin, due to excessive strain that is being placed on the limbs. The last two disorders are associated with the hock area. Studies by Thompson and Herring (1994) on the effect of horseshoe calks on foot kinematics led to the conclusions that calks change the joint angulations in a way that could lead to joint damage; no differences were detected in stride length, frequency or duration compared to regular horseshoes. Concentration of excessive pressure on the heel may result in development of sheared heels; similar change may result from a horseshoe with a trailer.

Padding Material

Benoit et al. (1993) compared the damping effect of steel horseshoe with that of polyurethane covered horseshoes, and of horseshoes fitted with plastic, leather or rubber pad. The horses were tested on asphalt. The results showed that all types of padding material dissipate shock significantly better than steel horseshoes. Marks et al. (1971) calculated a reduction of 19 percent in concussion for horseshoes fitted with a pad and molding compound applied to the solar surface. They also observed an improvement in horn quality in horses shod with the cushioning material, and speculated that this may be attributed to improved hoof circulation. Pardoe et al.(2001) indicated that plastic shoes may reduce the incidence of impact-associated stress (jarring) injuries in horses exercised on roads, by providing better slippage properties in comparison to metal and rubber horseshoes.

Wedge Pads

In a study on a group of ponies fitted with egg-bar shoes, strain was decreased from the DDFT and increased in the suspensory ligament (SL) (Riemersa et al., 1996). The application of a 7° heel wedge resulted in decreased strain from the DDFT and inferior check ligament (ICL), but strain in the SL was increased. The application of a 7° toe wedge increased the strain on the ICL. Willemen et al. (1999) indicated that horseshoes with heel wedges reduce the force exerted by the DDFT on the navicular bone.

Chapter 9

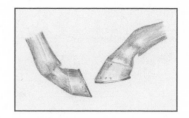

Foot Balance

THE PURPOSE OF BALANCING THE FOOT IS TO reduce strain and concussion from the limb in order to minimize lameness, increase the productive life of the horse and maximize its performance. Balancing the foot includes viewing the limb from two perspectives. The first is made from the side of the horse and is concerned with the dorsal-palmar/plantar balance of the foot. The second is made from the front (or rear) of the horse and is concerned with the medial-lateral balance of the foot. Dorsal-palmar/plantar imbalance may result from improper toe length and hoof angle, and by abnormal hoof conformation. Problems associated with this type of imbalance include *strain injuries* such as tendonitis and suspensory desmitis. In addition overstressing the flexor tendon is a predisposing factor for navicular disease, and injuries to the flexor area of the third phalanx. Medial-lateral imbalance may result from deviations of the hoof, digit or limb and unequal hoof wall length at the quarters and heels. Problems associated with this type of imbalance include *sprain injuries* such as collateral ligament desmitis. In addition, the digit is predisposed to development of sheared heels and side bone.

Hoof imbalance may result in abnormal concussion forces that may cause direct pain within the hoof or more proximally to it (Snow and Birdsall, 1990). In a study (Dyson, 1991) on a group of horses with DIP joint pain, a significant number of horses had imbalanced feet with some having toeing-in or toeing-out foot conformation.

Balancing the foot involves the correction of side-to-side and front to back imbalances. This is done by establishing proper foot and pastern axis. The *foot axis* is the inclination of the foot (or hoof) with reference to the ground surface as observed from dorsal and lateral perspectives. The *pastern axis* is the inclination of the segment of the limb between the fetlock and hoof with reference to the ground surface as observed from dorsal and lateral perspectives. When the foot is balanced, these axes form a straight line when viewed from the lateral and dorsal perspectives (Shively, 1982a).

DORSO-PALMAR/PLANTAR BALANCE

Dorso-palmar/plantar balance IS CONCERNED with the foot and pastern axes of the limb as viewed from the side of the horse. In this

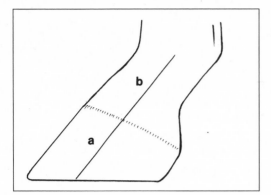

◆ **Fig. 9.1.** Dorso-palmar/plantar balance,
lateral view. The foot axis (a) and pastern axis
(b) in a balanced foot. (Adapted from Shively, M.J.
1982, fig. 3.)

view, the foot axis in essence is the hoof angle
(◆ fig. 9.1). In a properly balanced foot, the
dorsal hoof wall is parallel with the pastern
axis as viewed from their lateral planes
(Shively, 1982a; Balch et al., 1991a).
Concurrently, optimal hoof length should be
maintained. Dorso-palmar/plantar balance is
also concerned with palmar/plantar support
(see below). Factors that affect dorso-pal-
mar/plantar balance include excessive hoof
growth or wear, various foot disorders such as
laminitis and clubfoot, abnormal hoof conformation such as under-run heels, trimming
errors, horseshoes and horseshoe adjuncts.

One of the theories of foot balance,
described in many texts, indicates that ideal
dorso-palmar/plantar plane occurs when the
phalanges bones are aligned. Bushe et al.
(1987) indicated that regardless of the hoof
angle made to balance the foot, true axial
alignment does not occur because the pastern
joint is normally slightly overextended. In
addition, different alignments of the phalanges bones may result from individual variations among horses.

When the lines of the foot axis and the
pastern axis are not continuous when viewed
from the lateral side, the foot conformation is
described as *broken foot* (Shively, 1982a). Low
hoof angle, such as observed in long-toe low-
heels hoof conformation, causes a *broken
backward* foot axis (◆ fig. 9.2). Broken back-

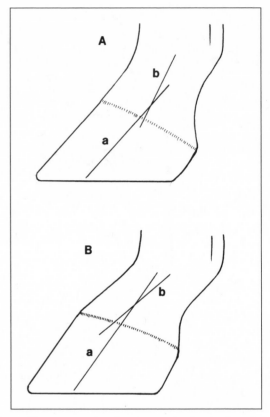

◆ **Fig. 9.2.** Broken foot axis. A. Broken backward
foot axis in low hoof angle. B. Broken forward foot
axis in high hoof angle. (Adapted from Shively, M.J.
1982a, figures 4A and 4B.)

ward foot axis has been associated with a
greater risk for breakdowns in racehorses
(Kobluk et al., 1990). High hoof angle, such as
observed in clubfoot, causes a *broken forward*
foot axis.

The goal of balancing the foot in a dorso-
palmar/plantar plane is to achieve an optimal
alignment of the phalangeal bones that falls
within a safe range. Correction of dorso-pal-
mar/plantar imbalance can be a challenge in
horses with a long-toe low-heels foot conformation that has a flat sole, which may indicate
previous history of laminitis. In these cases,
the heel may have proper height but trimming the sole is difficult. The solution to this
problem is to fit the hoof with wedged horseshoes or a horseshoe and a wedge pad that
raise the heels, and provides additional pal-

mar/plantar support. These cases should be shoed more often. Dubbing the toe in order to shorten the hoof lever arm in these cases should be avoided, as this will reduce the base area, and leave the foot axis broken.

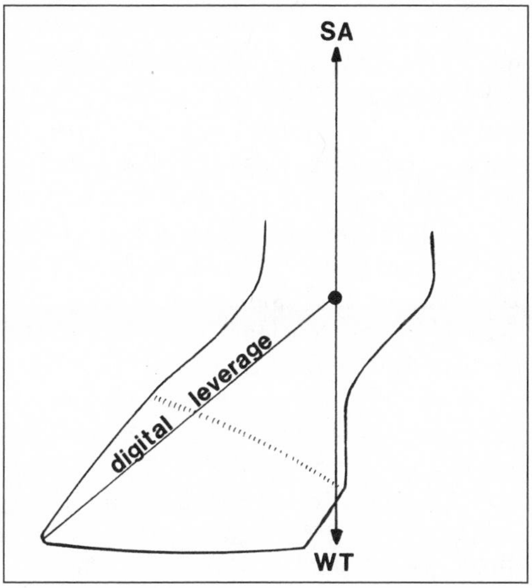

Palmar/Plantar Support

Palmar/plantar support describes the opposing action of the stay apparatus against forces that tend to collapse the digit. These forces act on the *digital leverage* which is formed by the slope of the digit. A line drawn from the fetlock joint to the tip of the hoof represents the digital leverage (◆ fig. 9.3). Various factors affect the ability of the stay apparatus to resist these forces, including foot and digit conformation, hoof growth and wear, and horseshoes and their adjuncts. Other factors include the weight of the horse and the strength of the suspensory apparatus. Decreased palmar/plantar support implies increased fetlock dorsiflexion (drop) toward the ground when the limb is loaded, thus more strain is placed on the suspensory apparatus and more force is required to rotate the foot forward. Any change that decreases the base distance, increases the load distance or increases the hoof lever arm affects palmar/plantar support.

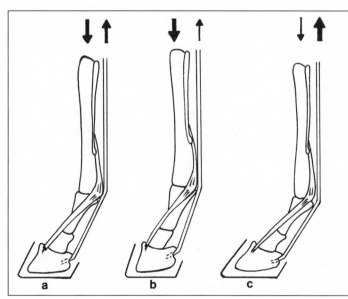

◆ **Fig. 9.3.** Palmar/plantar support. The horse's weight (WT) acts on the lever arm formed by the slope of the digit. This force is resisted by the stay apparatus (SA).

Another way to visualize palmar/plantar support is by comparing three conformation types of the digit: normal, upright pastern and slopping pasterns (◆ fig. 9.4). In the normal digit a balance between load and support, exist (if the horse is not tired or have long hooves etc.). With upright pasterns, there is good palmar/plantar support but the bony column receives too much weight. With slopping pasterns, palmar/plantar support is poor and the suspensory apparatus is overloaded (Brown Edwards, 1973).

◆ **Fig. 9.4.** Palmar/plantar support in three conformation types. Normal (a), upright pastern (b), and slopping pastern (c). The arrows represent the balance or imbalance between load on the bony column and support by the stay apparatus (represented by the suspensory ligament and deep digital flexor tendon). (Adapted from Brown Edwards G. 1973, page 165.)

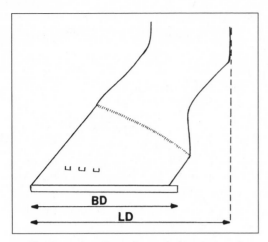

◆ **Fig. 9.5.** The effect of extended heels horseshoe on the support dimensions of the foot. BD=Base distance, LD=Load distance.

Once the horse is trimmed, the hoof continues to grow in a distal-dorsal direction. This growth increases the leverage placed on the digit, and consequently more strain is placed on the stay apparatus. Maintenance of optimal palmar/plantar support is an important principle of farriery. This is achieved by keeping regular trimming intervals; in cases where the horse is shod, the horseshoes should be fitted with the branches slightly extended. This, in essence, increases the base distance and provide more palmar/plantar support (◆ fig. 9.5). Some horses may be trimmed at a slightly higher hoof angle to compensate for development of low heels toward the end of the shoeing interval.

Hoof Angle Manipulations

Modifying the hoof angle changes the angulations of the digital joint and consequently the orientation of the foot axis. In a study that tested the effect of hoof angle on the digital and fetlock joints, one degree elevation of the hoof angle resulted in flexion of the DIP joint by 0.9°, flexion of the PIP joint by 0.3°, and extension (dorsiflexion) of the fetlock joint by 0.1° (Bushe et al.,1987) (◆ table 9.1). Similar results were obtained by Crevier-Denoix et al.

(2001). This data shows that manipulation of the hoof angle affects primarily the DIP joint. Thus, a slight change in hoof angle can lead to misalignment of the foot axis and pastern axis (Frandson et al., 1976). The hoof angle may be manipulated as part of the treatment of several foot disorders. This may include raising or lowering the hoof angle to vary the tension in the stay apparatus. Raising the hoof angle is commonly practiced to reduce tension from the DDFT in navicular disease cases in order to reduce pressure from the navicular bone. Lowering the hoof angle is commonly practiced to increase tension on the DDFT in contracted DDFT in foals.

Lochner et al. (1980) measured strain values in the stay apparatus in horses with hoof angle ranging between 40° to 70°. High hoof angle resulted in decreased mean tendon strain in the DDFT at standing. No significant difference in the level of strain was found in the SDFT or SL when the hoof angle was raised or lowered at standing and walking. Thompson (1998) indicated that DDFT strain decreased by 59 percent when the hoof angle was increased from 55° to 78°. At high hoof angle, significant increase in strain developed in the extensor branches of the SL. He proposed that the pull on the extensor branch may aid in stabilizing the third phalanx bone in laminitis cases.

Viitanen et al. (2003) showed that elevating the heels by 5° was associated with increased DIP joint intra-articular pressure and localized articular contact at the dorsal aspect of the joint. They indicated that this change might be detrimental to the joint in the long term. Crevier-Denoix et al. (2001) noted that heel elevation is strongly indicative for navicular disease cases because of the relief of DDFT tension, but heel elevation in cases of fetlock injuries is contraindicated in most cases because of the resulted fetlock dorsiflexion.

Hoof Length

As the hoof grows in a distal-dorsal direction, the *hoof length* becomes an important factor

Table 9.1 ◆ **The effect of hoof angle change on DIP joint angulation.**

Hoof Angle	JOINT ANGLE		JOINT ANGLE CHANGE	
	Range (°)	Mean (°)	Range (°)	Mean (°)
45	159 - 181	169.4	0	0
50	166 – 187	174.45	1 – 11	5.05
55	168 – 189	179.5	2 – 18	10.1
60	175 – 196	183.8	5 – 25	14.4
65	181 – 196	187.85	7 – 25	18.45
70	184 - 202	192.35	13 - 31	22.95

Reprinted with permission from Bushe, T. et al. 1987, table 3.

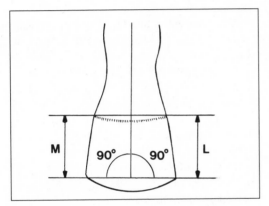

◆ **Fig. 9.6.** Medial-lateral balance in an ideal limb conformation, dorsal view. The bottom of the foot forms 90° to the vertical line drawn at the toe. The lateral (L) side of the foot is equal in height to the medial (M) side. (Adapted from Finnegan, D. and Rumph, J. 1991, p. 14.)

the navicular bone by the DDFT during breakover is increased. These effects increased with long-toe low-heels conformation that is commonly observed in horses. Therefore, proper dorso-palmar/plantar balance should include the maintenance of proper hoof length by trimming horses at the proper time.

 MEDIAL-LATERAL BALANCE

Medial-lateral balance IS CONCERNED WITH THE foot and pastern axes as viewed from the dorsal or palmar/plantar perspective (◆ fig. 9.6). In a properly balanced foot, the foot axis should be perpendicular to the ground surface, and the dorsal plane of the pastern axis should form a continuous line with the dorsal plane of the foot axis (Shively, 1982a; Adams, 1974). Factors that alter medial-lateral balance include conformational faults, trimming errors and uneven hoof wear.

Medial-lateral imbalance may result in uneven foot placement and increased pressure between joints at the high side of the foot and increased tension on the collateral ligaments at the low side of the foot (◆ fig. 9.7). Imbalance can lead to development of side bone (Dyson, 1988), ring bone (Butzow, 1961), sheared heels, quarter cracks and chronic heel soreness (Moyer and Anderson, 1975b), laterally distorted hooves (Lungwitz, 1891),

in balance. With hoof growth, the base distance moves away from the center of the limb and palmar/plantar support is reduced. Concurrently, the hoof lever arm is increased; therefore, the leverage over which the hoof pivots at the end of the stance phase is increased (Balch et al., 1996). The increased leverage amplifies the torque on the distal portion of the limb and delays breakover (Clayton, 1989; Balch et al., 1991b; Clayton, 1987; Balch et al., 1996). Therefore, excessive hoof length places abnormal tension on the stay apparatus of the limb (Moyer, 1981). In addition, the pressure on

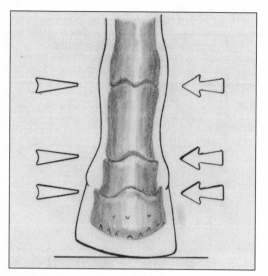

◆ **Fig. 9.7** Medial-lateral imbalance. Imbalance places abnormal pressure on the digital joints at the higher side (arrows), and abnormal tensional forces on the digital collateral ligaments at the lower side (arrowheads).

and chronic inflammation of the fetlock joint (Balch and White, 1985). Excessive strain to the lateral or medial collateral ligament, caused by hoof imbalance or abnormal footing, predisposes the horse to collateral ligament desmitis or inflammation of the collateral ligament of the DIP joint (Turner and Sage, 2002).

There are two methods for establishment of medial-lateral balance. In the first method, the hooves are trimmed level in order to establish equal distances from the ground at the medial and lateral aspects of the hoof. Hence, the lateral wall must be left a little longer than the medial wall (Butzow, 1961). A *trim gauge* can be applied to check the hoof wall height for levelness. Traditionally, most horses are trimmed according to this method regardless of their limb conformation. When this method is applied to horses with ideal limb conformation, the foot and pastern axes form a continuous line that is perpendicular to the ground. Ideal limb conformation is characterized by limb straightness, proper angulations of all joints, and a stance that is neither base-wide nor base-narrow (Balch et

al., 1991b). Following trimming, the heels may land simultaneously and the distribution of vertical forces between the medial and lateral hoof may remain within a normal safe range. When this method is applied to horses with less than ideal limb conformation (i.e. toeing-out), the medial and lateral aspects of the hoof remain perpendicular to the foot axis but not to the pastern axis. In this case, the heels may not land simultaneously during motion (Balch et al., 1991b). Because vertical force distribution within the foot is not a symmetrical event (Ratzlaff, 1988; Lochner et al., 1980, Balch et al., 1991b), the distribution of vertical forces in horses with less than ideal conformation is generally tolerated. Denoix (1999) showed that when the digit is asymmetrically loaded, the digital bones rotate and slide sideways relative to each other. He indicated that this response might be a normal protective response of the digital bones against uneven ground pressure.

In the second method used for establishment of medial-lateral balance, the hoof is trimmed in order to affect the landing pattern. The horse is observed during motion, and each hoof is trimmed until it lands simultaneously on both heels (Balch et al., 1991a). According to Moyer and Anderson (1975a) this method results in more even distribution of weight at both sides of the hoof. Balch et al. (1991a) indicated that the use of this technique to equalize weight bearing on the medial and lateral aspects of the hoof appears to be biomechanically incorrect. Finnegan and Rumph (1991) pointed out that horses trimmed to land flat often do not have a level foot. They indicated that in general, stress-producing lameness would be reduced if the foot is trimmed level and not so that it will land flat. Several authors indicated that the second method is often more successful in treating lameness (Moyer and Anderson, 1975a; Balch and White, 1985; Balch et al., 1991a). The disadvantage of this method is that it is more time consuming since the horse has to be observed during motion and each hoof may have to be re-trimmed (Balch et al., 1993).

Part 3 The Foal

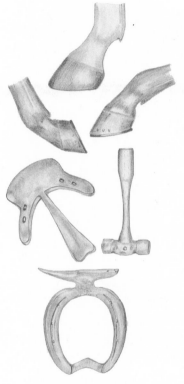

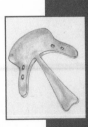

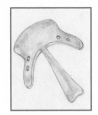

Chapter 10

The Foal's Foot

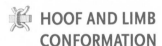 **HOOF AND LIMB CONFORMATION**

THE NEWBORN FOAL HAS HOOVES THAT ARE covered with soft tissue called *perinychium*. The perinychium protects the uterus and birth canal during gestation and labor (◆ fig. 10.1). As the foal begins to walk, this tissue wears off and the hooves become exposed to the environment.

The hoof of the young foal has a narrow and pointed outline; as the foal grows, the fore hooves become more rounded. Hoof growth is accompanied by development of a thick ring of horn parallel to the coronary band. This ring represents normal replacement of the "foal hoof" that grows out between four to five months of age (Ellis, 1998). Hoof growth rate in foals is 7 to 12 percent faster than that of mature horses (Butler, 1977).

Bone Growth

Foals reach 90 percent of their mature height at one year of age (Lewis, 1982). The highest growth rate and greatest elongation of bone

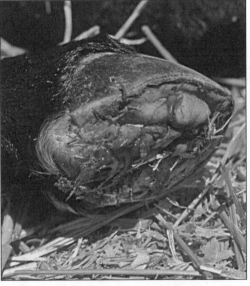

◆ **Fig. 10.1.** The perinychium in a foot of a six-hour-old foal. Some wear can be observed. (Photo by author.)

occurs during the first few months (Hintz 1978). Bone elongation take place at the *growth plates* located near the ends of the long bones (◆ fig. 10.2). The growth plate is made from a cartilaginous disc; bone elongation occurs by continuous division of cartilage

73

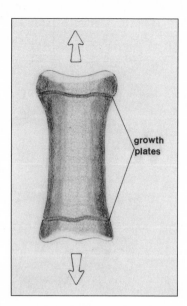

◆ **Fig. 10.2.** Growth plates in long bones are responsible for bone elongation (arrows).

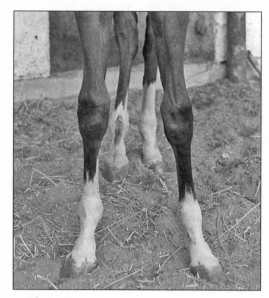

◆ **Fig. 10.3.** Placement of a foal in deep sand causes the foal to stand base wide, which leads to development of toeing–out conformation. (Photo by author.)

cells that ossify (change into bone). Lengthening of the first and second phalanges occurs from one growth plate located at their proximal end. Bone growth of the third phalanx occurs from an *ossification center,* not from a growth plate.

Lengthwise growth of the limb ceases when the growth plate "closes" or becomes ossified. "Closure" time of the growth plates varies according to each bone. Ossification of the growth plates in the first and second phalanges bones occurs at six to nine months of age. The distal metacarpal bone "closes" at 7½ to 13 months of age and the distal metatarsal bone "closes" at 9 to 14 months of age (Adams, 1974).

Banks (1986) indicated that application of normal, even and sustained pressure upon the growth plates results in even growth of the plate with proper spatial orientation of the bone. Application of abnormal compression to one side of the growth plate can retard growth of bone on that side and cause limb deviation (Banks, 1986; Stashak, 1987). This response may be used to correct deviations of the digit in foals. Trimming one side of the hoof results in increased ground pressure at the opposite side; the increased pressure results in slower bone growth on that side. Careful manipulation of the hoof is an important part of corrective trimming of foals, providing it is done before closure of the growth plates.

Environmental Effect on Limb Conformation

The physical environment where the foal is raised can have a major effect on limb growth and conformation. Hard ground or deep soft sand predisposes the foal to orthopedic disorders (Williams and Pugh, 1993). The increased impact caused by hard ground may place excessive pressure on the bones, joints and growth plates. Soft sand may lead to outward deviation of the toe by interfering with normal stance (◆ fig. 10.3). Williams et al. (1989) indicated that the use of forced exercise in horses that are less than one year of age might be detrimental to bone or cartilage development. Stall confinement with inadequate exercise can be detrimental to the growth plates (White et al., 1984). Negative effects of the environment may be enhanced in foals that already have conformational faults such as toeing-out or contracted tendons.

FOAL NUTRITION

Nutrition PLAYS AN IMPORTANT RULE IN THE development of the musculoskeletal system of foals. Inadequate nutrition, increased body size and muscle mass can lead to conformational and musculoskeletal abnormalities in growing horses (Williams and Pugh, 1993; Cymbaluk et al., 1990). Foals that nurse from mares that are heavy milkers or fed a creep feed ration high in protein and carbohydrates are predisposed to flexural limb deformities (Flecker and Wagner, 1986).

Proper nutrition for growing horses should start by feeding the pregnant mare a balanced ratio diet (Pugh and Williams, 1992; Pugh and Schumacher, 1993). Knight et al. (1990) indicated that supplementation of dietary *copper* to mares during late gestation, appears to reduce the prevalence of cartilage lesions in foals. Ingestion of locoweed by pregnant mares in New Mexico resulted in birth of foals with various limb disorders including flexural and angular limb deformities (McIlwraith and James, 1982).

Some mares may produce insufficient quantities of milk. In this case, supplementary artificial milk should be fed (Hinz, 1983; Carter, 1990). Milk production and milk quality begins to decline two to three months after foaling. At this time, foals should receive *creep feeding* (Pugh and Williams, 1992). Creep feeding generally begins when the foal is two to four weeks of age (NRC, 1989). When mares and foals are placed in high-quality pasture such as alfalfa, the foal may not require other feed until it is three months of age (Lewis, 1982). Good quality forage should always be available to foals (Cunha, 1991). *Legume hay* contains more protein, calcium, vitamin A and lysine com-

pared to *grass hay* and is preferred (Lewis, 1982).

The grain source in creep feeds usually includes oats, corn or barley. Rations based on a large amount of grain fed once or twice a day may be more detrimental than a diet of high-quality legume hay consumed over the course of the day. The grain to hay ratio should not exceed 60:40 for weanlings and 50:50 for yearlings (Williams and Pugh, 1993).

Correct *calcium-phosphorus ratio* in the diet of foals is important for proper bone development (NRC, 1989). The recommended range of calcium to phosphorus ratio is 1:1 to 3:1. Grains contain high levels of phosphorus but are deficient in calcium (Lewis, 1982). Boren et al. (1987) indicated that excessive protein intake does not appear to have an adverse effect on musculoskeletal development of growing horses.

HOOF TRIMMING

Hoof trimming OF FOALS SHOULD BE A ROUTINE procedure in foal management. Hunting (1898) stressed the importance of maintaining the hooves of foals short in order to prevent twisting of the foot. Ellis (1998) recommended that foals have their feet inspected and trimmed beginning from age four to six weeks. The trimming intervals vary according to the condition of the hooves or the presence of orthopedic disorder that requires corrective trimming. Foals with good limb conformation that are raised in appropriate environments wear their hooves evenly. These foals may require hoof trimming once as a weanling and once as a yearling; some foals may not require hoof trimming at all. Foals with a tendency for developing toeing-out conformation require corrective trimming every two to three weeks as a preventative measurement. Foals raised on green pasture and foals that are not exercised enough require more frequent hoof trimming compared to foals raised on dry and rocky ground.

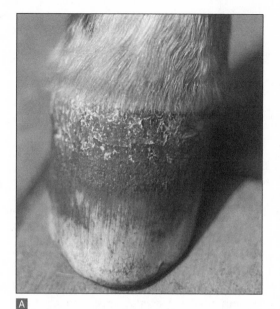 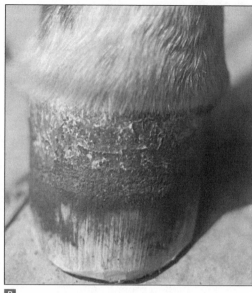

◆ **Fig. 10.4.** Hoof trimming of a foal. A. The hoof prior to trimming, note the pointed toe.
B. The hoof following trimming, the toe wall was rounded with racetrack hoof nippers held at
45° to the outer margin of the toe wall. The toe wall becomes smooth within a few days by
natural wear. (Photos by author.)

Trimming principles of the foal include trimming the hooves to the proper hoof angle and toe length and rounding the toes (◆ fig. 10.4). Establishment of foot and pastern axes is similar to that of adult horses; in most foals, hoof trimming requires the removal of excessive horn growth without changing the hoof angle. The tools used to trim the foal's hooves include a short blade hoof knife, horseshoeing file and racetrack hoof nippers. Most foals can be trimmed with a hoof knife alone.

The sole should be trimmed minimally, only to remove direct ground pressure from it. The frog and bars should be left intact. Uneven wear at one side of the hoof-bearing surface should be corrected (Ellis, 1998). Following trimming of the wall, the distal margins of the toe wall is rounded slightly with a file or with a hoof knife. The reason for rounding the toe is to encourage the foal to walk straight and breakover at the center of the toe. In hooves with a pointed outline, breakover may take place at the medial aspect of the hoof, causing uneven wear at that side,

which predisposes the foal to development of toeing-out. Enough toe wall thickness should remain in order to protect the white line. Weanlings and yearlings can be trimmed with racetrack hoof nippers. The distal toe wall is rounded with the same nippers or with a horseshoeing file. Hooves with thick horn ring nearing the distal toe wall are trimmed, and the toe is leveled with the rest of the hoof wall surface in order to prevent splitting of the toe (Ellis, 1998).

Handling the Foal

Since most foals are not halter broken, trimming procedures should be done in a well-padded stable. Prior to trimming, the foal should be placed on a level floor where its general conformation, limb conformation and foot balance can be evaluated. Stanley (in Tearney 2006) emphasized the importance of observing the foal in motion in order to see how it uses the legs. Trained foals may be observed by walking them away and toward the farrier, whereas untrained foals may be

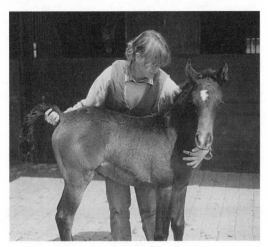

◆ **Fig. 10.5.** Handling the foal. Holding the foal as shown discourages it from bucking or jumping forward during trimming. Trimming should be done in a well-padded stall with the dam held next to the foal. (Photo by author.)

observed by leading the mare and letting them follow her.

During hoof trimming, young foals may be held by one person, by cradling the foal with one arm around the chest and one arm around the rump (Vaughan and Allen, 1987) (◆ fig. 10.5). Foals are generally more cooperative when the hind hooves are trimmed first. The foal should be placed parallel to the stable wall, facing a corner. This position discourages the foal from jumping forward. If the foal is quite, both hind hooves may be trimmed without turning the foal. The fore-hooves are trimmed by placing the foal parallel to the stable wall with its buttocks close to a corner; this position discourages the foal from bucking. Following trimming of one leg, the foal is turned and the opposite hoof is trimmed.

Corrective Trimming

Corrective trimming of foals involves trimming the foal's hooves in order to prevent, correct or improve limb deviations (Graham, 1965a). Hoof trimming may be used to alter the dorso-palmar/plantar plane, medio-lateral plane, or both. In some cases, hoof trimming may be the only treatment required, whereas in others it may be combined with application of corrective shoes or orthopedic devices. Some cases may require surgical correction.

Regular inspection of the foal's limbs and routine foot care are important in *prevention* of orthopedic disorders. Many foals develop good limb conformation with minimal foot care provided they have a good genetic base. However, some of these foals may develop problems due to environmental factors. Since it is difficult to predict which foal is going to develop a problem, a good foot-care management program is required. For orthopedic disorders in foals and methods of corrective trimming and shoeing, see chapter 11.

Chapter **11**

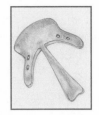

Farriery of Orthopedic Disorders in Foals

 TOEING-OUT

Toeing-out IS A VERY COMMON CONFORMATIONAL fault observed in foals and adult horses. Toeing-out is characterized by an outward deviation of the digit at the level of the fetlock joint or at the level of the pastern joint (Hermans, 1987). In some cases, the entire limb may be rotated outward. Toeing-out may be congenital (seen at birth) or acquired. The degree of toe deviation may be affected by environmental factors. Toeing-out in mature horses may cause interference between opposite limbs and uneven distribution of forces within the foot.

Predisposing factors for toeing-out include pointed toes, narrow chest, base wide conformation, cow-hocks conformation, and raising the foal on sand (see ◆ fig. 10.3). Ellis (1998) indicated that the normal foal tends to have a toeing-out stance, predisposing the hoof to excessive wear on the medial bearing surface. This stance may be related to the pointed toes commonly observed in young foals.

Increased wear at the medial bearing surface leads to limb deviation. The deviation may be self-corrected in foals with good limb conformation that are raised on firm ground. The increased pressure on the lateral aspect of the growth plates stimulates bone growth on that side, which maintains straight limb growth. The opposite effect may result in foals with poor limb conformation or foals that stand on deep sand. The pressure across the growth plates may be excessive enough to slow the bone growth at the lateral side. Once the *self-correction mechanism* is disturbed, the toes may deviate further, thus starting a cycle that worsens the condition. Excessive toeing-out conformation predisposes the foal to *fetlock valgus* or inward deviation of the fetlock joint.

Corrective Trimming of Toeing-Out

Corrective trimming of toeing-out includes lowering the lateral bearing surface of the hoof wall and rounding the toe. The hoof wall is trimmed until it tapers gradually from heel

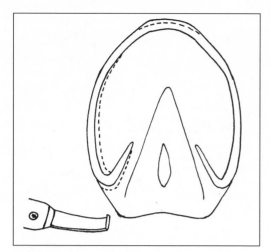

◆ **Fig. 11.1.** Corrective trimming of toeing-out, schematic illustration. The medial bearing surface of the hoof wall is lowered until it tapers from heel to toe and the toe is rounded (dashed lines).

Corrective trimming of toeing-in includes lowering the medial bearing surface of the hoof wall and rounding the toe. The medial hoof wall is trimmed until it tapers gradually from heel to toe, the medial heel should be 2 to 3 mm lower than the lateral heel. Hoof trimming should be repeated every two to three weeks. Corrective trimming of toeing-in should be done on foals with active growth plates. An attempt to correct the condition after that period will result in lameness.

CONTRACTED DEEP DIGITAL FLEXOR TENDON

Contracted flexor tendons IS A CONGENITAL (seen at birth) or acquired disorder that most commonly involves the forelimbs. The congenital disorder may be *developmental* (i.e. intrauterine malposition) or *heritable* (genetic) in origin (Wagner, 1994). The disorder is described as a *flexural deformity* because it affects joint angulations in the dorso-palmar/plantar plane. Contraction involves the shortening of the musculotendinous unit rather than the tendon itself (O'Grady, 1995a).

Contracted flexor tendons may involve the deep digital flexor tendon (DDFT), superficial flexor tendon (SDFT), or both. Causes of contraction include intrauterine malposition (McGaddery, 1992), stall confinement with limited exercise (Fessler, 1977; Owen, 1975), hard ground (McGaddery, 1992), nutritional imbalances (Wagner et al., 1985b; Wagner et al.1982; Williams and Pugh, 1993; McGaddery, 1992), overfeeding (Williams and Pugh, 1993; Rooney, 1974a) and genetic predisposition (Fessler, 1977). Both DDFT and SDFT contraction appear to be associated with high-energy diets with imbalance ratios fed to foals with a genetic potential for rapid growth (Fackelman, 1979; Fessler, 1977). Contracted DDFT is common in Quarter horses and Arabian horses. The disorder was observed in one breeding line of Arabian horses with more frequency in the right forelimb. These observations suggest that contracted DDFT has an heritable base.

to toe (◆ fig. 11.1). The lateral heel should be 2 to 3 mm lower than the medial heel. Lowering of the hoof wall excessively will cause lameness (Graham, 1965a). The distal toe wall is carefully rounded to encourage breaking over at the center of the toe. Hoof trimming is repeated at two to three weeks.

The foal should be kept on firm ground such as green pasture, paddock with packed soil or padded stable with a wooden floor. Corrective trimming of foals kept on deep sand is ineffective. The foals should be inspected regularly for signs of over-correction, which may lead to toeing-in conformation.

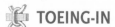 TOEING-IN

Toeing-in IS CHARACTERIZED BY AN INWARD deviation of the toe at the level of the fetlock or PIP joint; in some foals, the condition appears to have a genetic base. Toeing-in may develop in foals as a result of over-correction of toeing-out. Toeing-in places excessive strain on bones and ligaments and predisposes the foot to development of crooked hoof and sheared heels (see ◆ fig. 17.2).

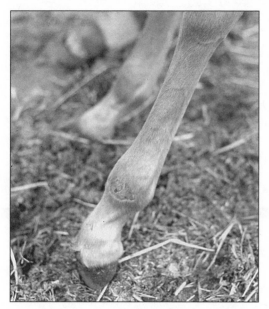

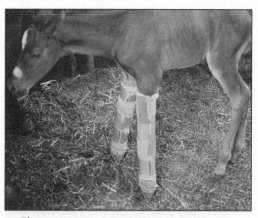

◆ **Fig. 11.3.** Splinting the forelimbs in the case shown in previous figure. The limbs were wrapped with a support bandage and two PVC splints were placed along each limb, at the dorsal and palmar sides. (Photo by author.)

◆ **Fig. 11.2.** Severe bilateral congenital DDFT contraction of the forelimbs in a one-week-old foal. (Photo by author.)

Congenital Contraction of the Deep Digital Flexor Tendon

Congenital contraction of the DDFT affect newborn foals, the condition may result from uterine malposition of the fetus (Rooney, 1974a). The disorder is not uncommon and may be bilateral or involve all four limbs (Wagner and Waltrous, 1990b). In most cases, contraction is mild; the heels are raised slightly above the ground and the fetlock joint is bent forward a little. Mild cases resolve spontaneously in the first few hours of life. In moderate cases, the heels elevate above the ground and may remain raised after the opposite limb is held up. In severe cases, the foal may walk on the dorsal part of the digit, thus predisposing it to pressure sores and septic fetlock joint (Johnson, 1973). The extreme flexion of the limb may result in rupture of the common digital extensor tendon (Meyers, 1976) (◆ fig. 11.2).

Treatment of congenital contraction of the DDFT includes splinting the limbs in an extended position. Splints made from 15 cm

diameter PVC pipe cut into 10 cm wide sections should include the affected joint(s) (◆ fig. 11.3). The splint should be replaced every three hours in order to prevent circulation impairment. This treatment can be very rewarding if done when the foal is less than one day old. Occasionally the condition will regress and splinting will be needed for an additional few days (Johnson, 1973).

Acquired Contracted Deep Digital Flexor Tendon

Most cases of *acquired contracted DDFT* develop between six weeks and six months of age (Wagner et al., 1982). Acquired DDFT contraction may result from increased bone growth relative to tendon length (Flecker and Wagner, 1986). The disorder is associated with growth of the third metacarpal bones, which occurs during the first eight months of life (Schmutzer et al., 1988). Other causes of DDFT contraction include pain and disuse of the limb (Rooney, 1977c; Metcalf et al., 1982). Steindler (1955) indicated that pain caused by arthritis and periarticular lesions can result in reflex muscle spasms that lead to contracted muscles. Similarly, disuse of the limb can leads to contraction of the flexor muscles.

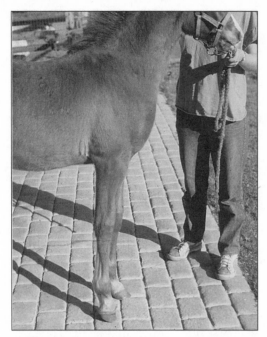

◆ **Fig. 11.4.** Contracted deep digital flexor tendon. Affected right foreleg in a four-month- old Arabian colt. (Photo by author.)

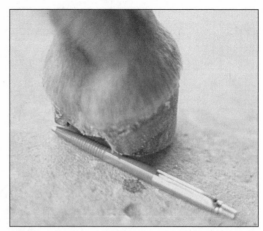

◆ **Fig. 11.5.** Contracted deep digital flexor tendon. A pen was placed under the heels to show the space between the heels and ground. (Photo by author.)

Sønnichsen (1982) indicated that shortening of the musculotendinous unit of the DDFT prevents normal extension of the DIP joint. The pull of the DDFT on the third phalanx results in raised heels and a broken forward foot axis (◆ figs. 11.4, ◆ 11.5). As a result, the gait become short and stiff. In cases with SDFT involvement, the pastern angle approximates the hoof angle but both appear steeper than normal (Schmotzer et al., 1988; Metcalf et al., 1982).

Contracted DDFT is classified into Grade I and Grade II contracture (Stashak, 1987). In Grade I, the angle formed by the toe wall and the ground is less than 90°. In Grade II, this angle exceeds 90° (◆ fig. 11.6). The severity of contraction can be assessed by lifting the opposite limb and observing the change in distance between the heel and the ground. The condition is more severe in cases where the heels do not drop; the lack of yield may be caused by the tensed DDFT and loss of DIP joint flexibility.

Mild cases of contracted DDFT may become complicated if not treated early.

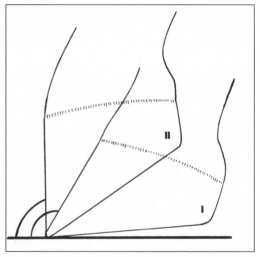

◆ **Fig. 11.6.** Grade I and Grade II deep digital flexor tendon contraction, schematic illustration.

Initially, the affected foot may become slightly steeper than the opposite foot, but this change may not be noticed. The pull of the DDFT may raise the heels a few millimeters above the ground with more pressure being placed on the toe. This pressure results in widening of the white line and development of bruised sole (Avisar, 1997). As the case progresses, the affected hoof begins to contract from lack of normal contact with the ground (Flecker and Wagner, 1986), causing the coro-

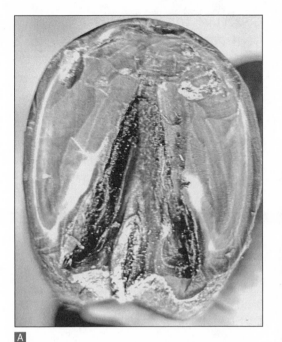

A

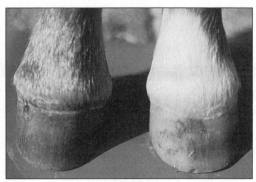

B

◆ **Fig. 11.7.** Mild contraction of the DDFT.
A. Solar view shows separation at the white line,
and discoloration at the sole caused by excessive
pressure on the toe wall. B. Dorsal view in a
unilateral case shows a contracted right hoof. Note
the slight prominence at the coronary band. (Photos
by author.)

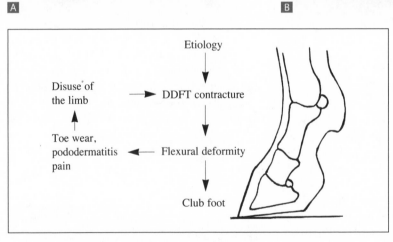

◆ **Fig. 11.8.**
Pain-contraction cycle.
The flow chart shows
the development of
clubfoot in the foal. The
abnormal position of
the toe begins a cycle
that complicates flexural
deformity. (Reprinted
from Avisar, Y. 1994,
fig.1.)

nary band to appear more prominent (Ellis, 1998); concurrently the heel lengthens, the toe wears, and the hoof angle may increase by 5° to 10° (◆ fig. 11.7). In advanced cases, the toe wall may become dished and the hoof may achieve the boxy appearance of clubfoot (see below). The sole and the hoof wall at the toe become very thin and bruises and abscesses may develop in this area (Fackelman, 1980).

Complications that may result from the increased pressure on the toe wall include dished toe, seedy toe, rotation of the third phalanx, resorption at the tip of third phalanx (Arnbjerg, 1988; Kaneps et al., 1993) and sole abscess (Fackelman et al., 1983a). In addition, the increased tension in the DDFT can lead to tendonitis (Curtis, 1992). In severe cases, the foal may walk on the dorsal hoof wall (Metcalf et al., 1982). Complications that lead to pain and lameness (Metcalf et al., 1982; Schmotzer et al., 1988) may initiate a *pain-contraction cycle* (Fackelman, 1980) (◆ fig. 11.8). The pain causes the foal to place less weight on the limb. Consequently, the disuse of the limb worsens the contraction (Fackelman, 1979).

Clubfoot in Foals

Clubfoot is characterized by flexed DIP joint, heels that are raised above the ground and excessively worn toe (Sønnichsen, 1982; Stick et al., 1992) which might appear dished (Schmotzer et al., 1988). In most cases, the heels touch the ground but remain abnormally long.

Clubfoot develops as a result of prolong DIP joint flexion caused by DDFT contraction, resulting in permanent stiffening of the joint capsule (joint envelope). The joint stiffness causes severe limitations in joint movement (McIlwraith and Fessler, 1978; Stick et al., 1992) that may cause stumbling during motion. Clubfoot has been classified into four grades according to degree of severity (Redden, 2003b). The prognosis for clubfoot is guarded if the problem is severe or of long duration (Metcalf et al., 1982) (for clubfoot in adult horses, see page 215).

Surgical Correction of DDFT Contraction

The surgical method for correction of DDFT contraction involves severing the inferior check ligament. The surgery is termed *desmotomy, which* means cutting a ligament. The principle of the surgery includes relieving tension from the DDFT by lengthening its musculotendinous unit (Sønnichsen, 1982; Lysholt and Sønnichsen, 1969). This is achieved by severing the check ligament, which attaches the DDFT to the third metacarpal bone. Good results were reported when treatment included desmotomy of the inferior check ligament and postoperative corrective horseshoeing (Arnbjerg, 1972; Wagner et al., 1982b; Rooney, 1977; Lysholt and Sønnichsen, 1982; Fessler 1977; McIllraith and Fessler, 1978; Lose et al., 1981b). It may take two to three weeks before resolution of the problem is achieved. (Sønnichsen, 1982). Correction of Grade II DDFT contraction may require severing the DDFT; this may result in limited use of the foal when it grows to maturity.

Corrective Trimming of DDFT Contraction

As soon as signs of DDFT contraction begin to develop, feed intake should be reduced, concentrated feed should be withheld and the mineral content of the feed balanced (Flecker and Wagner 1986; Wagner and Waltrous, 1990b).

Corrective trimming of DDFT contraction may be the only treatment required in mild and early cases (Metcalf et al., 1982). Results of trimming can be very rewarding if started early. Early signs of contracted tendons include the appearance of small splits at the bearing surface of the toe wall and widening of the white line. Early conservative measures include bandaging the limb(s) with a cotton bandage in order to promote relaxation of the DDFT and normal realignment of the DIP joint (Wagner et al., 1982). Some foals may require protection of the toe wall region with bandage material held by elastic adhesive tape.

Farriery principles of DDFT contraction include lowering the heels, protecting the toe and application of toe leverage when required. Pressure on the toe wall may be relieved by trimming a curved section from the bearing surface of the toe. The heels are lowered by 3 to 5 mm at each hoof trimming (◆ fig. 11.9). Lowering the heels increases the tension in

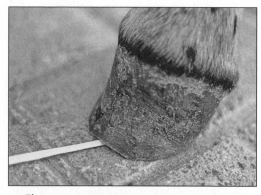

◆ **Fig. 11.9.** Hoof trimming of a mild case of DDFT contraction. The heels were lowered and a curved section from the distal toe wall was trimmed. A piece of straw was placed under the toe to show the trimmed area. (Photo by author.)

the DDFT and consequently the tension in the flexor muscles. Continuous tension on the muscles causes them to lengthen as a protective response against excessive tension (Guyton, 1986; Breazile, 1970); this response is better in younger foals (Kelly et al., 1987). Within a few days after trimming, the heels may drop gradually to the ground (Avisar, 1997). Hoof trimming is repeated each time the heels reach the ground. Corrective trimming continues until a hoof angle of 50° to 55° is established. Excessive trimming of the heels should be avoided as it predisposes the third phalanx to increased concussive forces and increased strain on the DDFT (Lochner et al., 1980; Kaneps et al., 1993). A limited amount of exercise to encourage stretching of the flexor muscles is important. The foal may be placed in a green pasture or hand-walked on soft ground.

Early recognition of complications is important. The sole and white line should be inspected regularly for changes in coloration, crevice formation, thrush, and abscess development. These lesions should be debrided; the exposed toe should be treated with pine tar and bandaged. The foal should be kept on a wooden floor or rubber mat in order to prevent further trauma. Damage to the toe wall may result from gravel or coarse ground. Placement of foals with contracted tendon on sand may worsen the condition, as the feet tend to rotate forward into the sand.

Cases that do not respond to trimming alone may require one or more of the following procedures: toe-wall reconstruction, application of toe extension, therapeutic horseshoes and surgery.

Toe Wall Reconstruction and Toe Extension

Toe wall reconstruction in foals is a procedure used to restore the normal conformation of the hoof by application of acrylic resin (Ferguson, 1994; O'Grady, 1995a). The acrylic resin protects the toe wall against excessive wear and increases leverage that promotes

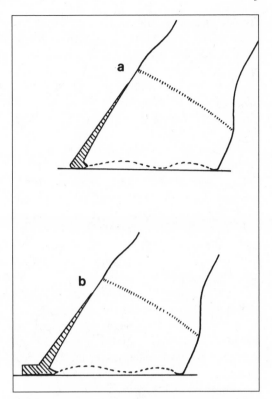

◆ **Fig. 11.10.** Toe wall reconstruction, schematic illustration. Reconstructed toe wall (a), and the addition of toe extension (b). The striped area represents the acrylic resin.

lowering of the heels (Ellis, 1998). Toe wall reconstruction may be the only treatment required in mild cases of DDFT contraction. In more advanced cases, the procedure may be combined with the addition of a toe extension or the application of a therapeutic horseshoe. The procedure should be delayed in cases with infected toe wall until the area is completely dry and cornified.

Toe wall reconstruction can be done conveniently with the foals under general anesthesia. Prior to application of the resin, the hoof is trimmed and the toe area is sanded lightly. The hoof is degreased with denatured alcohol and allowed to dry. An assistant applies the acrylic repair material. Low heat producing acrylic resin should be applied in order to prevent thermal injury. If excessive heat is produced, the foot should be cooled immediately with cold water. Application of resin to the sole should be avoided as it may cause bruising during weight bearing. In order to prevent that, the sole should be packed with Play dough prior to application of resin. The toe wall is built from the distal third of the toe downward until the normal length of the hoof is achieved. Additional resin is applied in moderate to severe cases in order to form a toe extension; this extension forms a leverage arm that encourages stretching of the DDFT and dropping of the heels. The length of the toe extension should be 1 to 2 cm and it should be parallel to the ground (◆ fig.11.10). The strength of the extension can be increased by incorporating synthetic fabric with the resin (Moyer and Sigafoos, 1993).

Arnbjerg (1972) and Sønnichsen (1982) described the application of acrylic material for construction of complete foal-clog glued to the hoof. The clog can be made with an extended toe (Sønnichsen, 1982). Low heat producing resin should be applied in order to prevent thermal injury to the foot.

Farriery of DDFT Contraction

The application of therapeutic horseshoes to foals with DDFT contraction is aimed at protecting the toe wall and increasing tension on the DDFT. Horseshoeing may be combined with toe wall reconstruction or surgical correction. The type of horseshoe applied to treat this condition depends on the age of the foal and the severity of the case. Early mild cases

in young foals are treated with synthetic glue-on shoes that provide protection for the toe wall. A simple glue-on shoe made from a flat pad can be constructed and glued to the hoof with Super Glue (see below). The horseshoe should remain in place for several weeks until the toe wall grows sufficiently. Rolling several layers of duct tape around the tabs secures the horseshoe further.

Foals that are three to four months old may be fitted with glue-on shoes, full metal horseshoes or tip shoes (Wagner et al., 1982). Synthetic glue-on horseshoes made from a flat pad as described above can be used. Alternatively, a glue-on shoe made from a commercial kit can be constructed (see below). Number 3 race nails should be used when applying nail-on horseshoes. The horseshoes outline should fit the "missing" outline of the hoof (◆ fig. 11.11). Ellis (1998) indicated that horseshoes that restrict hoof expansion might lead to development of narrow feet. Shoeing the healthy opposite limb in unilateral cases is not required in most cases. Horseshoes should be reset every two weeks; at each reset the heels are lowered by 3 to 5 mm until a hoof angle of 50° to 55° is established.

Cases that do not respond to trimming or simple shoeing alone require additional leverage on the toe wall. Leverage may be increased with a tip shoe or toe extension horseshoe. Either a glue-on shoe or metal horseshoe can be fitted with a toe extension. Horseshoes adequate for older foals include tip shoe or wedged-tip shoe nailed to the hoof

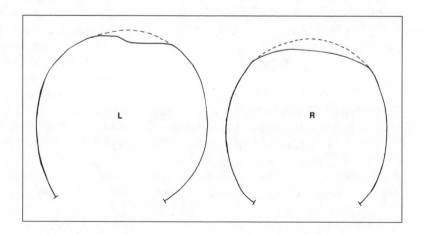

◆ **Fig. 11.11.**
The hoof outline of the forelimbs of four-month-old Quarter Horse foal with DDFT contraction at the right limb. Both hooves have a broken section at the distal toe wall (dashed lines). Note the differences in size between hooves. Drawing has been reduced.

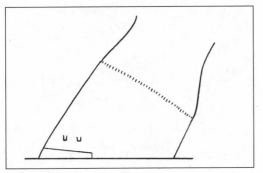

◆ **Fig. 11.12.** Wedged-tip horseshoe, schematic illustration, lateral view. (Adapted from Metcalf et al. 1982, fig. 2B.)

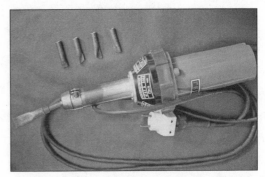

◆ **Fig. 11.13.** Hot air blower for plastic welding and nozzles. The nozzle fits into a tubular nozzle supplied with the instrument. Various nozzles made from copper pipe are shown. (Photo by author.)

(Flecker and Wagner, 1986; Schmotzer et al., 1988). Metcalf et al. (1982) described the use of a wedged-tip shoe made from round or square steel bar stock; the wedged-tip shoe raises the toe when it is not possible to lower the heels by trimming (◆ fig. 11.12).

Schmotzer et al. (1988) described the application of a wedged-tip mushroom shoe for prevention of heel contractures in foals following severing of the inferior check ligament. Fackelman et al. (1983a) recommended the use of beveled horseshoes to promote hoof spreading following surgery. Clubfoot cases may be fitted with a tip shoe following surgical resection of the check ligament; the tip shoe protects the toe wall-bearing surface and encourages toe growth.

All treated foals should be observed for signs of complications caused by excessive strain on the DDFT or check ligament. Signs may include reduced activity, pointing the limb, and lameness. Foals fitted with metal horseshoes should be observed closely for signs of lameness caused by a close nail; suspect nails should be removed.

Construction and Application of Glue-On Shoes for Foals

The construction and application of a glue-on foal shoe from a commercial kit is described as follows. The horseshoe is constructed from polyurethane and is attached to the hoof with tabs glued to the hoof wall. Construction of

the horseshoe requires some plastic welding skills and a hot-air blower; welding is performed at working temperature of 270 °C (500°F) and is used for connecting the tabs to the horseshoe (◆ fig. 11.13).

Once the affected hoof is trimmed, the hoof outline is traced on a cardboard while the foal is standing on it. Depending on the type of orthopedic disorder, a toe extension (contracted DDFT), palmar/plantar extension (flaccid tendons) or side support (ALD) is drawn; a 1 to 2 cm extension is appropriate for most cases. The drawing is transferred to the polyurethane pad provided with the kit and the pad is cut along the outer margins of the drawing line, using a jigsaw or band saw.

Three types of tabs are supplied with the kit: an angled tabs for toe or side extensions, regular (straight) tabs, and heel tabs. The planned position of each tab is marked on the cut pad with a permanent marker. The pad is placed in a vise and the uppermost toe tab is held at an open angle over the mark. The tabs should be welded perpendicular to the pad in order to prevent overlapping of the tabs during application of the horseshoe. The two parts are welded by heating the edge of the pad and the base of the tab simultaneously. The tip of the welder is held 3 to 5 cm from the welding field and hot air is applied. After 20 to 30 seconds, the plastic surface begins to liquefy and appear clear; the two parts are

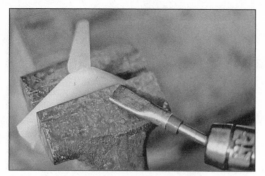

◆ **Fig. 11.14.** Heating a tab and a pad with a hot air blower. (Photo by author.)

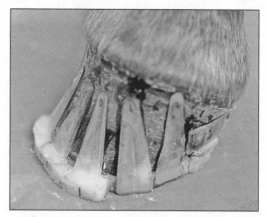

◆ **Fig. 11.15.** Completed glue-on shoe with a toe extension glued to the hoof of contracted DDFT case. (Photo by author.)

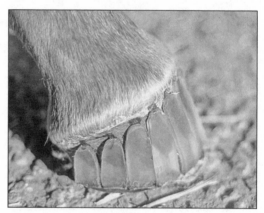

◆ **Fig. 11.16.** Glue-on shoe. A combination of plastic glue-on shoe made from a flat pad and a metal horseshoe with a toe extension. (Photo by author.)

pressed tightly for several seconds (◆ fig. 11.14. Excessive heat will churn the plastic and change its color to brown; this will result in a weak bond that is inadequate.

Prior to application of the horseshoe, the hoof wall is sanded lightly and degreased with denatured alcohol and allowed to dry. Small holes or crevices at the white line area should be debrided and filled with a hoof pack. The inner surface of the tabs is degreased with denatured alcohol and the horseshoe is left to dry. The horseshoe is fitted over the hoof and the limb is placed on the floor. Then, the opposite limb is lifted in order to achieve good hoof and shoe contact. A wooden or plastic wedge may be placed beneath the heels in cases where the heels do not reach the ground. Starting from the back tabs, each tab is pulled and one to two drops of glue provided with the kit are placed at the upper end of the tab and allowed to dribble to the bottom of the tab. Then the tab is pressed against the hoof wall for 10 seconds. The least the amount of glue used, the stronger the bond that is formed. To prevent thrush, pine tar is poured between the hoof and horseshoe (◆ fig. 11.15).

The horseshoe should remain in place between the shoeing intervals. In cases where the tabs become loose, the foal's owner should be instructed to clean the loose tabs and hoof wall with alcohol, and glue the tabs again with few drops of Super Glue. Alternatively, the tabs can be held in place by several layers of duct tape wrapped around the hoof; the wrap should not include the heel bulbs as this may interfere with circulation. The horseshoe may be reset until it become too small.

Alternatively, a synthetic glue-on shoe combined with a metal horseshoe can be constructed from a flat plastic pad. The hoof outline is drawn on a plastic pad, the shapes of the tabs are added to the drawing, and the drawing is cut with heavy scissors; the pad is immersed in boiled water until it soften and each tab is bent to the desired angle (◆ fig. 11.16). A metal horseshoe forged from a 4 x 15 mm bar stock is connected to the plastic shoe with copper rivets (◆ fig. 11.17). Other types of glue-on foal shoes that have been

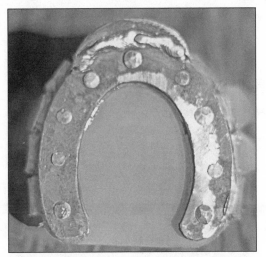

◆ **Fig. 11.17.** Solar view of the same glue-on shoe shown in fig. 11.16. Copper rivets were used to connect the pad to the horseshoe. (Photo by author.)

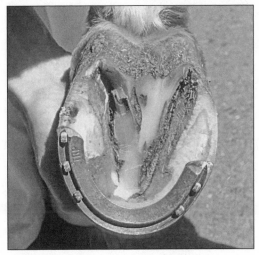

◆ **Fig. 11.18.** Tip shoe made from a training plate. (Photo by author.)

described include a shoe constructed from PVC plumbing pipe (Painter, 1996; Painter and Schumacher, 1997), and a shoe with a toe extension made from ABS plastic sheeting that is bonded to the hoof with acrylic adhesive (Bruggink and Sigafoos, 1997).

Tip Shoes

The *tip shoe* (toe tip, tips, toe plate, half-shoe) is a half-horseshoe that fits the bearing surface of the toe wall. The horseshoe is applied to foals with contracted flexor tendons, and to clubfoot cases in foals and mature horses. Stanley (2004) described the application of a half-shoe fitted with a full pad for treatment of sore feet. Tip shoes may be applied to pastured yearlings in order to protect their hooves; the horseshoe allows better hoof function and growth compared to a full horseshoe (◆ fig. 11.18). In cases of DDFT contraction, the tip shoe protects the toe wall and increases tension on the flexor tendons. Other indications for tip shoes include young horses in training, and adult horses, that overreach.

Tip shoes can be constructed from a training plate or light half-round horseshoe cut at the quarters, alternatively aluminum or

light iron bar stock can be used. The horseshoe thickness should be minimal in order to prevent gait alterations. Tips can be applied to foals that are three to four months old that have enough hoof wall thickness to accommodate size 3 race nails. The horseshoe is attached with two nails on each side. Additional nail holes should be added in order to allow alternate placement of nails at each reset; this practice decreases splitting in the wall and allows the renewal of horn.

Tip shoes used in the farriery of DDFT contraction are fitted over the bearing surface of the toe wall in order to increases tension on the flexor tendon. In all other cases, the tip shoe is set in level with the bearing surface of the hoof (Rich, 1907), unless they are pastured on soft ground. Fitting the tip shoe level is done by marking the position of the branches on the hoof, and stepping the bearing surface of the toe with a file until the horseshoe accommodates in the depression. This method can be used when there is enough horn that can be filed.

Tip shoes tend to concentrate pressure on the toe wall. This could lead to separation at the white line and to convexed toe, especially in overgrown hooves. Therefore, tip shoes should be reset at two to four week intervals.

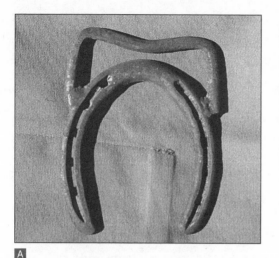

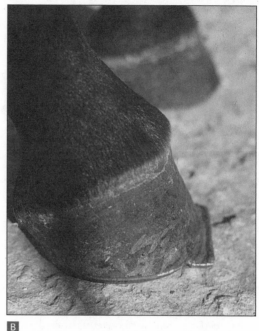

◆ **Fig. 11.19.** Toe extension horseshoes. A. Toe extension was made from 6 mm round iron bent into an M-shape and welded to a light half-round horseshoe. B. Toe extension made from a flat bar stock. (Photos by author.)

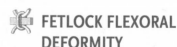

Toe Extension Horseshoe

The *toe extension horseshoe* is applied to cases of DDFT or SDFT contraction. The horseshoe delays breakover during motion and stretches the tendons more than normal (Flecker and Wagner, 1986; McIllwraith and Fessler, 1978; Wagner et al., 1982; Lose et al, 1981b; Schmotzer et al., 1988). In addition, it forces the heels to the ground when the foal is bearing weight (Schmotzer et al., 1988).

The toe extension horseshoe can be made from a light half-round horseshoe or from a light iron bar stock. The horseshoe is fitted to the hoof and a toe extension is welded to the horseshoe; in most cases, the toe extension is welded level with the ground surface of the horseshoe. In plastic glue-on shoes, the toe extension is a continuation of the pad. In order to prevent breakover at the sides of the toe, the extension is made into an M-shape (◆ fig 11.19). The length of the toe extension depends on the amount of leverage required; this can be from 1 to 4 cm. Short extensions can be made from a bar stock welded across the toe of the horseshoe. In order to encour-

age dropping of the heels the toe extension may angle towards the ground; the extension should raise the toe of the horseshoe by 0.5 to 1.0 cm. Johnson (1973) indicated that the pressure caused by the toe extension may lead to development of a toe crack at the coronary band.

🦮 FETLOCK FLEXORAL DEFORMITY

Fetlock flexoral deformity IS AN ORTHOPEDIC disorder caused by shortening of the musculotendinous unit of the superficial digital flexor tendon. The disorder, which is also termed contracted SDFT or knuckling over, commonly develops at 10 to 18 months of age. SDFT contraction is less common than DDFT contraction (Flecker and Wagner, 1986). The condition may be unilateral or bilateral and in most cases the forelimbs are affected (Fackelman, 1983b; Wagner et al., 1982). Fast growing foals that are on high concentrate diets are predisposed to fetlock flexoral deformity (Wagner et al., 1985b).

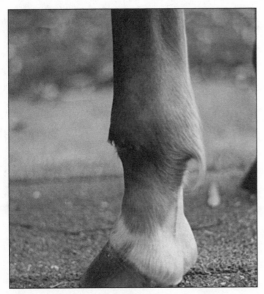

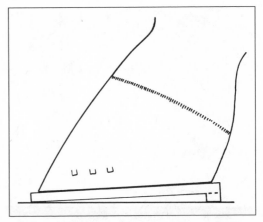

◆ **Fig. 11.21.** Horseshoe for SDFT contraction, schematic illustration. The horseshoe is fitted with a bar across the heels and a toe extension. (Adapted from Metcalf et al. 1982, fig. 7C.)

◆ **Fig. 11.20.** Bilateral fetlock flexoral deformity in a Quarter Horse weanling. Note the steep pastern and knuckling at the fetlock. (Photo by author.)

The SDFT is inserted into the first and second phalanges; therefore shortening of the musculotendinous unit of this tendon forces the fetlock forward (knuckle-over) and places the pastern in an upright position (◆ fig. 11.20). The heels may grow longer than normal but will remain on the ground. The hooves are generally not misshapen (Metcalf et al., 1982). SDFT contraction may be classified according to stage of development into Stage I or Stage II. In Stage I the fetlock may knuckle-over but it pops back into place, whereas in Stage II knuckling-over is constant (Wagner and Waltrous, 1990b). In severe cases, the DIP joint may subluxate (Metcalf et al., 1982; Wagner et al., 1985b). Knuckling-over may cause stumbling, and in unilateral cases, it results in the development of mismatched feet.

Corrective Trimming and Shoeing of SDFT Contraction

SDFT contraction is less amenable to correction compared to DDFT contraction (Wagner et al., 1982). Feeding should be restricted to a low carbohydrate diet as soon as the fetlock begins to show an upright position (Wagner et al., 1982; Flecker and Wagner, 1986).

Farriery principles of DDFT contraction include raising the heels and increasing the leverage on the toe wall. Raising the heels reduces tension from the DDFT and its check ligament (Metcalf et al., 1982). Thus, it forces the SDFT and the suspensory ligament to support weight, which stretches these structures (Flecker and Wagner, 1986). Mild cases respond favorably to hoof trimming alone; the hoof should be trimmed in order to establish a hoof angle of 58° to 60°. In moderate to severe cases; the heels should be raised with a wedge pad fitted to the horseshoe or with a square bar welded across the horseshoe branches (Metcalf et al., 1982) (◆ fig. 11.21). Leverage on the toe is achieved with a toe extension that increases tension on the superficial digital flexor muscle and suspensory ligament. In most cases, the toe extension should extend 2.5 to 5.0 cm from the center of the toe (◆ fig. 11.22). The elevated heels are effective when the horse bears weight, while the toe extension exerts its effect during motion (Fackelman, 1979).

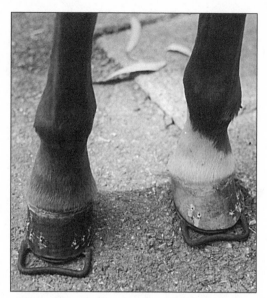

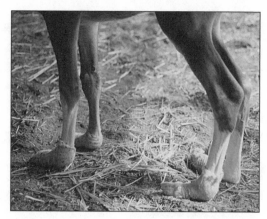

◆ **Fig. 11.23.** Extreme flexor tendon laxity in a newborn foal. The fetlock joints in all four limbs contact the ground. (Photo by author.)

◆ **Fig. 11.22.** Application of toe extension horseshoe to the same case shown in figure 11.20. In this case, the heels were not raised and no progress was made. (Photo by author.)

Farriery of SDFT contraction may be combined with surgical resection of the inferior check ligament (Flecker and Wagner, 1986; Wagner et al., 1985b) or of both the inferior and superior check ligaments (Blackwell, 1982; McIlwraith and Fessler, 1978). Exercise in the early postoperative period seems to improve the final result; hand walking is usually sufficient (Fackelman, 1979).

 FLACCID FLEXOR TENDONS

Flaccid flexor tendons IS AN ORTHOPEDIC disorder caused by weak flexor tendons. The disorder is seen primarily in newborn foals. The forelimbs are more commonly affected but all four limbs may be affected (Flecker and Wagner, 1986; Metcalf et al., 1982). Other names include slack tendons, weak tendons and flexor tendon laxity. In most newborn foals the condition is self-corrected within a few days.

Flaccid flexor tendons are characterized by weak flexor tendons that cause the foal to rock back on the bulbs of the heels with the

toe pointing upward. Foals kept on a rough surface may develop abrasions at the bulbs of the heels (Wagner and Watrous, 1990c; Flecker and Wagner 1986; Metcalf et al. 1982; Curtis and Stoneham, 1999). The heels of untreated cases may become under-run, thus forcing the foal to walk on the bulbs of the heels with worsening of the condition (Metcalf et al., 1982). In severe cases, tendon laxity is accompanied by extreme dorsiflexion of the fetlock that may touch the ground. The prognosis for these cases is poor (Stashak, 1987) (◆ fig. 11.23). Flaccid flexor tendons may be associated with sloped pastern conformation observed in older foals. These foals have weak suspensory apparatus that is not correctable.

Farriery of Flaccid Flexor Tendons

Most cases of flaccid flexor tendons are self-corrected during the first two days of life (Wagner and Watrous, 1990c). Cases that are not self-corrected within this time should be treated (Metcalf et al., 1982). Newborn foals with weak flexor tendons should be placed in a bedded stable. Shallow bedding that gives a firm-bearing surface is recommended (Wagner and Watrous, 1990c). In order to prevent bruising, the area of the bulbs of the heels may require the application of a protec-

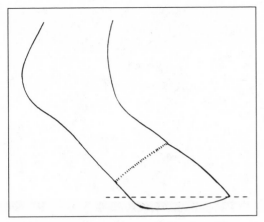

◆ **Fig. 11.24.** Trimming principles of a mild flaccid tendons case, schematic illustration. The dashed line shows the area that is trimmed in order to encourage solar contact.

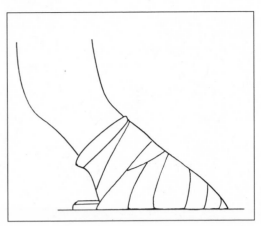

◆ **Fig. 11.25.** Application of heel extension in flaccid tendons, schematic illustration. See text for details. (Adapted from Adams O. R. 1974, fig. 6.165.)

tive bandage. The foot is wrapped with a self-adhesive bandage held in place with elastic adhesive tape. The legs should not be bandaged, splinted or casted as this may increase tendon laxity (Flecker and Wagner, 1986; Metcalf et al., 1982; Wagner and Watrous, 1990c). The amount of exercise should be limited (Flecker and Wagner, 1986).

Mild cases of flaccid flexor tendons may be treated by corrective trimming as the only treatment. Trimming principles include lowering the heels and leveling the hoof to provide a flat bearing surface, which brings the solar area into contact with the ground (◆ fig. 11.24). Corrective trimming is repeated once a week until the condition is corrected (Flecker and Wagner, 1986). One trimming may correct the condition in some cases.

Moderate cases of flaccid flexor tendons require increased palmar/plantar support. This is achieved with heel extensions that reposition the foot on the ground (Metcalf et al., 1982). The heel extension serves as a lever arm that lifts the fetlock when the foot is bearing weight (Flecker and Wagner, 1986). The extension is made from 3 mm thick aluminum bar. The bar should be slightly narrower than the hoof width, and extend 3 to 5 cm palmar/plantar to the heels (◆ fig. 11.25). Adams (1974) described the application of a

flat aluminum bar taped to the bottom of the foot with elastic adhesive tape. Alternatively, the bar can be glued to the hoof with low heat producing resin. Curtis and Stoneham (1999) described a case of severe flaccid tendons in the hind limbs treated successfully with heel extensions made from aluminum strips glued to the hoof with acrylic resin. Another method involves the application of an extended heel shoe made from plywood (Flecker and Wagner, 1986; Metcalf et al., 1982; Wagner and Watrous, 1990c) (see below).

One-to-two-month-old foals can be fitted with plastic glue-on shoes made with a palmar/plantar extension. In cases where the hoof wall is thick enough, an extended-heel metal horseshoe can be applied. The horseshoe is attached with number 3 race nails. Horseshoes are removed after one week and the condition is evaluated. The horseshoes may be reset if required.

Plywood Horseshoe

The *plywood horseshoe* is a foal shoe with extended heels used in the treatment of foals with flaccid flexor tendons (Metcalf et al., 1982; Wagner and Watrous, 1990c). The horseshoe is made from 6 mm thick plywood

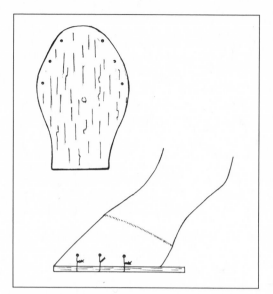

◆ **Fig. 11.26.** Application of plywood horseshoe, schematic illustration. See text for details. (Adapted from Metcalf S. et al. 1982, figures 1C and 1D.)

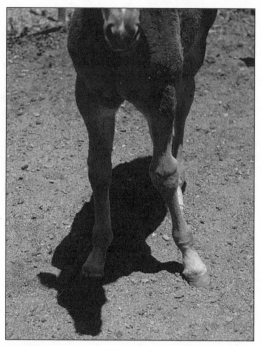

◆ **Fig. 11.27.** Carpus valgus in the left forelimb of a weanling. The carpal joint is deviated to the medial, and the limb distal to it deviated laterally, note the pressure rings on the medial aspect of the hoof. (Photo by author.)

and is connected to the hoof wall with stainless steel wire (◆ fig. 11.26).

Following trimming, the hoof outline is drawn on a plywood board; a 2 to 3 cm heel extension is "added" to the drawing and the plywood is cut with a jigsaw or a band saw. Three 2 mm holes are drilled on each side of the horseshoe margins. The horseshoe is placed over the hoof and equivalent holes are marked at the bearing surface of the hoof wall. A hand-held drill fitted with 1.5 mm drill bit is used to drill holes in the hoof wall. The holes are made at the marks and are directed proximally until they exit the hoof wall 10 mm from the hoof margins. The plywood shoe is connected to the hoof with 16-gauge stainless steel wire inserted through the holes. The two ends of the wire are coiled carefully in order to prevent cutting through the horn.

Alternatively, the horseshoe can be glued to the hoof with low heat producing acrylic resin. The resin should cover the margins of the horseshoes and part of the hoof wall. Application of resin over the solar area should be avoided in order to prevent bruising.

ANGULAR LIMB DEFORMITIES

Angular limb deformity (ALD) IS AN ORTHOPEDIC disorder characterized by joint deviations in the limb. Medial deviation of a joint is termed *valgus* and lateral deviation of a joint is termed *varus* (◆ fig. 11.27). ALD may be congenital (seen at birth) or acquired. Congenital factors for ALD include joint laxity, bone immaturity and uneven bone development (Auer and Martens, 1980; Auer et al., 1982). *Joint laxity* is associated with malposition of the fetal limbs within the uterus. Congenital ALD in most foals is self-corrected within two to four weeks of life.

Acquired ALD appears between one to six months of age; the condition may result from nutritional disorders (Coffman, 1973; Auer et al., 1983) such as imbalanced trace mineral intake (Messer, 1981), conformational faults and excessive exercise (Auer et al., 1983).

Abnormal weight distribution across joints caused by conformational faults may result in growth retardation in areas of stress concentration; the joint cannot be straightened manually (Auer et al., 1983). Predisposing conformational faults include narrow chest, cow hocks, toeing-out or toeing-in. ALD may develop from external trauma or infection to the growth plate (Auer et al., 1983; Wagner and Waltrous, 1990a). Failure to correct the causative problems results in worsening of the condition (Auer et al., 1983). Farriery of ALD may be combined with surgical treatment aimed at retardation of bone growth at the convex side of the joint and enhancement of bone growth at the concave side.

Treatment of ALD Associated with Joint Laxity

Treatment of joint laxity involves confining the mare and foal to a stall and immobilizing the limb. Exercise should be avoided as it may worsen the condition by creating uneven pressure across the joint that can lead to bone deformation (Auer et al., 1982).

The limb is wrapped with a support bandage, then a splint made from PVC pipe that was cut in half is placed over the concave side and wrapped with elastic adhesive tape. Prior to application of the splint, the limb is straightened manually. The length of the splint should be long enough to include the affected joint(s).

Alternatively, the limb is placed in a cast. Following curing the cast is cut into two half-shells along its dorsal and palmar/plantar planes and removed. The limb is wrapped with a support bandage; the two half-shells are placed over the bandage and wrapped. The bandage should be changed every three to four days and treatment should continue for three to four weeks (Auer et al., 1982).

Farriery of ALD Caused by Conformational Faults

Trimming principles of ALD caused by conformational faults include lowering the hoof

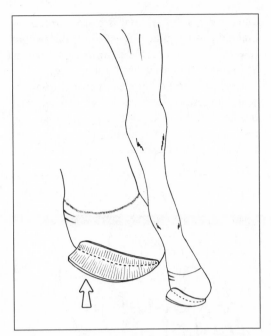

◆ **Fig. 11.28.** Side-support made with acrylic resin in carpus valgus case, schematic illustration. The resin increases the pressure at the convex side of the limb (arrow).

wall at the concave side of the limb and in some cases providing side support at the convexed side of the limb. Treatment of mild cases includes stall rest for at least one month combined with frequent corrective trimming. The bearing surface of the foot that rotates outward (valgus) should be lowered slightly at the lateral aspect with a hoof rasp every two to three weeks. This results in minimal inward rotation of the foot and helps disperse pressure across the carpus and tarsus. When this procedure is carried out over a period of time, both toeing-out and ALD might be corrected (Auer et al., 1983). In cases where the foot is rotated to the inside (varus), the medial aspect of the hoof is rasped.

Farriery of moderate cases of ALD includes lowering the unworn side of the hoof and providing side support by direct application of acrylic resin to the side of the hoof (O'Grady, 1995a). A low-heat-producing acrylic resin should be used (◆ fig. 11.28). Alternatively, the hoof may be fitted with a side-support glue-on horseshoe. For valgus deviation, the side support is placed on the medial side and for varus deviation; it is placed on the lateral side (◆ fig. 11.29). By shifting the weight toward the center of the limb, the hoof is encouraged to grow level (Ellis, 1998). The horseshoes should be reset every two to three weeks following inspection and trimming of the hooves. A metal side support horseshoe may be applied to weanlings and yearlings with severe foot deviations.

Correction of ALD may take several months; attempts to correct these deformities too rapidly may result in complications such as abnormal foot shape (Auer et al., 1983). Farriery may be combined with the application of a support bandage and a splint. Some foals require surgical correction in order to straighten the limb.

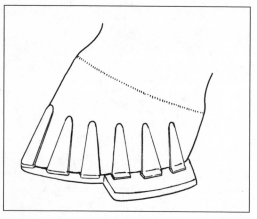

◆ **Fig. 11.29.** Side-support glue-on foal horseshoe, schematic illustration.

Part 4 Farriery Techniques

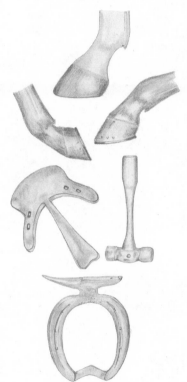

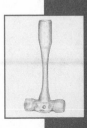

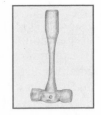

Chapter 12

General Considerations

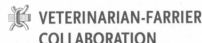 VETERINARIAN-FARRIER COLLABORATION

GOOD *veterinarian-farrier collaboration* IS essential for successful execution of foot care procedures. Issues that may be discussed prior to the intended procedure include the temperament of the horse, how much horn can be removed, the risk of supporting limb complications, use of resins, types of therapeutic horseshoes that may be applied, and the use of foot nerve blocks and tranquilizers. Once these issues are addressed, a treatment plan can be made and presented to the horse owner. In cases where extensive foot debridement is required, the horse owner or trainer should be informed of possible prolonged healing time.

A proper *ethical relationship* between farriers and veterinarian is mandatory. An excellent source of information on the relationship between farriers and veterinarians can be found in "The Farriers Guide" published by the British Farrier Registration Council (1986) or later editions. Both veterinarians and farriers should check their state laws that govern foot care procedures. These laws may vary between states and countries. By follow-

ing these laws, collaboration between farriers and veterinarians can be greatly enhanced.

In general, any foot procedures that do not involve standard farriery requires veterinary supervision. Non-standard farriery includes corrective farriery and invasive farriery. *Corrective farriery* includes reshaping abnormal hoof conformation without entering sensitive structures within the foot. *Invasive farriery* involves the entry into the hoof capsule. The farrier should be aware that he or she is not protected against liability suits that may arise from performing foot care procedures, other than standard farriery, without veterinary supervision. The veterinarian should be aware that he or she might not be protected against malpractice suites if he or she was not present during non-standard farriery procedures, even if permission was given to the farrier to carry out the procedure. The farrier should make sure that a veterinarian is present during any foot care procedure that requires reshaping of the hoof capsule, hoof debridement, exposure of dermis, hoof repair, and application of therapeutic horseshoes and orthopedic devices. In addition, the veterinarian is responsible for the medical aspects of each case including the use of diagnostic equipment, regional anesthesia of the foot, tourniquet application, foot surgeries, administration of drugs, topical medication and bandages. A veterinarian or a farrier who does not have the training or experience to carry out foot care procedures should refer the case to someone with appropriate training and experience.

HOOF CARE MANAGEMENT

PROPER *hoof care management* OF BOTH HEALTHY and diseased feet requires the consideration of various physiological and environmental factors. These factors may include horn moisture level, hoof growth, stable conditions, hoof dressings and horseshoes.

Following trimming, moisture loss from the horn causes the hoof to contract; this loss may increase with hot shoe fitting, environmental salts and dry bedding. In addition, the horseshoes may interfere with normal hoof function and as a result, the hoof may contract. In order to function properly, the horn has to reabsorb moisture and expand back. Application of a hoof poultice over the solar area can prevent moisture loss following trimming; moisture may be provided by keeping the horse in green pasture or by digging a waterhole in the paddock. Stabled horses should have access to a mud puddle.

Many hoof dressings (including hoof paints) tend to dry the hooves. Therefore, horse owners and breeders should be advised to use substances shown to be beneficial to the hoof; these substances include water, low-salt hoof poultice, and pine tar.

Hoof growth between trimming intervals affects the biomechanics of the foot and limb; as the hoof grows, the hoof lever arm, support dimensions of the foot, and palmar/plantar support are altered. These changes may affect the stay apparatus of the limb, particularly if the horse is being used in strenuous competition. One of the most pronounced changes observed is the tendency of the hoof angle to decrease between the trimming intervals. This change, which occurs in shod and bare-

foot horses, can be minimized by keeping proper trimming intervals.

Horseshoes can have significant effects on the hoof, including alteration of foot kinetics, kinematics and conformation. Ill-fitted horseshoes may affect the foot even if the horse is not working. Most of these problems can be prevented by adhering to proper horseshoeing principles, including the application of plain and light horseshoes with adequate palmar/plantar support. The use of horseshoe adjuncts should be avoided whenever possible. These principles may be modified in the farriery of lameness cases, as some horses may require the application of horseshoes or devices with odd shape.

Factors Affecting Hoof Health

The veterinarian and farrier have to recognize the different factors that affect *hoof health*. These factors should be considered in the prevention and treatment of foot and limb disorders. The following section describes various management factors that have a beneficial effects on the foot:

hoof trimming. Trimming the hoof at the proper time, and establishing optimal dorsopalmar/plantar balance, medio-lateral balance and hoof length can prevent many lameness cases.

barefoot. Keeping horses barefoot for various periods of time can improve hoof quality by permitting natural interaction between the hoof and the ground. In addition, it provides a "resting" period for the hoof from the effects of horseshoes and horseshoe nails.

rocky environment. Placement of horses in rocky fields for an extended period of time (i.e. one year or more) improves hoof quality. Although it is difficult to get an objective assessment on the degree of improvement, it could be significant.

grit. When a rocky environment is not available, large corrals covered with grit can be used to improve hoof quality. The grit wears

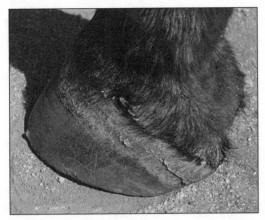

◆ **Fig. 12.1.** Placement of barefooted horses on fine grit results in consistent wear of the hooves. (Photo by author.)

down the hooves, maintains their length and reduces the incidence of thrush (◆ fig. 12.1).

exercise. Exercise improves the quality of hooves by increasing circulation, which provides nutrients to the foot and moisture to the hoof horn.

stable hygiene. Proper stable hygiene is important for prevention of horn damage.

straw bedding. Straw bedding does not draw moisture from the hooves, as do other types of bedding (i.e. wood shavings).

outside source of moisture. In arid areas, hydration of the hoof horn may be aided by making a waterhole where the horses are kept, or letting them stand in a puddle. The puddle can be created by a leaking water trough. Alternatively, a poultice may be applied periodically to the hooves. Absorption of excessive moisture should be avoided in periods of excessive rain.

pine tar. Periodic application of pine tar to the solar area prevents the development of thrush. The pine tar may be applied once or twice a week following hoof picking. Application of pine tar following hydration of the hoof reduces water loss.

hay. Feeding only hay to horses reduces the incidence of laminitis compared to feeding hay and concentrate feed (grain). Grain is not a natural feed for horses.

biotin. Continuous supplementation of biotin results in improvement of hoof substance in some horses. Biotin may be the only supplement with proven beneficial effect on hoof quality.

padding material. Placement of cushioned material between metal horseshoes and the hoof (i.e. rim pad) reduces shock and improves contact between the two surfaces.

THE HORSESHOEING SHOP

TREATMENT OF DISEASED HOOVES and application of therapeutic horseshoes is more conveniently done in a *horseshoeing shop* (◆ Fig. 12.2). The horseshoeing shop should have a large door opening that allows safe in and out movement of horses. The door should have a gate that keeps foals from bolting out. A door size of 2.5 m wide by 2.6 m high is adequate. The height of the shop ceiling should be at least 3 m; the ceiling should be fitted with strong fluorescence lights and a quiet ceiling fan that keeps flies away from the horses, thus, keeping them calm during shoeing. The floor of the horseshoeing shop should be made from a non-slippery material such as roughened cement.

The shop should have a safe *shoeing station* with a level floor covered with a rubber mat. A station size of 2.35 m wide by 2.5 m length is adequate. Ideally, the mat is fitted into a comparable depression made in the concrete floor; the mat is glued to the floor. The rubber mat prevents slippage and protects the hooves from wear caused by pawing. The surface of the mat should have a rough pattern, preferably one that can be swept easily. Each side of the shoeing station should be fitted with extra strong, 10 cm diameter horizontal pipe that confines the horse and provides an escape route for personnel. The

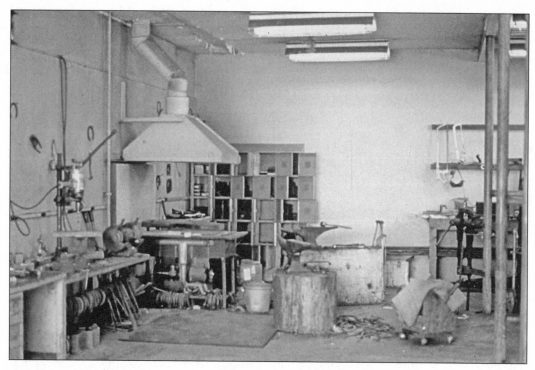

◆ **Fig. 12.2. Horseshoeing shop.** See text for details. (Photo by author.)

height of the pipe should be 1.2 m. Each end of the shoeing station should be fitted with a cross-tie ring placed at a height of 1.9 m. For added strength, the metal ring plates should be anchored to the wall with 20 mm bolts that pass through the wall into equivalent plates placed on the outer wall.

Horse Restraint

The amount of *restraint* (Vaughan and Allen, 1987) applied during foot-care procedures depend on the extent of the injury and the horse's predisposition. Some horses may require general anesthesia for foot debridement while others may stand quietly with a nose twitch and regional foot anesthetic.

Horse restraining during farriery procedures may be achieved by one or more of the following techniques: holding the horse with a lead rope, keeping flies away, bringing another horse for company, using a nose twitch, administering a tranquilizer, and/or

administering regional foot anesthesia. Some horses may strike violently with a foreleg when a twitch is applied, hence the horse handler should never stand directly in front of the horse. Tranquilized horses can kick; hence, these horses should be approached carefully, especially when lifting the hind limbs. Avoid loud sounds and sudden movements as these can awaken the horse. Tranquilized horses should not be tied.

During farriery procedures, a competent handler should hold the horse; the handler should stand on the same side that the farrier is working. This way the horse's rear end can be moved away from the farrier by pulling its head toward the handler. The horse may be cross-tied if trained for that; cross-tie should be reserved for non-painful procedures such as standard trimming and shoeing. The cross-tie ropes should be fitted with a quick release snap (◆ fig. 12.3).

Trimming young foals is best done in the corner of two smooth walls on a non-slippery

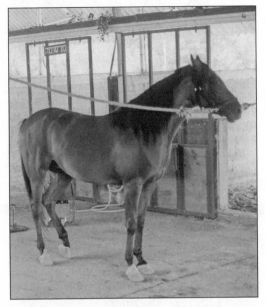

◆ **Fig. 12.3.** Cross-tie. A convenient restraint method for horseshoeing. (Photo by author.)

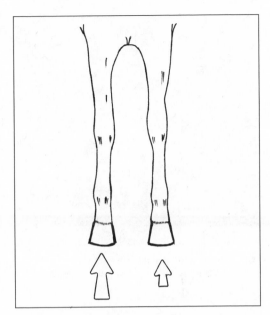

◆ **Fig. 12.4.** Uneven weight distribution between the forelimbs caused by lameness (arrows), schematic illustration.

rubber mat. Nervous, untrained foals should be trimmed in a well-padded stable and not in the shop. (See page 76.)

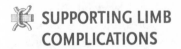 **SUPPORTING LIMB COMPLICATIONS**

DURING THE RECOVERY PERIOD FROM FOOT AND stay apparatus injuries, and other lameness conditions, the healthy opposite limb begins to carry excessive weight (◆ fig. 12.4). The increased weight dorsiflexes the fetlock joint and strains the flexor tendons and suspensory ligament. The added weight placed on the bony column increases tension in the laminar bonds, thus increasing the risk of third phalanx rotation. Redden (2003a) showed that excessive weight placement on a limb reduces blood flow to the area of the dorsal laminae. Acute laminitis in the supporting limb is a serious potential complication in lameness conditions (Wheat and Pascoe, 1980; Peloso et al., 1996; Redden, 2003a). Peloso et al. (1996) reported that the mortality rate of hors-

es with *supportive limb laminitis* can reach 50 percent, and the clinical manifestation of laminitis typically comes three to six weeks post-injury.

Prevention of supporting limb complications should begin by pulling the horseshoe, trimming, and balancing the hoof. In cases where the horse bears weight on the affected limb and is able to walk, the opposite healthy limb is fitted with a horseshoe in order to prevent spreading and chipping of the hoof. In more serious lameness conditions, the sole of the supporting limb should be fitted with solar or frog support pads in order to support the third phalanx and relieve some tension from the laminae. Frog support pad, custom support foam or a heart-bar shoe provides solar support (see Laminitis, chapter 16). Redden (2003a) recommended that the supporting foot in cases of non-weight-bearing lameness be supported as soon as possible after the injury by raising the heels and supporting the sole. This can be achieved with a commercial solar support boot designed to raise the heels; solar support is achieved by the application of elastic polymer between the

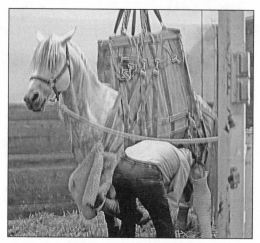

◆ **Fig. 12.5.** **Horse sling.** The sling was used to support a horse with severe laminitis. (Photo by author.)

pad and sole. Raising the heels relieves the DDFT and reduces the pulling force on the third phalanx. Wheat and Pascoe (1980) recommended fitting the healthy opposite limb with a horseshoe and wedge pad. The space between the sole and pad should be filled with soft acrylic resin. In addition to sole support, the supporting limb should be fitted with a heavy support bandage in order to reduce strain from the suspensory apparatus. Some horses may require the support of a sling (see below).

Stokes et al. (1998) described the application of an elevated hoof boot used for raising the healthy limb in cases where the opposite limb is fitted with a cast (page 176). The raised boot allows the horse to walk better and encourages more even use of both limbs. In cases where supporting limb laminitis is suspected, the foot boot should be fitted with a wedged-shaped wood that raises the heels. The space between the hoof and boot should be filled with custom support foam or soft acrylic resin in order to provide solar support. Prior to application of the boot, the bulbs of the heels should be protected against pressure sores by wrapping the area with rolled gauze held in place with a self-adhesive bandage.

The Sling

The *sling* (Vaughan and Allen, 1987) is a device used to suspend the horse in order to remove weight from injured limb(s), and to reduce the risk for supporting limb complications (◆ fig. 12.5). The sling permits treatment and bandage replacement during convalescence and the application of horseshoes. Candidates for a sling include cases of non-weight bearing lameness, severe laminitis, complete hoof loss, traumatic rupture of the suspensory apparatus, and deep penetrating wounds of the foot. The sling is particularly useful for horses that don not lie down, and in some cases, the sling maybe the only method that enables the horse to stand. In order to prevent pressure sores, the sling should be well padded and fitted properly. Slinging should be alternated with rest by allowing the horse to lie down periodically on a well-bedded stable floor. Ideally, the stable floor should be covered with a rubber mat. In order to relieve the suspensory apparatus all the limbs should be fitted with a support bandage during slinging.

Chapter 13

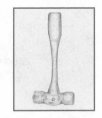

Foot Care Procedures

FARRIERY TERMINOLOGY

THE FOLLOWING LIST INCLUDES FARRIERY TERMS that appear in the text:

bar stock. Metal of various sizes that is used for forging horseshoes.

creasing. Making a groove along the ground surface of the horseshoe where the horseshoe nails are positioned or at other locations in order to increase traction.

extended branches. Extending the horseshoe branches behind the heels in order to increase palmar/plantar support.

full fitting. Fitting the horseshoe with the horseshoe branches gradually protruding from the quarters toward the heels. Full fitting provides an expansion surface for the hoof wall (see ◆ fig. 13.8; plate 21).

ground surface. The surface of the horseshoe that contacts the ground.

hoof surface. The surface of the horseshoe that is fitted against the hoof.

keg horseshoe. A manufactured horseshoe as opposed to forged or hand-made horseshoe.

nail position. The position of the horseshoe nail holes on the horseshoe. Nail position is determined by hoof wall thickness, or presence of defects in the wall.

pitch. Implies the angulation of the horseshoe nail holes, which correlate with the hoof wall angulation (Martinelli and Ferrie, 1998).

seated out. Concaving the solar edge of the horseshoe to prevent contact between the horseshoe and sole in order to reduce sole pressure (Martinalli and Ferrie, 1998) (◆ fig. 13.1).

set under. Setting back the horseshoe so the toe wall protrudes forward, as may be done in overreaching.

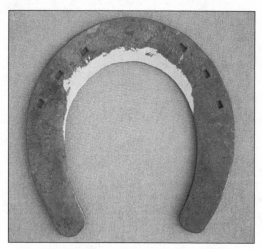

◆ **Fig. 13.1.** Seated-out horseshoe, the solar edge of the horseshoe was grinded in order to prevent sole pressure. (Photo by author.)

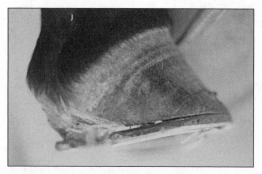

◆ **Fig. 13.2.** Sprung horseshoe. (Photo by author.)

sprung horseshoe. A bent horseshoe that is partially pulled, because of overreaching, treading and other causes (◆ fig 13.2).

web. The width of the horseshoe.

 TOOLS AND APPLIANCES

THE FOLLOWING SECTION PROVIDES a description of horseshoeing tools and appliances used in therapeutic horseshoeing:

modified alligator forceps. The modified alligator forceps is used as a stripping tool in hoof wall resection procedures. The tool is

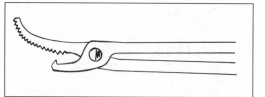

◆ **Fig. 13.3.** Modified alligator forceps made from a horseshoe nail clincher, schematic illustration. The lower jaw was shortened and filed to create a hook at the end.

made from a horseshoe nail clincher by adding an angled hook to the lower jaw (Pollitt and Daradka, 2004). Alternatively, the inner surface of the lower jaw is filed in order to make a hook at the end (◆ fig. 13.3). The hook is used to grasp the white line prior to hoof wall removal.

crease nail puller. The crease nail puller is used to remove the horseshoe without placing leverage on the hoof as occurs with pull-offs. The tool is especially useful for preventing trauma to the laminae in laminitis cases. Prior to removal of the horseshoe, the clinches are rasped, the hoof and horseshoe are held firmly with one hand and each horseshoe nail is removed individually.

creaser. The creaser is used to crease the horseshoe along the toe and quarters, and to make grooved horseshoes.

hoof gauge. The hoof gauge is used to measure the hoof angle. The tool is used for comparison between opposite limbs and for detecting changes in hoof angle caused by various foot disorders.

hoof knives. Hoof knives of various sizes and shapes are available for hoof trimming and debridement. Short-bladed knives are more convenient for trimming foals. A set of detachable blades of different types is commercially available. The set includes a digging knife that is very useful for deep debridement. Loop knives are useful for debridement and

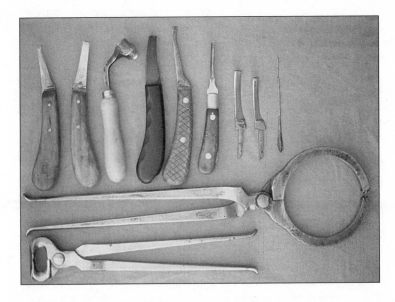

◆ **Fig. 13.4.** Tools used for hoof debridement. The tools include hoof testers, half-round hoof nippers, hoof knives, digging knife, loop knife, Swiss hoof knife and a blunt flexible metal probe. (Photo by author.)

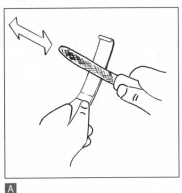
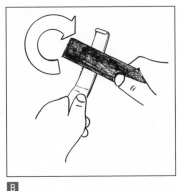

◆ **Fig. 13.5.** Sharpening the hoof knife. A. Prior to sharpening a new knife, the blade is thinned at the inner surface with a round steel file. B. Sharpening the knife is done with a triangular wet stone; the inner blade is sharpened by clockwise circular motions (for right-handed knives). The outer blade is not sharpened except for a few sharpening strokes that smooth its surface .

for grooving the hoof wall, and are available in various sizes (◆ fig. 13.4). Double-bladed hoof knives such as sage knives are not recommended because of the risk of pressing the upper blade with the thumb. Hoof knives may be sterilized (autoclaved) and used in aseptic surgical procedures of the foot. Maintaining sharp hoof knives is important for safety and precision use (◆ fig. 13.5).

flexible metal probe. A blunt metal probe is used for exploration of suspicious tracts within the hoof capsule, such as undermined sole and penetrating wounds. X-raying the foot while the probe is inserted into a tract is use-

ful in determining the depth and direction of the lesion.

half-round hoof nipper. The half-round hoof nipper is used for removal of sections of sole or wall during debridement procedures and in dorsal hoof wall resection of laminitis cases. The nippers permit the removal of horn sections under good control (◆ fig. 13.4).

hoof rasp. A hoof rasp may be used to thin the dorsal toe wall in laminitis cases; once the hoof wall is thinned, a hoof knife or a motorized burr is used to complete the removal of horn. A good quality hoof rasp should be used for hoof trimming and foot care procedures. A worn rasp tends to remove more wall than sole and as a result, the sole becomes bulged above the level of the hoof wall bearing surface. This may result in lameness caused by excessive sole pressure.

light driving hammer. A light driving hammer such as a race hammer is used to drive horseshoe nails in cases of sensitive foot. A light driving hammer or ball-peen hammer may be used to locate a painful area within the foot by carefully tapping the hoof wall and solar area.

hoof tester. The hoof tester is used to locate painful sites within the foot by applying pressure to the hoof capsule (Turoff, 1998; Anderson, 1992). Commercial hoof testers in several sizes and designs are available (◆ fig. 13.4). The tool can be constructed from 10 mm galvanized iron rods. Anderson (1992) recommended using a large hoof tester for examining the wall and sole and a smaller, adjustable hoof tester for examining the frog and across the heels. Examination of the foot should be systematic with constant application of pressure. Pressing a painful area will cause the withdrawal of the foot; this response should be repeatable (Turoff, 1998). A positive response may be noticed in horses with thin soles, although it may not be the source of lameness.

motorized burr. The motorized burr (Renchin et al., 1995) is used for removal of loose, broken and damaged hoof wall and for burring-out the hoof wall prior to the application of repair material (see ◆ fig. 16.63). The motorized burr can be fitted with various types of tungsten-carbide bits suitable for hoof wall debridement and undercutting (O'Grady, 2001b). Other types of bits that can be used include high-speed steel bits.

hot air blower. The hot air blower is used for welding plastic glue-on foal shoes (see ◆ fig. 11.13). The tool may be used to dry the hoof horn surface prior to application of acrylic resins, speed up curing of resins in cold ambient temperature, and for application of molded pads.

 HOOF TRIMMING

UNLESS THE CASE REQUIRES SOME MODIFICATIONS due to individual requirements, the principles of *hoof trimming* of diseased feet are similar to those of normal feet. Hoof trimming in most cases includes trimming the hoof to normal proportions, that is, proper hoof angle, toe length and medio-lateral balance. Specific trimming requirements for each case of foot or stay apparatus disorder should be considered. For example, leaving the heels in club-foot cases relatively high, or relieving one heel in cases of sheared heels.

Once the first hoof is trimmed, the toe length is measured with wing dividers. The wing divider is placed with one arm on a measuring evener placed under the hoof wall and the other arm at the hairline border of the coronary band, then the nut is tightened (◆ fig. 13.6). The accuracy of the measurement can be increased by using the *coronary rim* as a landmark; the coronary rim can be palpated as a distinct ridge at the end of the upper hoof wall (Balch et al., 1991a). The measured toe length is than "transferred" to the opposite hoof by placing one arm of the wing divider at the coronary band, using the same landmark as before. The lower arm is pressed into the toe wall in order to make a dent mark. The hoof is trimmed similarly to the first hoof and the solar area is rasped until the dent mark appears at the tip of the toe. At this point, both hooves have the same toe length. The hoof angles of both hooves are compared, and if necessary are corrected until both hooves have the same angle (◆ fig. 13.7).

Proper leveling of the hoof solar surface requires skill and experience as the farrier has to level the solar surface, establish medio-lateral balance, dorso-palmar/plantar balance and proper hoof height nearly at the same time. Following rasping the solar surface, the

EXAMINING THE FOOT

WHENEVER POSSIBLE, HORSESHOES SHOULD BE removed prior to examination of the foot. In cases where laminitis is suspected, the horseshoe should be removed with a crease nail puller and not with pull-offs. The solar surface is cleaned with a hoof pick and all loose and flaky horn is trimmed away. A hoof tester is applied to the hoof in order to detect sensitive areas. A light race hammer can be used to detect pain by tapping the outer hoof wall and sole. In cases where the hoof is the source of pain, the solar area is trimmed until fresh sole and frog horn is reached; the entire hoof is examined for evidence of pus, undermined sole, bruises, black spots, and discoloration and separation at the white line. Some subsolar abscesses may have very small drainage tracts that are difficult to see. Suspicious areas are examined by inserting a sterile flexible metal probe into them. In order to prevent the formation of false tracks, the probe should not be forced. The normal color of the white line is yellow-gray; reddening of the white line is common but may not be considered as a problem unless there are other clinical signs (Anderson, 1992). The coronary band should be observed and palpated carefully for evidence of pain, pus and foreign bodies. Once a suspected tract is located it should be explored and debrided.

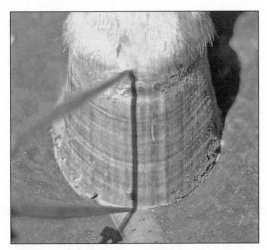

◆ **Fig. 13.6. Measuring toe wall length.** In order to increase the accuracy of the measurement, a measuring evener is placed under the bearing surface at the toe wall. (Photo by author.)

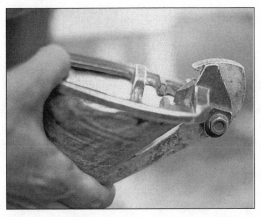

◆ **Fig. 13.7.** Measuring the hoof angle with a hoof gauge. (Photo by author.)

 ## HOOF DEBRIDEMENT

NEARLY EVERY FOOT REQUIRES SOME DEGREE OF debridement in order to prevent or treat a disorder. This may include scrapping "powdery material" from the white line in minor cases of white line disease, trimming deeper horn affected by thrush, or extensive removal of the sole in cases of suppurative pododermatitis. Debridement procedures may require prior disinfection of the foot, regional anesthesia, and application of a tourniquet. Treatment may be followed by the application of protec-

sole may bulge slightly above the level of the hoof wall-bearing surface. This bulging results from moisture loss from the hoof horn or from using a worn hoof rasp. The sole surface adjacent to the hoof wall should be concave in order to protect the sole from chronic bruising (Moyer, 1980; Balch et al., 1998b). Moisture loss from the hoof may be reduced by applying a poultice to the solar area immediately following hoof trimming.

tive horseshoes constructed specifically for the case.

Most cases of foot debridement can be done with a sharp hoof knife and a metal probe. Other tools that are commonly used include a hoof rasp, special knives such as a loop knife and a digging knife, half-round hoof nippers, and a motorized burr equipped with various bits.

Following the identification of a sensitive area within the foot, the hoof is trimmed and prepared for regular shoeing. This allows the fitting of the horseshoe that may be forged at this time, and avoids rasping a hoof that is bleeding or has a missing section of wall.

Prior to debridement, the affected area should be disinfected. Disinfection of sub-solar abscess cases can be done by application of alcohol over the solar area. Disinfection of deep penetrating wounds requires the sub-mersion of the foot in gauze soaked in alcohol for 24 hours. The gauzes are covered with a nylon stocking and a foot bandage is applied. Hennig et al. (2001) indicated that foot sub-mersion would not remove all the bacteria that are capable of causing wound infection, but their numbers can be significantly reduced if the hoof is trimmed and the super-ficial hoof wall is rasped prior to submersion.

During debridement only affected horn should be removed, and sensitive tissue should be left intact unless the dermis is affected. When performed carefully, most cases of foot debridement can be carried out without causing unnecessary bleeding. Once bleeding begins, it may be necessary to apply a tourniquet to the lower limb (see below).

Regional Anesthesia of the Foot

Regional anesthesia of the foot (foot block) is a common procedure used in painful foot pro-cedures. The anesthetized area may include part of the foot or the entire digit. Farriery of horses with loss of foot sensation requires special consideration. Hot shoes should be fit-ted briefly in order to prevent thermal injury and horseshoe nails should be driven with extra care. Once treatment is completed, the horse should be placed in a stable until the foot regains its sensitivity. Placing a horse with a foot block in a paddock or pasture can result in a serious fracture caused by miscal-culated foot placement.

Part of the foot may become permanently desensitized by foot lacerations involving the digital nerves, or following surgical transec-tion of the palmar digital nerves, a procedure done in some horses with navicular disease. The farrier should be notified about this condition so he or she can be more careful when driving horseshoe nails. These horses should be monitored closely for signs of developing infection within the hoof; signs may include swelling of the coronary band and pus secretions.

Tourniquet

A *tourniquet* may be applied to the limb dur-ing surgical procedures of the foot in order to control bleeding. The types of tourniquets used include a rubber tourniquet and a hand-powered pneumatic tourniquet. The tourni-quet may be applied over the mid-cannon bone or to the pastern area. Some horses resist the rubber tourniquet and may strike violently with the forelimb or kick. Appli-cation of the pneumatic type tourniquet per-mits monitoring of the desired pressure.

Once treatment is complete and the wound is wrapped with a pressure bandage, the tourniquet is removed; leaving a tourni-quet under the foot bandage can result in the loss of the horse due to *foot gangrene*.

Foot Disinfectants and Medication

Prior to deep debridement of the foot, the hoof should be trimmed and wrapped for 24 hours in gauzes soaked in 70 percent alcohol, secured under a foot bandage. Following debridement, the wound should be lavaged with non-irritating antiseptic solution. Valdez (1980) recommended using diluted povidone-iodine solution for wound lavage. The solu-tion is made by adding 1 to 2 ml 10% povi-done-iodine into 1000 ml of sterile saline.

Wound lavage should be done under high pressure. This can be achieved by using a dose syringe, or a disposable 60 cc plastic syringe fitted with an 18-gauge needle (Stashak, 1991). Deep foot wounds should be dressed with antibiotic ointment or with polydine ointment kept under a foot bandage.

Superficial wounds can be disinfected prior to debridement with 70 percent alcohol, 3 percent hydrogen peroxide or 5 percent povidone-iodine solution. Alternatively, the foot may be soaked for 30 minutes in a footbath made from saturated *magnesium sulfate* (Epson salts) in warm water. Following debridement, the wound is lavaged daily under pressure with diluted povidone-iodine solution. Superficial wounds can be dressed in the same manner as deep wounds or with pine tar.

Tetanus Vaccination

Horses are very sensitive to *tetanus* and many receive regular vaccination against the disease. Since the environment where horses live contains large numbers of tetanus spores, the vaccination status of the horse should be checked following injury to the foot, and the horse may be revaccinated according to the clinician's decision. In cases where a horseshoe nail was accidentally driven into sensitive tissue or the hoof was trimmed too deep, the horse owner should be informed so a decision regarding revaccination can be made (see page 160, horeshoe nail pricks).

🐾 FITTING THERAPEUTIC HORSESHOES

THE *principles of farriery* OF HORSES WITH FOOT disorders are similar to those for normal horses, with the exception that some cases may require horseshoe modification or the application of a therapeutic device not commonly used on normal horses. The construction of hand-made horseshoes for treatment of foot disorders is preferred (Butler, 1985). Hand-made shoes enable the farrier to determine

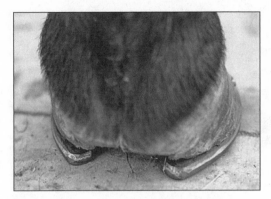

◆ **Fig. 13.8.** Fitting the horseshoes full, the horseshoe branches extend backward in order to increase palmar/plantar support. (Photo by author.)

the weight, web size and thickness of the horseshoe, the horseshoe design, nails position, nails pitch, and the addition of horseshoe adjuncts (Moyer, 1981). Horseshoes should be fitted full from the quarters back to the heels in order to form an *expansion surface* for the hoof (Luikart, 1993). The horseshoe branches should extend beyond the butters to provide palmar/plantar support (Butzow, 1961) (◆ fig. 13.8). The edges of the horseshoe branches should be ground smooth to reduce the possibility of the horseshoe being trapped or sprung (Balch et al., 1988b). In cases where the horse is being exercised, the opposite foot should be fitted with a horseshoe that has similar weight and dimensions.

A minimum number of horseshoe nails are used to attach the horseshoe to the hoof. Placing three nail holes on each side of a hand-made horseshoe is appropriate for most light horses. The position of the horseshoe nail holes in surgical horseshoes may be altered according to each case. Nail placement can be shifted toward the toe wall in cases of missing sections of wall at the quarters. Alternatively, the hoof wall can be reconstructed and the nails can be driven through the repair material. In cases of contracted heels, the horseshoe nails are positioned toward the toe in order to encourage hoof wall expansion at the quarters and heels. In chronic laminitis cases, the nail position is shifted

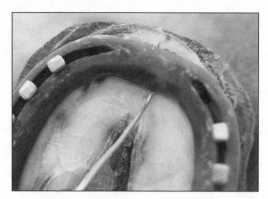

◆ **Fig. 13.9.** Seating out the horseshoe as indicated by a probe inserted between the sole and horseshoe. (Photo by author.)

toward the heels in order to relieve the toe wall. The farrier should be notified if the foot is desensitized, either by a nerve block or from an accident, so extra precautions can be taken when driving horseshoe nails.

Many of the horseshoe modifications that are used in therapeutic horseshoeing are being applied routinely in the farriery of normal horses; examples include squaring the toe in navicular disease, using tip-shoes in foals with contracted tendons, and seating the horseshoe in sole bruising and laminitis cases (◆ fig. 13.9). Some cases may require the application of horseshoes or devices with odd shapes such as an extended heels horseshoe. These horses should be kept stabled and should be hand-walked during the convalescence period. In unilateral cases, the opposite limb may be fitted with a regular horseshoe that protect the hoof. In cases where a thick pad is applied to the affected foot, the opposite foot should be raised to the same level. This can be achieved by fitting the horseshoe with an open pad of similar thickness. In cases where a flat, thin pad is applied, the healthy limb may be fitted only with a horseshoe.

Hot Shoe Fitting

Hot shoe fitting allows the farrier to examine the horseshoe for fitness without the need for cooling the horseshoe. This permits more rapid and precise shaping and leveling of the horseshoe. Prior to fitting, the horseshoe should be perfectly level and at *black heat.* The horseshoe should then be held against the hoof for a few seconds and checked for fitness. The charred areas formed over the solar surface indicate where more horn should be rasped in order to achieve a level bearing surface. Hot horseshoes should not be used for stamping the hoof in order to make the horseshoe fit.

In order to prevent thermal injury, hot shoe fitting should be applied only on horses with healthy hooves containing an adequate moisture level. Hot shoe fitting is contraindicated in foals, laminitis cases, thin sole cases, and missing sections of hoof wall. Russel (1878) indicated that burning the sole when fitting hot horseshoes can damage the sensitive laminae and sole, causing the hoof to become hard, dry, and brittle. Rick (1907) noted that the horseshoe and the sole can be made perfectly level without getting a hot shoe near the foot (see thermal injuries, page 202).

Moisture loss from the hoof following trimming and hot shoe fitting should be replenished by application of a hoof poultice applied over the solar surface. The poultice can be covered with waxed paper cut to fit the solar area. During that time, the opposite foot can be prepared for shoeing. Following shoeing, the solar area should be covered with pine tar in order to prevent additional moisture loss.

BAR HORSESHOES

Bar horseshoes AND THEIR MODIFICATIONS ARE the most common therapeutic horseshoe used for treatment of foot and limb disorders. The basic horseshoe has a bar that connects the horseshoe branches. Placement of the bar across the horseshoe branches increases the stability of the horseshoe and results in more even distribution of ground forces, thus relieving excessive pressure from the quarters and heels (Sprinhall, 1964). The bar may be used to load the frog in order to relieve weight

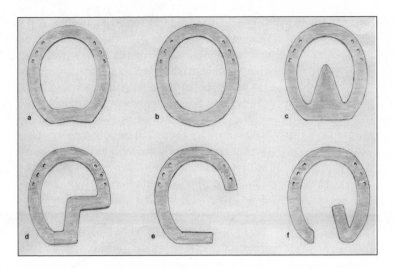

♦ **Fig. 13.10.** Examples of bar horseshoes, schematic illustrations. Straight-bar shoe (a), egg-bar shoe (b), heart-bar shoe (c), z-bar shoe (d), three-quarters-bar shoe (e), half-bar shoe (f).

from a quarter; in this case, the frog should be soft and well developed (Rich, 1907).

Bar horseshoes are classified according to the shape of the bar into straight-bar shoe, convexed bar shoe and egg-bar shoe. Modifications of the bar horseshoe include the heart-bar shoe, adjustable heart-bar shoe, wedged egg-bar shoe, navicular egg-bar shoe, half-bar shoe and double half-bar shoe, three-quarters-bar shoe, Z-bar shoe and the treatment plate (♦ fig.13.10). These horseshoes are described under the various foot disorders for which they are commonly used.

Bar horseshoes may be forged from iron or aluminum bar stock; commercial horseshoes made from iron, aluminum and titanium are available (Millman, 1998). Many synthetic glue-on shoes have a design similar to that of egg-bar horseshoe.

Bar horseshoes are used in the treatment of sheared heels (Moyer and Anderson, 1975), under-run heels, quarter and heel cracks, third phalanx fractures, corns, navicular disease (Moyer, 1980), white line disease (Kuwano et al., 1998), inflammation of the distal sesamoidean ligament (Moyer, 1982) and laminitis. The bar horseshoe protects the palmar/plantar area of the foot in cases of diseased frogs and bulbs of the heels. The additional support provided by the bar permits placement of horseshoe nails holes at different positions. The bar shoe stabilizes the hoof

and provides protection to painful areas and missing sections of hoof wall. The horseshoe permits normal growth of horn by removing pressure from specific areas of the hoof wall, and it permits exercising the horse during the convalescence period. Lungwitz (1891) indicated that the bar horseshoe allows better hoof deformation compared to the open horseshoe, and it is very useful for treatment of diseases and defective hooves.

Straight-Bar Shoe

The *straight-bar shoe* is a horseshoe with a bar across the horseshoe branches (fig. 13.10a). The horseshoe is used in horses with weak hoof wall, hoof wall cracks, missing sections of hoof wall, third phalanx fractures and for construction of a treatment plate. The straight-bar horseshoe can be made from a keg shoe by welding a bar across its branches or by forging it from various sizes of bar stock. The bar is positioned straight across the horseshoe branches, thus reducing the possibility of the horseshoe being pulled by a hind hoof.

Convex-Bar Shoe

The *convex-egg bar shoe* is a horseshoe that is fitted with a bar that is arched forward, this lessen the possibility of the horseshoe being pulled by a hind hoof.

Egg-Bar Shoe

The *egg-bar shoe* is an extended bar shoe that protects and supports the palmar/plantar aspect of the foot (fig. 13.10b). An egg-bar shoe may be applied to cases where additional palmar/plantar support is required. The horseshoe is used in cases of bruised heels, hoof cracks (Moyer, 1981; Evanse et al., 1966), chronic laminitis, missing sections of heel, dermatitis of the bulbs of the heels, and suspensory ligament desmitis or inflammation of the SL (Bennett, 2005). Moyer (1982) described the use of the egg-bar shoe and a rolled toe in cases of inflammation of the distal sesamoidean ligament. A wide-web egg-bar shoe provides excellent protection to the solar region of the foot and heels area. This horseshoe may be constructed from various sizes of bar stock or from a worn horseshoeing rasp. The egg-bar shoe is commonly used in the farriery of hoof wall cracks following repair of the defect. A wide-web egg-bar shoe should be applied to cases with extensive hoof wall loss in order to stabilize the limb and protect the hoof until repair is possible. A straight bar shoe or a convex-bar shoe should be used in cases where there is a risk of the horseshoe being pulled by the hind leg.

Chapter 14

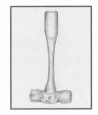

Acrylic Reconstruction

 ACRYLIC RESINS

THE APPLICATION OF *acrylic adhesives* FOR THE repair of hoof wall defects began about 40 years ago (Jenny et al., 1965; Evans et al., 1966) and has become an important part of the treatment of foot disorders. The hoof repair material combined with a therapeutic or keg horseshoe protects and stabilizes the hoof and permits normal hoof function during recovery. Jenny et al. (1965) recommended using the repair material for attachment of horseshoes without using nails.

Applications of acrylic materials in hoof care procedures include the repair of hoof wall cracks (Moyer, 1983; Moyer and Sigafoos, 1993), hoof wall loss, seedy toe, chronic laminitis, thin hoof wall (Moyer and Sigafoos, 1991), contracted tendons, deformed hooves, crooked hooves (Jenny et al., 1965) and under-run heels (Moyer and Sigafoos, 1991; Sigafoos, 1991; Bruggink and Sigafoos, 1997). Acrylic adhesives are commonly used to correct orthopedic disorders in foals. Farriers and veterinarians should become aware to the possibility that acrylic resins may cover up hoof defects, which could be difficult to detect during pre-purchase examinations.

The repair material is an *acrylic resin* called *polymethylmethacrylate* (PMMA). The acrylic resin has two components that when mixed together begin a rapid *polymerization* (curing) process. The optimal condition for the curing process is absent of oxygen (Jenny et al., 1965). Cold ambient temperature slows the curing process; the rate of curing can be increased by warming the resin with a hair dryer or hot air blower. Following curing, the repair material should have similar properties as the hoof horn.

Two types of acrylic resin products are available for hoof repair. The first type has powder and liquid components, and the second type has two paste components. The *powder-liquid type resin* requires careful measuring of the liquid and powder according to the manufacturer's recommendation. The liquid is poured into the powder and the two components are mixed with a wooden tongue depressor. The mixing begins the curing process. During this process, the consistency of the mixture begins to change from syrup to smooth paste, then it becomes rubbery and finally it changes into a solid. The resin should be applied to the hoof at the transition from syrup to paste consistency. A softer cured resin can be obtained by adding more liquid into the mixture. The cured resin of some products is too hard and may cause sub-solar bruising when applied to the sole. The advantage of the liquid-powder product is that no mixing tips or cartridges are used, there is less waste, which makes the product more environmentally friendly. The liquid portion has a limited shelf life, which can be significantly extended by refrigeration (Jenny et al., 1965).

The *paste-type resin* is supplied in a two-part cartridge that is fitted into a dispensing gun. The cartridge is fitted with a disposable mixer tip that mixes the two paste components during application. The resin is applied directly to the area that is being repaired or on glue-on shoes. Craig and Craig (2003) indicated that the optimal curing temperature for acrylic resins is between 20C° to 27C° (70°F to 80°F). They recommended placing the cartridge in a bucket of warm water prior to application of resin when the ambient temperature is cold, and storing the cartridge in a cool place during the summer. Prior to application of the resin, some material may have to be squeezed out until the correct mixing proportions are achieved. This results in wasted material. The advantages of the paste type resin include rapid application and convenience.

 ## RESIN APPLICATION SAFETY

THROUGHOUT THE APPLICATION OF ACRYLIC resins, the operator should wear latex or rubber gloves, and a mask fitted with an air filter that prevents inhalation of *hazardous fumes*. The procedure should be done outdoors in a well-ventilated area. The horse should be faced upwind in order to reduce exposure to toxic fumes. The gloves and mask should be worn during mixing and application of acrylic resins. A protective mask should also be worn when rasping the repair material after it cures, and when sanding or grinding any other synthetic materials. Failure to do this can result in inhalation of *hazardous chemical*

dust released from these materials (Bradley D. in Strickland, 2001).

During the polymerization process (curing process), the acrylic material releases a considerable amount of heat; some resins can reach 260°F and should not be used on hooves. The temperature within the mixture of resins used in hoof repair may reach 65°C (150°F) (Gauthier, 2001). Moyer and Sigafoos (1991) recommended using PMMA products that produce relatively low heat (see appendix A). The repair material should be applied in several layers, with each new layer applied over a cured layer. Excessive heat production should be monitored by placing the hand over the resin and observing the horse for signs of discomfort. In cases where excessive heat is produced, the hoof should be cooled immediately with cold water.

 ## HOOF CAPSULE REPAIR

THE STRENGTH OF REPAIR OF HOOF CAPSULE defects depends largely on meticulous preparation of the treated area. Any present infection has to be treated and allowed to heal, and the treated area should be completely dry and cornified (Evans et al., 1966). Repairing hoof wall defects too early may damage the tender epidermal germinal tissue by the heat of polymerization (Fessler, 1971a).

Prior to the repair procedure, the hoof is trimmed for shoeing, all loose horn should be removed and the affected area should be debrided. In order to increase the strength of the repair, the margins of the defect are undercut when possible in order to form a buttress along its edge (Jenny et al., 1965; Evanse et al., 1966)(see page 181). Undercutting the hoof wall at the quarters and heels may not be possible in horses with thin hoof wall. The strength of the repair may be increased by forming a stepladder pattern along its margins (see fig. 16.74); hoof wall cracks may be stabilized prior to the repair by several lacing techniques (see hoof capsule cracks, chapter 16). Acrylic resins should be reinforced with fabric material in order to increase the strength of the repair (see below).

In order to increase the strength of the bond between the hoof and resin, the surface around the defect should be sanded, and degreased with denatured alcohol or acetone. Following degreasing the foot should be kept clean and allowed to dry by placing it on a clean towel. The acetone must be pure in order obtain clean surface, this type of acetone can be purchase from car paint suppliers (Wilson and Pardoe, 1998). Alternatively, 90% alcohol may be used as a degreaser material. A hair dryer should not be used to dry the hoof following the application of flammable materials such as acetone (Wilson and Pardoe, 1998).

Once the hoof is dry, the first layer of resin is applied over the defect and allowed to dry, than the entire surface is sanded lightly (Sigafoos, 1991). When a liquid-powder resin is used, the cured layer should be swabbed with the fluid portion prior to application of a new layer (Jenny et al., 1965). Additional layers are added as required. Curing is facilitated by wrapping the entire foot with a nylon glove (the glove used by the operator can be inverted over the hoof) or with aluminum foil (Jenny et al., 1965; Moyer and Sigafoos, 1993). Detailed information on hoof wall repair techniques can be found in Moyer and Sigafoos, 1993.

Composite Lay-Up

The strength of the repair can be increased significantly by incorporating fabric material with the resin; the combined resin and fabric forms a *composite*. A fabric (webbing) material made of *polyethylene filament fabric* is commonly used (Moyer and Sigafoos, 1993; Moyer and Sigafoos, 1991; Sigafoos, 1991; Sigafoos, 1995; O'Grady, 2001). Alternatively, a *fiberglass sheet* (Sigafoos, 1995; Stanley, 2004) or *polypropylene fibers* (Wildenstein, 2004) may be applied.

Fabrics vary in their adherence, strength and resistance to wear. Thus, the selection of fabric should be based on the type and location of the repair, and the depth at which the

Table 14.1 ◆ Comparison of fabric properties of four materials.

Fabric Type	Adhesive Compatibility	Tensile Strength	Abrasion Resistance
S2 Fiberglass	Excellent	NA	NA
Kevlar[1]	NA	High	Poor
Spectra[2]	Poor	High	High
Carbon Fiber	Excellent	High	NA

1. Suitable for inner layers.
2. Suitable for outer layers.
NA= No information available.
Data from Sigafoos R. 1995.

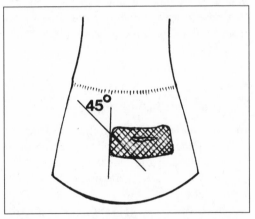

◆ **Fig. 14.1.** Fabric placement in hoof wall repair, schematic illustration. The strength of the repair is increased by placing the fabric with the direction of the braided fibers at 45° to the plane of the hoof.

fabric is placed (Sigafoos, 1995) (◆ Table 14.1). In addition, the direction of fiber yarn placement in relation to the hoof wall is important (Sigafoos, 1991); maximum reinforcement is achieved when the fabric is placed with the fibers at 45° to the long axis of the hoof (◆ fig. 14.1).

A strong composite is made by using two to three layers of resin-impregnated fabric. The first layer of resin is applied over the defect and allowed to cure. Then a fabric dressed with resin is added. Additional layers of composite are added as needed and the entire foot is wrapped in order to facilitate curing.

O'Grady (2001) described the reconstruction of a hoof wall defect with PMMA reinforced with three layers of fabric. Helms et al. (1994) described a similar procedure for toe wall reconstruction following surgical removal of keratoma. Pardoe and Wilson (1999) compared the mechanical properties of different fixation techniques used to stabilize quarter cracks. They concluded that acrylic adhesive repairs can resist shear forces like screw plate repair without the risk of screws being penetrated into sensitive structures. They indicated that the yield force of the repair was low in comparison to the forces applied to the hoof during motion; therefore, they recommended that the hoof be protected from localized or uneven loading with a protective horseshoe.

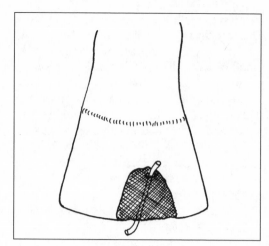

◆ **Fig. 14.2.** Establishment of drainage under the repair material, schematic illustration. See text for details.

Establishment of Drainage

In cases where the defect in the hoof is infected, the repair should be delayed until healing is complete and the defect area is dry and cornified. Alternatively, a *drainage tract* can be made between the wound and the repair material. Prior to application of resin, the infected area is covered with clay (or Play dough). A thin plastic tube with a 5 mm diameter is placed over the clay. The tube should protrude beyond the upper and lower ends of the wound (◆ fig. 14.2). The resin is applied and allowed to cure. Once curing is complete, the plastic tube is removed and the clay is flushed out (Moyer and Sigafoos, 1993). The upper opening of the drainage tract is used for daily flushing of the wound with a solution of diluted povidone-iodine in saline.

Hoof Repair Failure

Causes of *hoof repair failure* include inadequate debridement, presence of thrush,

incomplete degreasing of the affected area, excessive moisture, application of old and inert materials, development of shear forces caused by application of light horseshoes or strenuous work, glueing the hoof to the horseshoe, and failure to use reinforcing techniques such as fabrics and lacing. Other factors include insufficient surface preparation and movement prior to bond formation (Wilson and Pardoe, 1998).

Horseshoes Used in Hoof Repair

The type of horseshoes applied in hoof repair procedures depends on the extent of the repair and the type of activity done by the horse. A keg shoe, training plate, wide-web horseshoe or bar horseshoe may be applied. Bar horseshoes provide the best protection and stability and should be applied whenever possible.

The horseshoe may be applied before or after completion of the repair. Moyer and Sigafoos (1991) indicated that PMMA can be trimmed, rasped, and nailed like normal hoof wall. When the resin is applied to the hoof after the application of the horseshoe, the hoof surface of the horseshoe should be covered with thin plastic film, such as plastic

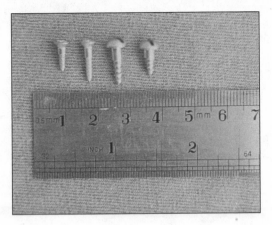

◆ **Fig. 14.3.** Examples of screw types used in hoof procedures. (Photo by author.)

food wrap, that prevents adherence of resin to the horseshoe. Adherence between the horseshoe and hoof may prevent normal expansion at the quarters and heels and could lead to abnormal shear forces and repair failure.

Application of Screws in Farriery

Screws may be used in hoof care procedures such as hoof wall repair, attachment of modified treatment plates, connection of support plates, and attachment of plastic patches. Screws may be incorporated in repair of hoof wall cracks in order to increase the strength of the repair; the screws are placed along the length of the crack and are connected with a stainless steel wire. The resin and fabrics are applied over the stabilized area.

Wood screws or sheet metal screws, 2 to 3 mm in diameter, should be used in the hoof wall (◆ fig. 14.3). Screws should be placed in hooves with adequate hoof wall thickness and should not be driven through more than 2/3 of the hoof wall thickness. Prior to application of a screw, the selected position is predrilled with a hand-held drill that is fitted with a drill bit with a diameter that is 1 mm smaller than the screw's largest diameter. Each screw is applied carefully with a hand-held screwdriver into the predrilled hole.

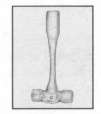

Chapter 15

Glue-On Horseshoeing

 APPLICATIONS

Glue-on horseshoes HAVE AN IMPORTANT PART IN therapeutic farriery of various foot disorders, abnormal foot conformation, and orthopedic disorders in foals (page 87). Synthetic glue-on horseshoes have important advantages over metal horseshoes, which include excellent shock absorption properties and allowance of hoof expandability.

Glue-on shoes are applied in the treatment of chronic laminitis (Craig and Craig, 2003; O'Grady, 2004), contracted heels, long-toe low-heels hoof conformation (Denson, 2004), hoof wall loss, fractures of the third phalanx, damaged heels (O'Grady and Watson, 1999), navicular disease, chronic bruising (Moyer, 1980), white line disease (Turner, 1998), and concussion-related lameness such as side bone and ring bone. The horseshoe may be applied to horses with missing sections of hoof wall where driving horseshoe nails could be risky.

Application of glue-on shoes should be done outdoors in a well-ventilated area. A low heat producing resin should be used to glue the horseshoe (see appendix A). The person that applies the horseshoes should wear rubber or latex gloves and an appropriate laboratory mask that prevents inhalation of toxic fumes (see Resin Application Safety, chapter 14).

 TYPES OF GLUE-ON HORSESHOES

SEVERAL TYPES OF GLUE-ON HORSESHOES, MADE with different materials and various designs, are commercially available. Currently, glue-on shoes may be divided into three general types: synthetic glue-on shoes, aluminum core shoes and metal horseshoes. The application of plastic and aluminum glue-on horseshoes has been described by Champagne, 1998; Juell, 1998; O'Grady and Watson, 1999; Ludford, 2004, and others.

Synthetic Glue-On Horseshoes

Synthetic glue-on shoes are made from acrylic polymers, *polyurethane* or *polyethylene* (Strickland, 2001). This horseshoe is commonly designed as a wide-web bar shoe, which makes it suitable for therapeutic applications. The plastic horseshoe absorbs energy efficiently, it is lightweight, and it permits expansion of the hoof (Moyer, 1980). The horseshoe is available in different sizes, and one company produce the horseshoe in 2 widths. One product is made from two plastic parts: a soft inner component that absorbs shock and a hard outer component that resists wear (Craig and Craig, 2003). The glue-on shoe is glued to the hoof with a fast-curing resin with similar final hardness as the hoof horn. Some glue-on horseshoes are available with horseshoe nail holes, so that nails may be used to increase the strength of horseshoe attachment.

Application of synthetic glue-on horseshoes requires specific preparation of the hoof for shoeing. In order to prevent contact between the frog and the horseshoe, the frog is trimmed level with the wall-bearing surface. The solar surface of the hoof is degreased with denatured alcohol and the hoof is placed on a dry towel. The hoof surface of the horseshoe is cleaned with denatured alcohol and allowed to dry. The resin is applied along the outer half of the horseshoe's web, from quarter to quarter. The height of the resin should be about 6 mm. The horse's limb is lifted and the horseshoe is placed on the hoof and held at the desired place. In order to prevent the glue from spreading out, the horseshoe should be held gently without pressing it too hard. Excessive glue is smeared around the horseshoe and hoof until it is smooth; the final layer of glue should be about 3 to 4 mm thick. In order to prevent weakening of the bond, the glue-on shoe should be held without movement until the resin cures. Depending on the external temperature, curing may take 90 seconds to 3 minutes. Curing can be checked by pressing the resin with a fingernail; once the resin is cured it can no longer be marked with the fingernail. At this point, the limb is placed carefully on the ground and the horse is kept in place for an additional five minutes before it can be walked (Craig and Craig, 2003). Horseshoe removal is done with regular pull offs.

Glue-On Horseshoe with Aluminum Core

The *glue-on horseshoe with aluminum core* is made from an aluminum horseshoe covered with polyurethane; the horseshoe has tabs that are used to glue the horseshoe to the hoof wall. The aluminum core provides rigidity while the plastic material absorbs shock.

The hoof is trimmed and the horseshoe is fitted to the hoof, a shaping device provided by the manufacturer is available. Prior to application of the horseshoe, the wall surface is sanded lightly and degreased with denatured alcohol and then the hoof is placed on a clean towel. The inner surface of the tabs are degreased with denatured alcohol and allowed to dry. The horseshoe is placed on the hoof, the leg is placed on the ground and the opposite leg is lifted by an assistant. The glueing process begins from the rear tabs on both sides of the hoof and continues forward. Each tab is pulled aside and few drops of glue provided by the manufacturer are placed on the top of the tab and allowed to trickle down. The tab is pressed firmly against the wall and held for 10 seconds. The process continues toward the toe tabs.

Glue-On Metal Shoes

Glue-on metal horseshoes may be applied to horses with broken hoof wall that are too weak to hold horseshoe nails. This horseshoe permits growth of new hoof wall while the horse continues to work. The hoof is trimmed and the horseshoe is fitted to the hoof.

The hoof wall-bearing surface is degreased with alcohol and the leg is placed on a clean towel. The horseshoe hoof surface is degreased with alcohol and allowed to dry. The inner web of the horseshoe is fitted with a *horseshoe liner* made from sticky neoprene strips. The strips prevent flow of resin to the solar area in order to prevent sole bruising. The resin is applied to the outer web of the horseshoe, the limb is lifted, and the horseshoe is applied as described for synthetic glue-on shoes. Horseshoe removal is done with regular pull-offs.

According to Stanley (2004), the application of glue-on metal horseshoes over a period of time results in heel contraction. This may result from limited heel expansion during weight bearing, caused by the restriction of the glue. Contrary to that, Craig and Craig (2003) measured gradual expansion of the hoof wall following application of synthetic glue-on shoes.

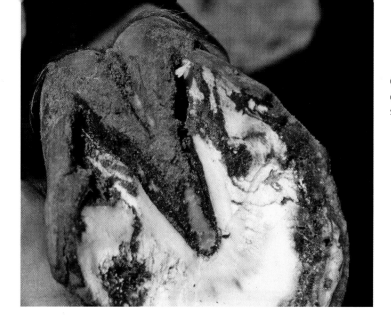

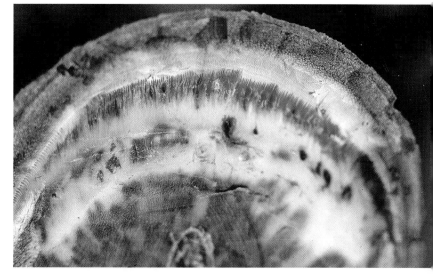

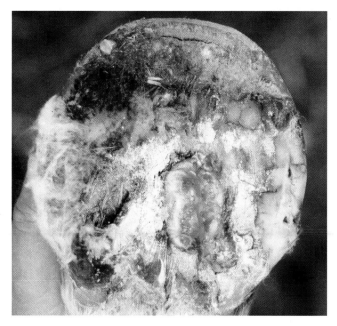

◀ **Plate 1**
Corn, dry form, appears as red discoloration at the angle of the sole.

▶ **Plate 2**
Chronic laminitis with widening and discoloration of the white line.

◀ **Plate 3**
Healthy granulation tissue over the frog area appears as pinkish tissue about seven days after surgical debridement of a penetrating wound.

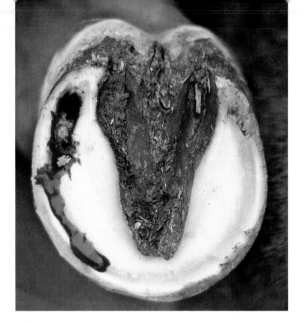

▶ **Plate 4**
Sub-solar abscess with a worm-like tunnel filled with thrush

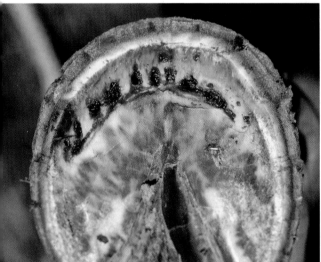

◀ **Plate 5**
Chronic laminits complicated by solar prolapse

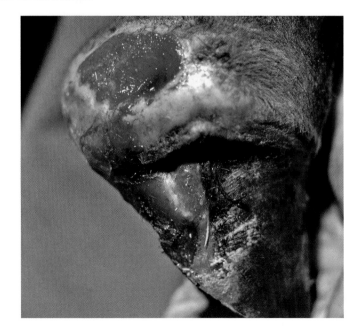

▶ **Plate 6**
Healing avulsion injury at the quarter area.

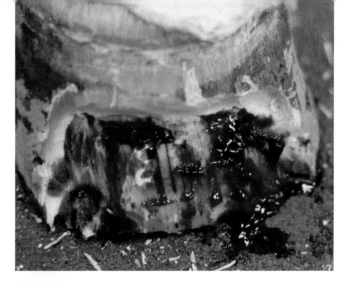

▶ **Plate 7**
Dorsal hoof wall resection in a chronic laminitis case.

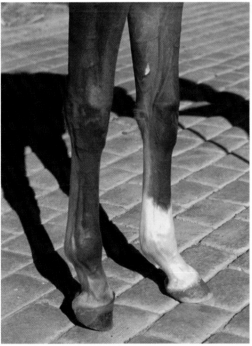

◀ **Plate 8**
Contracted deep digital flexor tendon in the right foreleg of a weanling Arabian colt.

▶ **Plate 9**
Extended egg-bar shoe used to protect diseased heel bulbs

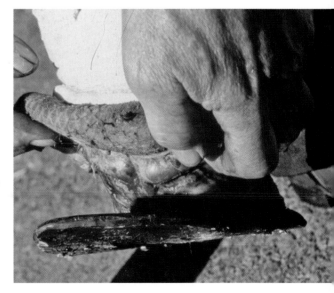

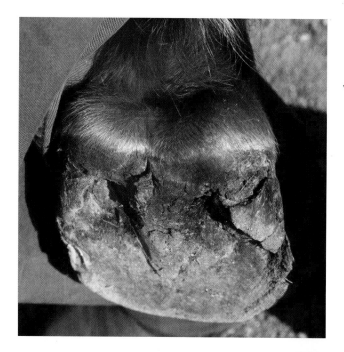

◄ **Plate 10**
Weak heels with horizontal cracks.

► **Plate 11**
Avulsion of a section of hoof wall in a case of neglected hooves.

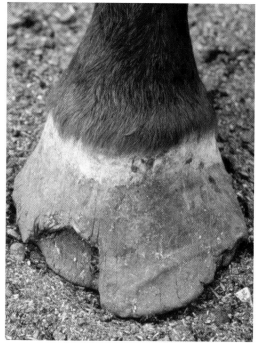

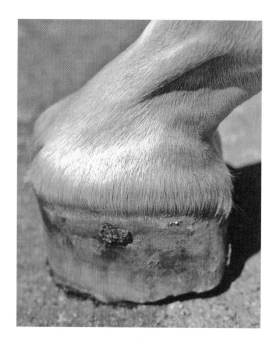

◄ **Plate 12**
Severe club foot.

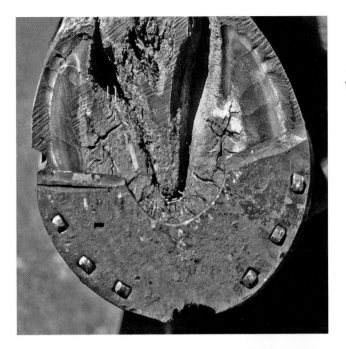

◀ **Plate 13**
Wide web tip shoe.

▶ **Plate 14**
Chronic laminitis with red pigment over the hoof wall.

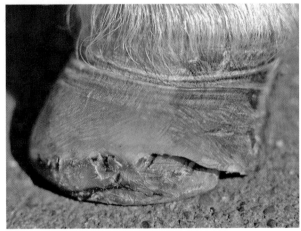

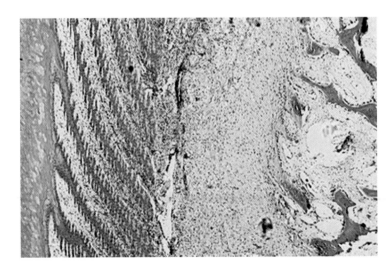

◀ **Plate 15**
Microscopic cross section of the laminae taken from a fetal foot. (Courtesy of Dr. C.L. Ownby, Oklahoma State University.)

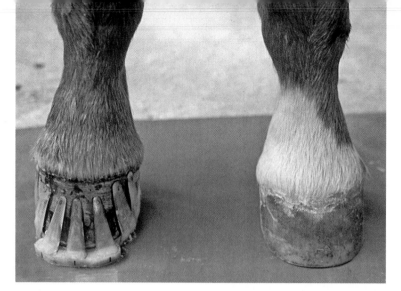

◄ **Plate 16**
Glu-on shoe in a foal with contracted deep digital flexor tendon.

► **Plate 17**
Reversed horseshoe and a wedge pad. The leather string was used to tie a piece of oakum to the pad.

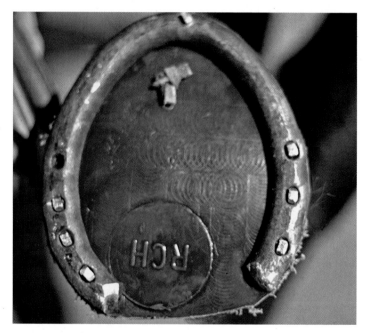

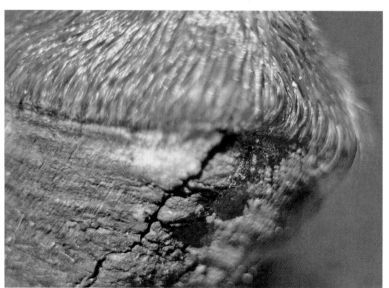

◄ **Plate 18**
Deep complete quarter crack.

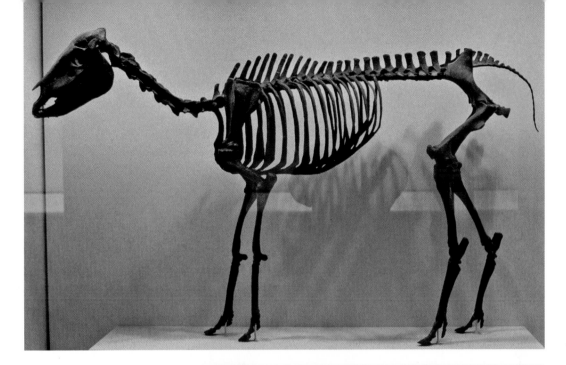

▲ **Plate 19**
Reconstructed skeleton of
Parahippus leonensis, a three-toed
horse that lived in the Miocene
epoch of Florida. (Courtesy of
Florida Museum of Natural
History, Gainesville.)

▶ **Plate 20**
Cornification of the laminar
surface in chronic laminitis case.
The laminae become covered with
new horn that protects the dermis
until growth of new hoof wall
is completed.

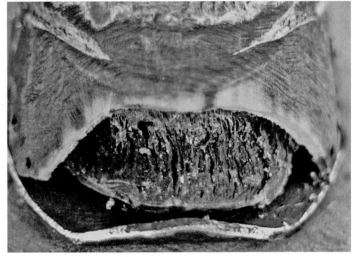

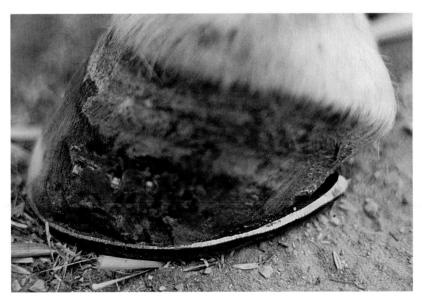

◀ **Plate 21**
Full fit of a
horseshoe.

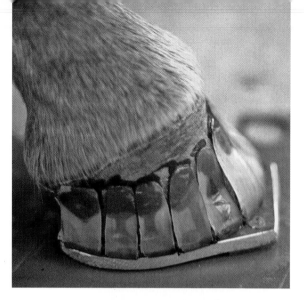

◀ **Plate 22**
Glue-on horseshoe made from a plastic pad and aluminum plate.

▼ **Plate 23**
Heel bulb contraction.

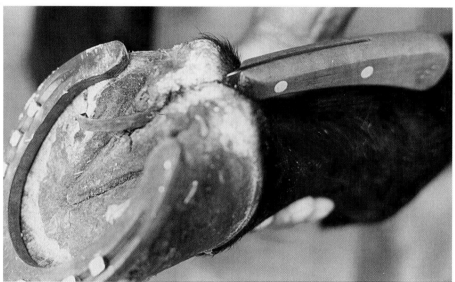

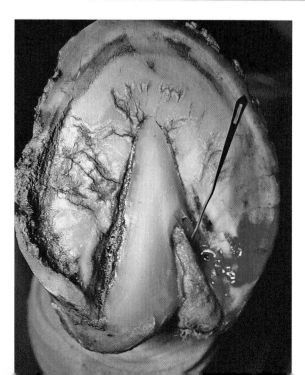

◀ **Plate 24**
A probe is inserted into the lesion of navicular bursitis case.

Part 5 Therapeutic Farriery

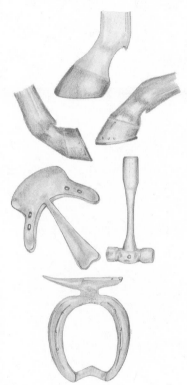

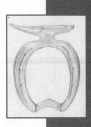

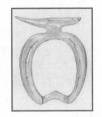

Chapter 16

Farriery of Foot Disorders

🦴 LAMINITIS

Laminitis IS A DISEASE OF THE FOOT characterized by inflammation and destruction of the laminae. The disease more commonly involves the forefeet, but in some cases, all four feet are affected. It rarely affects the hind feet only (Colles and Jeffcott, 1977). One study showed that the age group of affected horses is between four and ten years old, with similar sex distribution (Coffman et al., 1972). The disease has metabolic and mechanical forms, and it is associated with various conditions. These include grain overload, colic, retained placenta, generalized disease, steroid therapy, excess intake of cold water after hard exercise, grazing on lush spring grass, overfeeding, toxins, excessive weight bearing on one limb following an injury to the opposite limb, and work on hard ground (Linford, 1990). Laminitis may develop as a complication of *Cushing's syndrome* (Harman and Ward, 2001; Eustace, 2001a) and *obesity-related laminitis*; both causes are linked to excessive cortisol production (Eustace, 2001a). The disease may develop in horses with white line disease (Redden, 1990; Kuwano et al., 1998; Oke, 2003). Another cause includes exposure to black walnut shavings (True et al., 1978; Galey et al., 1991).

There are differences in sensitivity to development of the disease among horses; these differences may relate to obesity, nutrition, laminar bond strength, horn quality, working surface and type of work. Hood et al. (1994b) proposed that certain breeding lines of Quarter Horses might have a genetic predisposition for development of chronic laminitis.

Laminitis may be complicated by *secondary sepsis*, which may be accompanied by drainage sites at the coronary band and sole (Coffman et al., 1972; Johnson, 1972). Once the disease develops, the damage to the foot may be irreversible. Therefore, prevention of the disease is extremely important. Laminitis follows developmental, acute and chronic phases (Pollitt, 1999) and it may become refractory. Cripps and Eustace (1999) classi-fied the disease into laminitis, acute founder, chronic founder and sinker.

Garner et al. (1981) described the development of the *metabolic form* of laminitis caused by *carbohydrate overload*, which is the most common cause of laminitis in horses; the carbohydrate source may be from lush pastures or excessive grain. Pollitt (1999) proposed that laminitis is caused by a substance produced by hindgut bacteria following carbohydrate overload; this substance is capable of activating *laminar enzymes* that disintegrate the laminar architecture, thus causing detachment between the dermal and epidermal laminae with consequent displacement of the third phalanx within the hoof capsule. Grain overload can be prevented by gradual introduction of grain, feeding proper amounts, and preventing accidental access of the horse to grain bins.

Pastures may contain *fructan*, a carbohydrate that can accumulate in high levels in grass (Longland and Cairns, 2000), and predispose the horse to *grass laminitis*. Hay made from grass containing high fructan levels is another source. This type of laminitis can develop in horses that are considered resistant to the disease. Grass laminitis has been diagnosed in Przewalski's horses kept in a semi-reserve in Germany that contained high carbohydrate grass (Budras et al., 2001), and in mustang horses kept in a poor quality grass pasture in California. This type of laminitis is more difficult to control; the substance may accumulate in the stubbles of dead plants in pastures that appear brown. The accumulation of fructan depends on many factors including weather conditions (Watts in Nyland, 2006). This type of laminitis commonly develops more slowly, and it is the *sub clinical* form of laminitis (Walsh in Nyland, 2006). Prevention of grass laminitis includes testing samples of grass from suspected pastures, avoiding overgrazing, feeding low-sugar varieties of grass, and placing horses in dry paddocks during periods of high risk.

Mechanical tearing of the bonds between the sensitive and insensitive laminae causes the mechanical form of laminitis. Predisposing factors for this form of laminitis include excessive body weight (Coffman et al., 1969; Rooney, 1977a), long toe (Rooney, 1977a), traumatic induced laminitis caused by prolonged work on a hard surface or "road founder" (Peremans et al., 1991; Rooney, 1978a; Dart and Pascoe, 1988), supporting limb complications in opposite or diagonal limbs (Redden, 1986b; Dart and Pascoe, 1988) and lowering the heels in clubfoot cases. The disease, which is also called "pony founder," is common in Shetland ponies (Rooney, 1978a) and other pony breeds kept on lush grass. In this form of laminitis, lameness improves with rest but tends to reoccur during work. Treatment of laminitis includes medical, surgical and farriery care.

MECHANICS OF THIRD PHALANX ROTATION

The displacement of the third phalanx is affected by three forces: tearing force, driving force and pulling force (Coffman et al., 1970). The *tearing force* develops from ground pressure against the toe wall and is responsible for separation between the third phalanx and the toe wall (◆ fig. 16.1). The *driving force* develops by the weight of the horse on the digital bones and is responsible for sinking and rotation of the third phalanx. The *pulling force* develops by the pull of the deep digital flexor tendon on the third phalanx in a palmar/plantar direction, and is responsible for rotation of the third phalanx. Hence, the tearing force is increased with increased hoof lever arm, the driving force is increased by excessive weight

or load on the limb, and the pulling force increases with low heels. Once rotation begins, the driving force and the pulling force increase their effect due to the fulcrum formed by the digital cushion (Coffman et al., 1970). Leach (1983a) indicated that in order for the third phalanx to rotate, some attachments between the wall and the bone should remain in the heels and quarters area. A vital number of laminae are required for binding the third phalanx to the hoof (Pollitt, 1986). Once the laminar arrangement is disrupted, the third phalanx may rotate, or more rarely, displace downward (sink), ending in a serious lameness condition (◆ Fig. 16.2).

O'Grady (2004) indicated that two forms of rotation are observed in chronic laminitis. One form is *capsular rotation,* which is characterized by moderate rotation of the third pha-

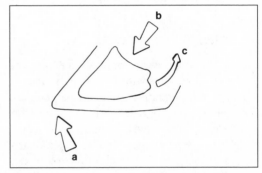

◆ **Fig. 16.1.** Forces that act on the third phalanx. Tearing force (a), driving force (b), and pulling force (c). (Reprinted by permission from Coffman et al. 1970, fig. 2. Illustration modified to text.)

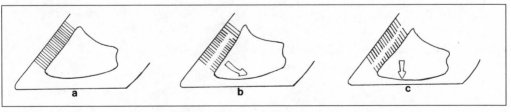

◆ **Fig. 16.2.** Third phalanx rotation and displacement, schematic illustration. Normal anatomic relationship between the third phalanx and the hoof capsule (a), third phalanx rotation (b) and distal displacement (sinking) (c). Rotation and sinking may occur simultaneously. The parallel lines represent laminar bonding.

lanx and pronounced dorsal displacement of the toe wall. The second form is *phalangeal rotation*, which is characterized by more pronounced rotation of the third phalanx and functional shortening of the musculotendinous unit of the DDFT. Capsular rotation is caused by torque that develops from long toes, work on hard pavement or constant pounding on the ground that weakened the laminae. Phalangeal rotation result from extensive destruction of the dorsal laminar surface. A combination of both forms with various degrees of severity develops in some cases. The farriery of each case depends on the type of changes that take place (O'Grady, 2004) (page 137).

Farriery principles of third phalanx rotation include reducing the forces that act on the bone, namely, shortening the HLA by dubbing the toe, supporting the third phalanx with padding material, and relieving tension from the DDFT by raising the heels.

NUTRITION OF LAMINITIS CASES

Jackson (1996) recommended feeding the acute laminitis case with a limited amount of soluble carbohydrates. This can be achieved by feeding a diet high in soluble fiber and low in starch. The source of fiber should come from good quality hay that is cut at early stages of maturity, has low lignin content and high leaf/stem ratio. Chronic cases of laminitis should be fed with a fat supplement instead of soluble carbohydrates (sugars). The protein requirements should be maintained in order to encourage hoof re-growth. A hoof supplement containing biotin (50 to 100 mg/day), methionine (9 gm/day) and chelated zinc (400-600mg/day) should be added to the diet. Budras Et al. (2001) recommended avoiding grazing of susceptible horses, such as overweight and/or chronic founder horses, on pastures rich in water-soluble carbohydrates. Additional information on low carbohydrate grass types suitable for horses may be obtained from the United States Department of Agriculture (USDA) or local agriculture extension office.

Acute Laminitis

PRIOR TO DEVELOPMENT OF CLINICAL SIGNS OF *acute laminitis*, some warning signs indicating that the horse is at risk may be observed. These signs include increased digital pulse and hoof surface temperature; the horse may not be lame. At this stage, aggressive preventative measures should begin and include removal of grain, administration of mineral oil and medical treatment. (O'Grady, 1993a). Pollitt (1999) indicated that the process that initiates the destruction of the laminae begins before the first clinical sign of laminitis.

The acute stage of laminitis is characterized by development of lameness. The horse may be reluctant to move, and when walked, the steps are short and weight is placed on the heels in order to reduce pressure from the painful toes. When the forelegs are the only limbs that are affected, the horse places its hind legs well under the body and the forelimbs are placed forward in a typical "sawhorse stance" (Redden, 1986) (◆ fig. 16.3). Other signs include strong digital pulse, increased hoof warmth, and positive reaction to hoof testers at the region of the sole. In an experimentally induced carbohydrate overload, it took 40 hours for the first clinical signs to appear (Garner, 1975). In severe

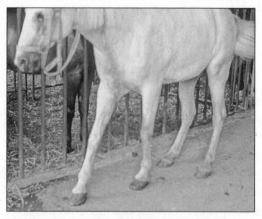

◆ **Fig. 16.3. Founder stance.** Stance of a mare affected by laminitis in the forelegs. The right limb that is more painful is placed farther forward with more weight placed on the heels. (Photo by author.)

cases, rotation may occur within 24 to 48 hours (Coffman et al., 1972), and in some cases, the third phalanx may penetrate the sole in 24 hours (Redden, 1986). In other cases, radiographic evidence of third phalanx rotation may not appear until the fifth day (Redden, 1986). Third phalanx rotation and/or sinking results in flattening of the sole. The pressure may be severe enough to cause *solar prolapse,* which is characterized by a crescent shape protrusion of solar dermis through the horny sole between the point of the frog and toe wall (Eustace and Caldwell, 1989b; Goetz, 1987) (see plate 5). Cripps and Eustace (1999) indicated that solar prolapse may result from slight sinking and considerable rotation of the bone, or from considerable sinking with minimal rotation. Third phalanx sinking is less common than rotation (Moore and Allen, 1995) and occurs when the laminae are entirely detached from the circumference of the hoof wall. Consequently, the sole appears flattened or convex and the coronary band becomes indented; the entire hoof may be slough (Marianne, 1986). Most cases of supportive limb laminitis involve sinking of the third phalanx (Peloso et al., 1996). The prognosis for cases with distal displacement of the third phalanx is poor (Baxter, 1986; Hunt, 1993; Cripps and Eustace, 1999).

RADIOGRAPHY OF LAMINITIS

Lateral radiographs of the foot, taken at the acute and chronic stages, are used to calculate the degree of third phalanx rotation and sinking in order to assess prognosis and methods of therapy. Prior to radiography, the hoof is marked with a metal marker that shows the location of the dorsal hoof wall and its proximal border; this gives the position of the third phalanx relative to the hoof capsule. Two important measurements that are obtained from the radiograph include the horn-laminar zone (Redden in Tearney, 2005) and founder distance (Cripp and Eustace, 1999) (◆ fig. 16.4).

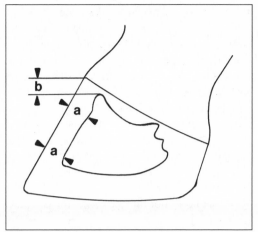

A

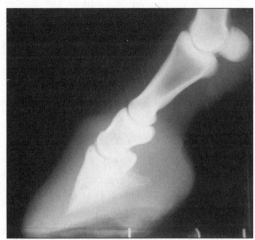

B

◆ **Fig. 16.4.** Radiography of laminitis. A. The horn-laminar zone (a), and founder distance (b), schematic illustration. B. Lateral radiograph of third phalanx rotation. Note that the dorsal aspect of the bone is not parallel with the dorsal hoof wall. (Photo by author.)

The *horn-laminar zone* is the distance between the dorsal border of the third phalanx to the outer hoof wall, measured below the extensor process and at the distal margin of the third phalanx. In the normal horse this distances should be equal, although their length may vary due to variations among horses (Redden in Tearney, 2005). Rotation of the third phalanx increases the distance of the distal horn-laminar zone. One study showed that horses with less than 5.5° rotation returned to former athletic function, whereas horses with more than an 11.5° rotation lost their usefulness as performance animals (Stick et al., 1982). Cripps and Eustace (1999) indicated that these measurements have a limited value in cases of distal displacement of the third phalanx due to minor bone rotation.

The *founder distance* is measured from the proximal border of the hoof wall to the proximal border of the extensor process, vertically. This distance increased with sinking of the third phalanx (Baxter, 1986; Redden, 1986). The founder distance has a significant prognostic value in acute laminitis cases; the greater the distance the poorer the prognosis becomes (Cripps and Eustace, 1999; Eustace, 2001b). For detailed description on radiography of laminitis see Redden (1986).

Emergency Treatment of Acute Laminitis

Since it is difficult to predict the outcome of acute laminitis, all cases should be treated immediately and aggressively (Redden, 1986). The first measure includes pulling the horseshoes from the affected hooves by filing the nail clinches and removing the nails with crease nail pullers. Pulling the horseshoe with pull-offs should be avoided as it may cause laminar tear. Creaseless horseshoes can be removed by loosening the horseshoe slightly with pull-offs, then tapping the horseshoe back into place with a light hammer. This loosens the nails and permits their individual removal.

Following removal of the horseshoes, the hooves are trimmed if overgrown; the hoof angle should not be altered and the sole should be preserved. Linford (1990) recommended leaving the foot axis unchanged and dubbing the toes to decrease the effect of the lever arm. At this stage, the heel should not be lowered as this causes the DDFT to tense, possibly causing further detachment of the third phalanx (Chapman and Platt, 1994). Fol-

lowing trimming, the sole should be supported in order to prevent further detachment of the third phalanx. This can be achieved by placing the horse on deep sand (Colles and Jeffcott, 1977, Coffman et al., 1970; Marianne, 1986) or mud (Colles and Jeffcott, 1977). Harman and Ward (2001) recommended placing the horse on washed river sand, as this type of sand shifts best under the horse's weight. They also recommended keeping the hooves soft and pliable in order to relieve pressure from the inner hoof capsule. A study by Van Eps and Pollitt (2004) showed that placing the limb in iced water markedly reduced the severity of acute laminitis. Walking the horse at this stage of the disease can increase lamellar tearing (Redden, 1986), and third phalanx detachment (Cripps and Eustace, 1999).

Several authors recommended elevating the heels in acute laminitis cases in order to reduce the pulling force of the DDFT (Redden, 1992; Moor, 1916; O'Grady, 1993a). Harman and Ward (2001) indicated that cases with tight tendons will often stand with the toes rotated into the ground, and this can provide a good indication as to how to shoe the horse. Redden (1992) described the application of wedge pads that elevate the hoof angle by 18°. Thompson et al. (1992) indicated that raising the heels reduces the pull of the DDFT markedly, and increases the tension in the extensor branch of the suspensory ligament, which helps stabilize the third phalanx.

Some cases may require resection of the toe wall in order to drain and relieve pressure from the affected area. Resection should be performed in cases with extensive separation, serum accumulation, suppuration and necrotic tissue. Less severe cases may benefit from burring several holes through the affected wall to promote drainage and reduce pressure (Redden 1988).

One of the most important principles of treatment of acute laminitis is to provide mechanical support to the third phalanx by increasing *solar support* (♦ fig. 16.5). Several methods for providing solar support are available. These include the application of a frog support pad, solar support pad or solar support boot. The frog support pad can be used in

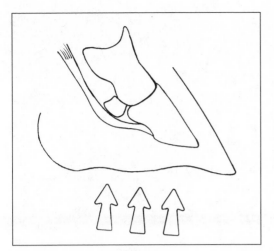

◆ **Fig. 16.5.** Solar support, schematic illustration. The position and direction of support are indicated by the arrows. Shifting the support backward places pressure on the digital cushion, which may rotate the third phalanx further. Shifting the support forward may place excessive pressure on the margins of the third phalanx.

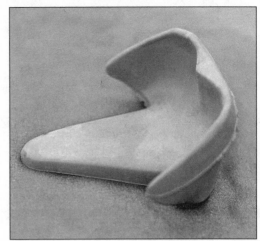

◆ **Fig. 16.6.** Frog support pad. (Photo by author.)

emergency treatment of acute laminitis by applying it against the frog and taping it to the hoof with adhesive tape. In cases where commercial pads are not available, a pad can be made from 2 to 3 cm thick natural rubber cut into a triangular shape. The pad should protrude 0.5 to 1.0 cm above the level of the hoof wall-bearing surface. It is important to position the frog support pad correctly in order to provide proper support for the third phalanx (see below). Eustace and Caldwell (1989b) recommended using a piece of leather or plastic as a temporary frog support device. The material is cut to the shape and size of the frog and taped over the frog, protruding above the level of the wall. Harman and Ward (2001) used 5.0 cm (2") thick Styrofoam taped to the bottom of the hoof. Solar support should be maintained for one to two weeks, and progress of each case should be monitored. Moyer and Redden (1989b) indicated that the placement of resilient padding material in the shape of the frog might not prevent rotation or sinking of the third phalanx if sufficient laminar damage exists.

FROG SUPPORT PAD

The *frog support pad* is used to support the frog in cases of suspected or acute laminitis, and for prevention of supporting limb laminitis. The pad may be applied to hooves with extensive wall loss following dorsal hoof wall resection, or debridement of white line disease. Frog support pads are available commercially or can be made from 2 to 3 cm thick natural rubber cut into triangular shapes; the thickness of the pad used depends on the size of the frog and desired support (◆ fig. 16.6). The pad is fitted against the frog with adhesive tape or duct tape so it shares weight bearing with the hoof wall. The pressure exerted by the pad should provide frog support without causing discomfort to the horse.

Correct positioning of the frog support pad is important. The pad should extend from the bottom of the bulbs of the heels to 1 cm palmar/plantar to the apex of the frog; placing the pad too close to the apex of the frog may compress blood vessels at the sole and cause pain (Goetz, 1987). Positioning the pad too far palmar/plantar places excessive pressure on the digital cushion, which may result in further rotation of the third phalanx.

Hood et al. (1995) indicated that frog support pads used in chronic laminitis cases may increase pain, and the frog is not a good indicator for placement of the pad.

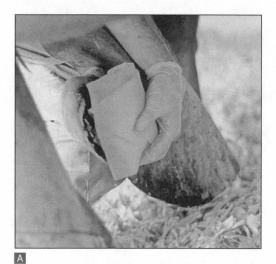

A

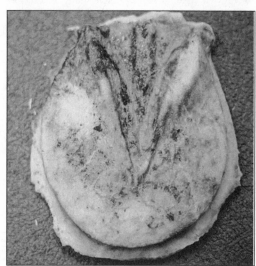

C

SOLAR SUPPORT PAD

The *solar support pad* is used to support the sole and frog in laminitis cases. The pad can be made from *padding foam,* which is a cast padding material available in 3" packed rolls. The foam is applied to the solar area and held in place with elastic adhesive tape (◆ fig. 16.7). The padding foam molds into the sole and frog, thus forming a cushion with a close anatomical fit. The pad can be removed for examination of the foot and reapplied again (Colahan, 1994a). Alternatively, a *silicone impression material* may be applied. Two equal parts of the material are mixed by hand and applied over the solar area. The hoof is placed on a clean towel until the impression material is cured. Additional layers of impression material may be added as needed in order to achieve adequate solar support. Both types of solar support pads can be used with solar support boots.

SOLAR SUPPORT BOOT

Redden (1986) describes the application of a *solar support boot* in acute laminitis cases. The boot is fitted with a frog wedge that resembles the mirror image of the frog, and with a wedge pads that raises the heels; thus, it provides solar support and relieves tension from

◆ **Fig. 16.7.** Application of padding foam in laminitis case. A. A roll of foam is unrolled and folded into a square; the foam is immersed in water and placed over the sole so it protrudes about 3 cm above the level of the hoof wall-bearing surface. B. The foam is wrapped with elastic adhesive tape and the limb is placed on the ground. C. Following curing, the foam achieves the imprint of the solar surface of the hoof. (Photos by author.)

the DDFT. The device, which is commercially available, can be taped, glued or nailed to the hoof. The solar support boot may be applied to a healthy opposite limb in order to prevent supporting limb laminitis.

In cases where a commercial boot is not available, a regular hoof boot fitted with a wedge pad connected with screws to its bottom may be applied; two or three 3° pads may be required to lessen tension from the DDFT. Prior to application of the boot, the solar area should be packed with padding foam or silicone impression material.

Farriery of Acute Laminitis

Shoeing the acute laminitis case with conventional horseshoes is contraindicated, as hammering will increase laminar tear (Linford, 1990; Marianne, 1986; Redden, 1986; Moyer and Redden, 1989b). Redden (1986) indicated that application of devices that place excessive pressure on the sole and frog may disrupt blood supply to the sole dermis. Goetz (1987) noted that application of full pads, casts or treatment plates during a period of active rotation or sinking may compromise blood circulation in the sole. Eustace (1999) indicated that fitting a reversed horseshoe in acute laminitis seems to induce contraction of the DDFM to an abnormal degree, which could lead to development of refractory laminitis.

Mild cases of acute laminitis may be fitted with synthetic glue-on shoes. The glue-on shoe protects the foot, absorbs concussion and provides solar and palmar/plantar support.

DORSAL HOOF WALL RESECTION

Following rotation of the third phalanx, a wedged space is formed between the dorsal bone surface and inner hoof wall. This space is filled with blood and serum (Redden, 1987) that is gradually being replaced by new horn, which is similar in structure to the white line (Kuwano et al., 2002). The wedged material, which is also described as epidermal wedge (Roberts et al., 1980) or laminar wedge (Dart 1988), places pressure on the third phalanx and obstructs blood supply to the laminae (◆ fig . 16.8).

Dorsal hoof wall resection is aimed at reducing tissue damage caused by serum and blood accumulation (Redden, 1987), and re-establishment of normal circulation and spatial orientation between the third phalanx and hoof (Goetz, 1987; Peremans et al., 1991). The procedure is recommended for severe cases of laminitis (Coffman et al., 1969; Redden, 1987), and it is done in acute or chronic cases (Goetz, 1987; Chapman and Platt, 1994). In one study on a group of 21 ponies with laminitis, 11 ponies underwent dorsal hoof wall resection and regained complete soundness, whereas only 2 of the 10 ponies treated conservatively recovered completely (Peremans et al., 1991).

Dorsal hoof wall resection may be carried out by thinning the hoof wall with a hoof rasp or half-round hoof nippers, followed by the

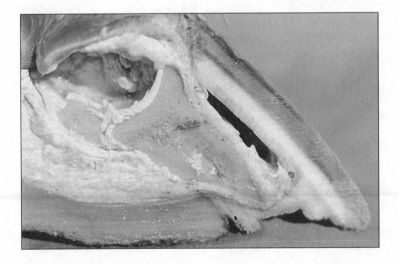

◆ **Fig. 16.8.** Longitudinal section through a foot with laminitis showing a wedge-shaped space that developed between the third phalanx and inner toe wall. (Photo by author.)

use of an electric burr. Alternatively, a wall strip procedure, described by Pollitt and Daradka (2004), can be performed (page 195). The hoof wall is removed until a soft, spongy to the feel, and pinkish-white tissue is exposed. Necrotic brown-colored laminae should be removed (Goetz, 1987). The area that is included in the resection should extend 1 to 2 cm distal to the coronary band to the bottom of the hoof; approximately one third of the hoof wall circumference may be removed. Peremans et al. (1991) indicated that only loose horn should be removed until firm attachment reappears between dermal and epidermal laminae. Redden (1987) recommended rasping the dorsal hoof wall until the sensitive laminae is exposed and then using a hoof knife to "square up" the edges of the defect. He indicated that if hemorrhage and sensitivity is noticed when the rasp penetrates the laminar tissue, the resection should be delayed. Alternatively, the dorsal hoof wall can be removed with half-round hoof nippers, and the edge of the defect "squared up" with an electric burr (Ferguson, 1994) (see plate 7). Following completion of the procedure, the exposed area is covered with sterile gauze pads soaked with povidone-iodine solution and a foot bandage is applied. Treatment is continued with daily warm Epsom salts soaks and daily bandage changes (Redden, 1987).

Redden (1988) indicated that the loss of hoof wall following resection may result in hoof capsule instability, followed by excessive movement of the third phalanx and delayed healing. Therefore, cases that undergo extensive toe wall removal should be fitted with a stabilizing metal plate combined with a wide-web bar horseshoe and side clips (Pollitt and Daradka, 2004) (see ◆ fig. 16.85). Cases that undergo partial length resection can be fitted with a wide-web horseshoe alone.

Refractory Laminitis

Cases of *refractory laminitis* include recurrent episodes of third phalanx rotation or sinking. Hood et al. (1994a) indicated that blood circulation in the hoof of refractory cases is worse than that of treatable cases. A predisposing factor for refractory laminitis includes contraction of the DDFT with consequent pull on the third phalanx. This complication may require the surgical incision of the check ligament of the DDFT (Chapman and Platt, 1994).

Treatment of refractory laminitis cases in an attempt to salvage the horse may require severing the DDFT (tenotomy) in order to stabilize the third phalanx. The hoof should be fitted with an extended heels horseshoe (Allen et al., 1986; O'Grady, 1993a; Cripps and Eustace, 1999) or with an egg-bar shoe (O'Grady, 1993a) in order to provide palmar/plantar support until new flexor support develops (Allen et al., 1986). Jann et al. (1997) described the application of a modified trailer shoe in horses that underwent tenotomy of the DDFT. This horseshoe, which is similar to the egg-bar horseshoe, should extend about 3-5 cm beyond the heels. They recommended applying the horseshoe prior to the surgery in order to reduce stress from the affected limb(s).

Chronic Laminitis

Chronic laminitis OR FOUNDER is characterized by stabilizing of the third phalanx and improvement in the degree of lameness (Yelle, 1986). Hoof growth is commonly abnormal, and the affected hoof may develop a convexed toe, high heels, flat or dropped sole (Baxter, 1992) and widening of the white line at the toe wall (see plate 2). Chronic laminitis is commonly accompanied by reduced horn growth at the toe wall and faster growth at the heels (Goetz, 1987; Curtis et al., 1999a); this growth pattern may be a result of alterations in the vascular supply to the foot (Ackerman et al., 1975; Goetz, 1987) with consequent development of *laminar rings* on the hoof wall surface, characterized by closer rings at the toe wall that diverge toward the heels (◆ fig. 16.9). Weakening of the white line combined with ground pressure against the toe wall predisposes the hoof to development of convexed toe. A wide, flaky white line and a curling dorsal hoof wall is a common hoof conformation in chronic laminitis

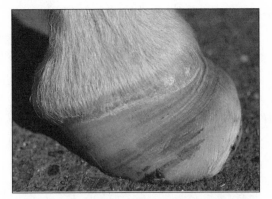

◆ **Fig. 16.9.** Chronic laminitis. Irregular hoof growth resulted in development of laminar rings, convexed toe and high heels, note that the rings diverge from the toe toward the heels. (Photo by author.)

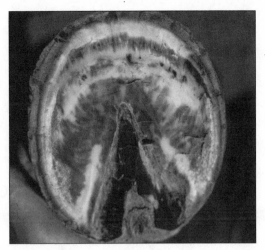

◆ **Fig. 16.10.** Chronic laminitis. Note the abnormal widening of the white line. (Photo by author.)

(White and Baggett, 1983) (◆ fig. 16.10). Some cases may become complicated by *pododermatitis* or foot infection characterized by subsolar suppuration (pus) (Johnson, 1972; Marianne, 1986). Severely neglected cases may develop abnormal corkscrew shaped hooves, accompanied with severe damage to the third phalanx (Verschooten, 1994).

Farriery of Chronic Laminitis

Farriery of chronic laminitis is aimed at protecting the foot and establishment of normal hoof conformation. The outcome of farriery may be affected by various factors such as intact laminar surface area, laminar bond strength, hoof quality, body weight, concurrent infection and alterations in the third phalanx position.

Trimming principles of chronic laminitis with capsular rotation include trimming the toe wall, dubbing excess toe, and lowering the heels (◆ fig. 16.11). Dubbing the toe shortens the HLA and reduces the effect of the tearing force; removal of excess toe wall and lowering the heels places the third phalanx in a more natural position relative to the hoof capsule. Lowering the heels should be done gradually over a period of several trimmings in order to prevent excessive tension on the DDFT. The sole should not be trimmed in order to prevent sore feet. Chronic laminitis cases with

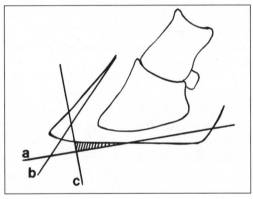

◆ **Fig. 16.11.** Trimming principles of chronic laminitis with capsular rotation, schematic illustration. The three lines represent the area where the hoof is trimmed in order to establish normal hoof conformation and third phalanx position. Lowering the heels (a), trimming excess toe wall (b), and dubbing the toe wall (c). Reposition of the third phalanx may result in a space under the toe wall (striped area). (Adapted from Moyer W. 1980. Corrective Shoeing. The Veterinary Clinics of North America, large Animal Practice, Vol. 2, No.1. pp 3-24, figure 1.)

phalangeal rotation are trimmed as described above, but the heels should be raised again with wedged horseshoes in order to reduce tension from the DDFT (O'Grady, 2004). Hoof trimming may be combined with *coronary grooving*, a method described by Rit-

meester and Ferguson (1996), which is aimed
at improving toe wall growth associated with
chronic cases (Ritmeester et al., 1998). Lowering the heels in cases that develop from excessive concussion should be avoided, especially
in horses with clubfeet. Horseshoes used for
chronic laminitis cases should have adequate
palmar/plantar support that shifts some of
the load from the toe wall toward the heels
(Curtis et al., 1999). In order to prevent sole
pressure, the inner web of the horseshoe hoof
surface should be well seated out. Moor (1919)
recommended rolling the toe of horseshoes
in laminitis cases. Curtis et al. (1999) recommended unloading the dorsal hoof wall in
order to encourage growth that is more normal. This is done by leaving a small space
between the horseshoe and toe wall. In severe
third phalanx rotation, a space between the
toe wall bearing surface and the horseshoe
develops following trimming, leaving the toe
wall suspended; in this case the application of
acrylic resin may be required in order to build
the toe wall (see ◆ fig. 16.11).

Mild cases may be shod with plain horseshoes, glue-on horseshoes, square-toed horseshoes, reversed horseshoes or egg-bar shoes.
Cases that are accompanied by pododermatitis should be debrided and treated daily in a
footbath containing mild antiseptic solution
such as diluted povidone-iodine or Epsom
salts. Once the solar area heals, it is packed
with oakum and pine tar, and a wide-web
horseshoe with a protective pad is applied.

Farriery of more severe cases with a risk
for further third phalanx rotation should have
solar support; these cases include horses with
missing sections of hoof wall, obese horses,
and horses with thin hoof wall and small feet.
Application of horseshoes without solar support may produce transient improvement by
removal of direct solar pressure. This may be
followed by displacement of the third phalanx
with worsening lameness (Taylor et al., 2002).
Redden (1986a) recommended using a modified treatment plate fitted with a frog support
pad (◆ fig. 16.12). Several authors recommended the use of a heart-bar shoe in order to provide frog support (Moore and Allen, 1995;
Butler, 1983; Chapman and Platt, 1994).

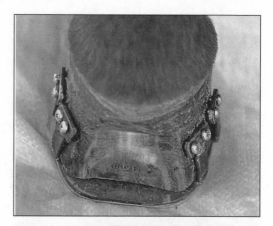

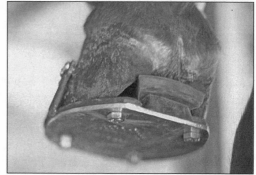

◆ **Fig. 16.12.** Modified treatment plate, dorsal
and solar-palmar views. The horseshoe is attached
to the hoof with wood screws placed through the
clips; the pressure of the plate against the pad
maintains frog support. (Photos by author.)

Other types of horseshoes that are
described in the literature for chronic laminitis include a reversed horseshoe with a leather
pad (White and Baggett, 1983), glue-on shoes
(Peremans et al., 1991; Craig, 2005), a horseshoe and leather pad applied with pine tar
and oakum (Coffman et al., 1969) and a
wedged reverse horseshoe (Tanaka et al.,
2002). Curtis et al. (1999) described the use
of a W-horseshoe, which is a reversed horseshoe with a frog support bar similar to the
heart-bar shoe. Goetz (1987) described the
application of an adjustable heart-bar shoe
designed to provide support for the third phalanx. In some cases, it may take several trials
until the proper protective horseshoe is
found; then the same horseshoe type should
be maintained until new hoof growth replaces

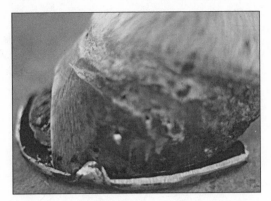

♦ **Fig. 16.13.** Shoeing a chronic laminitis case with a wide web horseshoe, side clips, rocker toe and extended heels. Note the space between the cornified laminar bed and horseshoe. (Photo by author.)

the injured tissue and the horse is no longer lame. The horseshoes should be reset every four to six weeks; at each reset, the hooves are trimmed as described above.

Stabilized cases of chronic laminitis with toe wall separation are treated by resection of the undermined wall and careful debridement of the margins of exposed area. The missing section is left open in order to keep the area dry and permit cornification of the laminae. The hoof is fitted with a wide-web horseshoe that protects the sole and enables the horse to walk (♦ fig. 16.13). A stabilizing bar added across the toe wall in cases with extensive hoof wall loss provides additional security. Once the exposed area is dry and cornified, the toe wall may be reconstructed with a resin.

Chronic laminitis horses should be hand walked daily, for 5 to 10 minutes, in order to increase blood circulation to the foot and stretch the DDFT musculotendinous unit. Exercise should be increased gradually and the horse should be observed for signs of lameness. The space between the horseshoe and the sole should be examined regularly for a decrease in distance, which may occurs in refractory cases. Refractory cases should have their horseshoes removed and the hooves fitted with some form of solar support; then the case should be reevaluated.

REVERSED HORSESHOE

The *reversed horseshoe* (backward horseshoe, open-toe horseshoe) is a keg or forged horseshoe that is fitted and placed at 180° to the hoof. When using a keg horseshoe, additional nail holes are made at the horseshoe branches (♦ fig. 16.14). The reversed horseshoe removes pressure from the toe wall and provides palmar/plantar support. This horseshoe is used in the treatment (White and Baggett, 1983) of mild cases of chronic laminitis with stable third phalanx. The reversed horseshoe may be fitted with a thick leather pad that protects the sole. The pad is connected to the horseshoe with copper rivets. Prior to application of the horseshoe, the sole is packed with

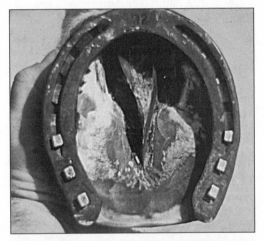

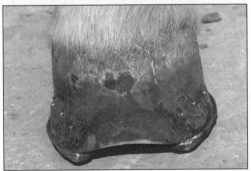

♦ **Fig. 16.14.** Reversed horseshoe, solar view and dorsal views. Following application of the horseshoe, the toe wall that protrudes over the horseshoe is trimmed with hoof nippers and the lower half of the toe wall is squared with a hoof rasp. (Photos by author.)

pine tar and oakum. The reversed horseshoe may be applied to cases of distal toe cracks following debridement of the crack. This application is adequate for non-working horses that are stabled or pastured. The horseshoe may be modified into a W-horseshoe by adding a heart-bar for frog support.

Tanaka et al. (2002) described the application of a wedged reversed horseshoe that was used to raise the heels in a case of chronic laminitis with solar prolapse; in addition, the horseshoe was fitted with sole cushion support material (Redden, 1998).

MODIFIED TREATMENT PLATE

The *modified treatment plate* is designed to provide frog support in laminitis cases. The main advantage of this device is that no horseshoe nails are applied (Redden, 1986b). The modified treatment plate is constructed from an open horseshoe fitted with T-shaped clips that are used to secure the horseshoe to the hoof wall with screws (see ◆ fig. 16.12). The horseshoe is fitted with a plate attached to the ground surface with bolts. A frog support pad is placed between the frog and plate; the pressure against the frog is adjusted by altering the thickness of the pad.

The device is made from a horseshoe forged from a 0.5 x 2.5 cm bar stock (◆ fig. 16.15). The horseshoe is fitted to the hoof. Four T-shaped clips made from 3 x 12 mm bar stock are welded to the horseshoe. Two holes, 3 mm in diameter, are drilled in each clip; the clips are bent with pliers until they fit snug against the hoof wall. The device is attached to the hoof wall with wood screws while the horse bears weight on it. The frog is fitted with a triangular pad cut from natural rubber; the pad should extend from the bottom of the bulbs of the heels to 1 cm palmar/plantar to the apex of the frog. A plate made from 3 mm thickness sheet metal is connected to the horseshoe with three 3/8" bolts.

HEART-BAR SHOE

The *heart-bar shoe* is commonly used in the treatment of chronic laminitis cases. This

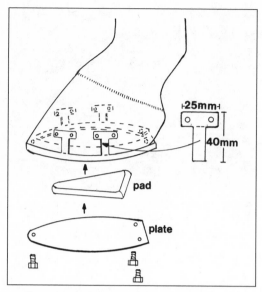

◆ **Fig. 16.15.** Construction of a modified treatment plate, schematic illustration. See text for details. (Adapted from Redden R.F. 1986a, figures 7 to 9.)

horseshoe is a modified egg-bar shoe fitted with a triangular metal plate positioned along the frog. The plate provides frog support and prevents third phalanx rotation (Goetz, 1987; Eustace and Caldwell, 1989a). The egg-bar provides additional palmar/plantar support. The toe may be squared or rolled to ease breakover (Ritmeester et al., 1988). The heart-bar shoe may be applied as a preventative measure against supporting limb laminitis or cases with missing sections of hoof wall (◆ fig. 16.16).

Eustace (1989) described the treatment of ten horses with chronic laminitis, most of them had solar prolapse. The treatment, which included dorsal wall resection and application of heart-bar shoes, resulted in the recovery of seven of the subject horses. In a different study, application of heart-bar shoes to chronic laminitis cases resulted in significant improvement of dorsal laminar blood flow (Ritmeester et al., 1998).

The heart-bar shoe may be forged or made from an egg-bar shoe by welding to it a triangular metal plate. The plate should have

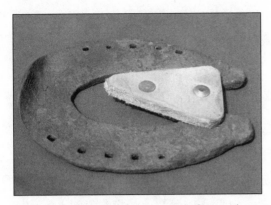

◆ **Fig. 16.16.** Heart-bar shoe made from wide-web rocker-toe horseshoe, fitted with frog support plate covered by leather pad. (Photo by author.)

a minimum of 4 mm thickness. The supporting plate should extend 2 cm palmar/plantar from the apex of the frog (Eustace and Caldwell, 1989a). Turner (1998) indicated that the supporting plate should underlie about 63% of the solar length of the third phalanx, which is usually about one cm. palmar/plantar to the frog's apex. Radiographs are used to locate the location and position of the bone. Placing the plate over the point of the frog may cause pressure necrosis beneath the frog and sole (Moore and Allen, 1995; Goetz and Comstock, 1985). Eustace and Caldwell (1989a) indicated that the frog support achieved should leave the horse comfortable following nailing of the horseshoe. They recommended adding a leather or plastic pad between the supporting bar and the frog in cases where the frog is atrophic and recessed. The pad can be made from natural rubber or soft acrylic resin. The resin is poured over a triangular mold that is placed over the supporting plate and allowed to cure (Podoll, 2005). The triangular mold is available commercially or can be made from a used kitchen cutting board. The degree of pressure against the frog is tested by placing the horseshoe over the sole and pressing it downward. In cases where the horse resents the pressure, the supporting plate should be set farther from the frog (Chapman and Platt, 1984). Cooke (2006) described the application of a G-bar shoe to a chronic laminitis case with missing sections of hoof wall at the medial quarter and heel. This horseshoe, which is similar to a three-quarter bar shoe, was fitted with a frog support bar, and the affected area was protected with acrylic resin.

Redden (1986b) indicated that heart-bar shoes that are not made and fitted properly can accelerate laminar damage. Cripps and Eustace (1999) showed that incorrect positioning of the frog support plate resulted in pain, whereas application of the horseshoe to cases of sinking third phalanx may result in damage to sensitive tissue (Tanaka et al., 2002). Linford (1990) indicated that frog support horseshoes continue to put pressure on the frog when the horse is recumbent, and this can lead to *sub-solar necrosis*. Moyer and Redden (1989b) pointed out that heart-bar shoes do not stabilize or improve the condition of the foot in cases with significant laminar damage.

Cases accompanied by solar prolapse should be protected by raising the hoof with a rim pad placed between the hoof and the horseshoe (Eustace and Caldwell, 1989b). Horses fitted with heart-bar shoes should not be walked on rocks as this could bend the plate against the frog and result in lameness.

ADJUSTABLE HEART-BAR SHOE

Goetz and Comstock (1985) described the construction and application of *adjustable heart-bar shoe* for treatment of laminitis. The device is fitted with a hinged frog support plate that permits adjustment of the amount of pressure against the frog. Horses that were fitted with this device instantly walked better, or became slightly lamer for 24 to 72 hours and then improved significantly. In some cases, improvement may take weeks to months.

The device is made from a keg shoe or forged horseshoe with a thickness of 10-12 mm (◆ fig. 16.17). The horseshoe is fitted to the hoof. A hinge made from 8 mm iron rod is cut to fit between the horseshoe branches; the hinge is fitted into an iron pipe with the same inner diameter, and the rod is welded to the horseshoe branches. The horseshoe is placed over the hoof and measurements for the frog support plate are taken. The tip of the sup-

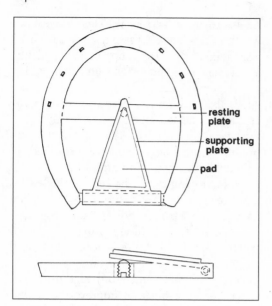

◆ **Fig. 16.17.** Adjustable-heart bar shoe, hoof surface and profile, schematic illustration. Frog support is adjusted by tightening or loosening the Allen screw against the supporting plate. See text for details. (Adapted from Goetz T.E. and Comstock C.M. 1985, figures 1 to 6.)

porting plate should be 2.0 cm palmar/plantar from the tip of the frog. This position may be determined from radiographs. The plate is made from 4 mm flat metal cut to fit the shape of the frog. A resting bar made from 6 x 18 mm bar iron is welded across the horseshoe where the ends of the supporting plate rests. The supporting plate is welded to the iron pipe of the hinge, and the resting bar is drilled and tapped to fit 5/8" inner Allen screws. The supporting plate should be padded with natural rubber or soft acrylic resin as described for heart-bar shoe.

The advantages of this device are that pressure on the frog can be fine-tuned, and the direction of pressure is rotational rather than directly upward. The disadvantages of the device include continuous placement of pressure on the frog, even when the horse is lying down, and excessive pressure that may result from accidentally stepping on an object such as a stone. In addition, the construction of the device is relatively difficult.

GLUE-ON HORSESHOES

A synthetic glue-on bar shoe can be applied to cases of chronic laminitis. The glue-on shoe eliminates pounding with a hammer, protects the solar area, reduces concussion and provides solar and palmar/plantar support. The comfort provided by the horseshoe encourages the horse to walk and enhances healing; the flexibility of the horseshoe improves foot circulation and stimulates new horn growth (Craig, 2005). The synthetic horseshoe may be applied to mild cases of acute laminitis. Peremans et al. (1991) describes the use of glue-on shoes with aluminum core and tabs in ponies with laminitis.

The application of synthetic glue-on horseshoes includes hoof trimming and preparation of the hoof for glueing (see chapter 15). Prior to application of the horseshoe, the solar area is packed with *silicone impression material*. The opening at the center of the horseshoe is fitted with a plug provided by the manufacturer. In order to relieve the toe wall, the resin is applied at the quarters and palmar/plantar surface of the horseshoe. The horseshoe is positioned palmar/plantar to the toe in order to shorten the hoof lever arm and reduce pressure on the toe wall. In cases where the heel has to be raised, more resin is added to the palmar/plantar aspect of the horseshoe and the horseshoe is placed at an angle to the hoof (Craig and Craig, 2003; Craig, 2005). In cases with bulging sole, additional resin can be applied in order to relieve pressure from the sole; alternatively, the hoof surface of the horseshoe can be concaved with a grinder. The horseshoe is removed by loosening it carefully with pull-off, the hoof should be held firmly in order to reduce strain from the laminae, prior to that the glue may be cut carefully along the margins of the horseshoe and hoof using a short-blade utility knife.

TOE WALL RECONSTRUCTION

Toe wall reconstruction of chronic laminitis cases (Graham, 1965b; Jenny et al., 1965; Coffman et al., 1969) protects the foot, stabilizes

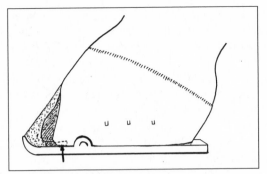

◆ **Fig. 16.18.** Toe wall reconstruction, lateral view, schematic illustration. The illustration shows the wooden wedge (arrow) and reconstructed toe (dotted area). See text for details.

the hoof capsule and improves its cosmetic appearance. The reconstruction procedure is performed on cases that have undergone toe wall resection or partial debridement. The procedure should be done in cases where the third phalanx is stable. The resin should be applied on cornified laminae that are dry and free of infection (Fessler, 1989). Coffman et al. (1969) recommended undercutting the hoof wall to strengthen the bond between the repair material and horn. Once the toe wall is prepared, the hoof is fitted with a wide-web horseshoe (Avisar, 1996). A small wooden wedge is inserted between the horseshoe and the sole; this raises the toe, and prevents the hoof from rocking as the horse shifts weight on the limb (◆ fig. 16.18). The toe area is filled with acrylic resin; two to three layers of synthetic fabric should be incorporated with the resin. In order to prevent solar pressure, the repair material should not contact the sole. Once the resin is cured, the wooden wedge is removed.

Coffman et al. (1969) described the application of bar shoes and repair material for the treatment of severe chronic laminitis cases. The toe was reconstructed with hard plastic material and the sole was supported with soft plastic material. Jenny et al. (1965) described a similar procedure, but in this case, they used a horseshoe with two to three clips glued to the hoof. They recommended covering the entire frog and sole with soft plastic to sup-

port the third phalanx and provide a cushion for the sensitive foot.

Prevention of Laminitis

Prevention of laminitis is extremely important because of the extensive damage to the feet and lack of specific therapy for the condition. Preventative measures involve monitoring the environment, the activity of the horse, the nutritional plan, and related disorders. This monitoring may include maintenance of proper trimming intervals, avoiding working on hard ground, disposal of black walnut shavings, pasturing horses on low carbohydrate grass pastures, preventing obesity, providing minimum amount of concentrates, locking the feed bin, and treating horses with retained placentas, infectious diseases and colic with the aim of reducing the risk of developing laminitis. In addition, the selection of hardy horses with good quality hooves may reduce the incidence of the disease, although these horses can develop laminitis just as easily if they become fat or exposed to excessive carbohydrates.

 WHITE LINE DISEASE

White line disease (WLD) IS A FOOT DISEASE characterized by progressive separation between the hoof wall and laminae. Other names for the disease include seedy toe and hollow wall. The disorder affects all breeds of horses throughout the USA, Europe and other countries, and it is more prevalent in hot and humid areas (Redden, 1990). In a study that included 1781 Thoroughbred racehorses in Japan, 204 · (11.5%) of the horses were affected, with most incidences occurring in the forelegs (Kuwano et al., 1999). White line disease may not cause lameness, but it predisposes the foot to infection, and potentially to third phalanx rotation.

WLD begins as a crumbling and mealy white horn between the hoof wall and laminar dermis (Jenny et al., 1965). The most common site for the disease is the dorsal quarter area

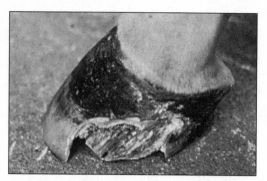

◆ **Fig. 16.19.** White line disease. The affected area involves the lateral quarter of the hind foot. (Photo by author.)

(Redden, 1990; Kuwano et al., 1999). Initially, the only noticeable change is a powdery area at the sole-wall junction. If left untreated this area develops into a fissure; in some cases extensive separation between the hoof wall and horny laminae may develop. The extent of the lesion can be determined with a metal probe, or by hearing a hollow sound when the hoof wall is tapped lightly with a shoeing hammer (◆ fig. 16.19). The cavity that is formed beneath the hoof wall becomes filled with soil, small stones and manure. Exposure of the white line predisposes the hoof to sub-mural abscess that may break out at the coronary band. Extensive hoof wall separation may result in the inability of the hoof wall to support the third phalanx and consequently in the rotation of the bone (Redden, 1990; Kuwano et al., 1998; Oke, 2003).

The exact cause(s) of the WLD is not clear but factors that appear to be associated with development of the disease include some types of inflammatory process in the wall matrix, mechanical trauma, nutritional problems, hereditary vulnerability (Young and Monticello, 1989), and wet and polluted environments (Redden, 1990). Tjalsma and Van Mauric (1995) indicate that fungi may be a factor in the development of WLD. Certain bacteria and fungi have been isolated from affected hooves but it is not clear whether they digest horn (Redden, 1990). In one case study (Kuwano et al., 1996), large quantities of fungus were isolated from the white line. The most susceptible region for fungal invasion

was the terminal horn, the horn tubules were markedly damaged. In a different study (Kuwano et al., (1998) isolated fungi from 10 percent of the cases investigated. White line disease might be caused, or become complicated by onychomycosis or fungal disease of the hoof (page 199). Budras et al. (1998) indicated that insufficient stall hygiene reduces the horn quality and allows keratolytic (horn destroying) bacteria and fungi to initiate decay. The intensity of horn destruction increases with the level of moisture in the tubular horn of the white line. Higami (1999) found a correlation between low zinc and copper diet and WLD in a group of horses that received a deficient diet for prolonged time.

Farriery of White Line Disease

Kuwano et al. (1999) indicated that proper foot management can prevent many cases of WLD. This includes examining the hoof at each shoeing interval for the presence of powdery white line lesions. These areas should be debrided with a hoof knife and disinfected with tincture of iodine. The hoof wall should be left intact unless the lesion is extensive. Larger lesions should be debrided thoroughly until healthy horn is reached. In some cases, the section of hoof wall that covers the defect has to be removed in order to expose the lesion. Removal of hoof wall can be achieved with half-round hoof nippers. Debridement of WLD should be complete as leaving infected horn will result in continuation of the disease process (Redden, 1990). The debrided area should be disinfected twice a day with tincture of iodine and left open to dry. In cases with extensive hoof wall loss, the hoof should be fitted with a frog support pad. Prior to debridement, the hoof is trimmed and prepared for horseshoeing. The horseshoe may be forged and fitted at this stage. The tools that were used for hoof trimming and debridement should be disinfected with 90% alcohol after their use.

Farriery of WLD includes the application of a protective horseshoe. Horseshoeing may be combined with hoof wall reconstruction. The type of horseshoe applied depends on the extent of the lesion, the strength of the hoof wall and the type of work performed by the horse. Bar shoes, aluminum bar shoes (Kuwano et al., 1998) and wide-web horseshoes (Young and Monticello, 1989) have been recommended. In cases where a large section of hoof wall is missing the frog should be supported with a heart-bar shoe; large clips may be welded to the horseshoe and used to connect the horseshoe to the hoof with the use of screws. In order to allow for attachment of the horseshoe an artificial wall can be created with the application of fiberglass casting material around the hoof (Turner, 1998). The addition of a stabilizing plate may be required in cases that are left open (see ◆ fig. 16.85). O'Grady (1993b) described the application of a heart-bar shoe fitted with a T-shape *supporting brace* used in cases with extensive hoof wall loss (◆ fig. 16.20). Cases with little hoof wall loss may be fitted with a bar shoe and a pad. Prior to shoeing, the sole area is packed with pine tar and oakum. Kuwano et al. (1999) recommended reducing pressure from the toe with a horseshoe that eases breakover. A glue-on horseshoes may be applied to horses that are too sore footed for nailing (Turner, 1998).

Prior to hoof wall reconstruction, the lesion should be completely dry and cornified. The repair should be delayed in cases where the lesion contains drainage tracts or exposed

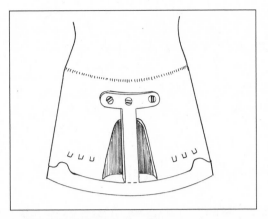

◆ **Fig. 16.20.** Supporting T- brace, schematic illustration. The brace is shaped to fit the contour of the hoof wall above the defect, the brace is welded to the horseshoe and connected to the hoof wall with screws. (Adapted from O'Grady 1993b, fig. 8.)

dermal laminae (◆ fig. 16.21). Preparation for repair includes removal of loose horn, trimming the edges of the lesion, undercutting the defect in the hoof wall, sanding and degreasing the hoof wall. The edge of the lesion may be "squared" with a hoof knife, loop knife, or with a motorized burr. The horseshoe may be applied prior to the repair. In this case, it should be wrapped with thin plastic that prevents adherence of resin to the horseshoe hoof surface. This is particularly important when the defect is located at the

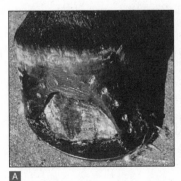
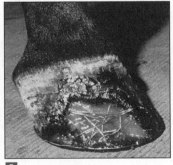
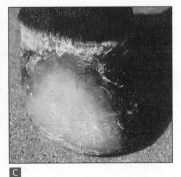

◆ **Fig. 16.21.** Hoof wall reconstruction of white line disease case. A. The hoof wall over the undermined area was removed, the edge of the defect was undercut and several holes were drilled along the defect margin; the hoof was shod with a training plate. B. A scaffold for the resin was made by inserting copper wire through the holes in the defect margin and the first layer of resin was applied. C. Completed hoof repair. Stronger repair is obtained by incorporating synthetic fabrics with the resin and avoiding glueing the horseshoe to the hoof. (Photos by author.)

quarters or heels area. Glueing the hoof to the horseshoe in these areas interferes with hoof expansion and results in abnormal strain at the repaired area. The sole area next to the lesion should be packed with Play dough to prevent adhesion of resin to the sole. The resin should be combined with two to three layers of synthetic fabric.

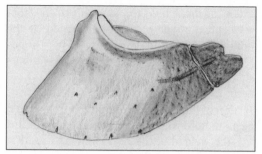

◆ **Fig. 16.22.** Third phalanx bone fracture involving the wing of the bone.

THIRD PHALANX FRACTURES

Third phalanx fractures MAY RESULT FROM penetrating foreign bodies, racing injuries (Sparks, 1970), infection of the third phalanx, flexural deformities (Honnas et al., 1988a), and traumatic insults (Gerring, 1980) such as caused by running on hard surfaces, stepping on stones or kicking hard objects. Fractures of the third phalanx are more common on the forelimbs (Gabel and Bukowieki, 1983) and are more common in Thoroughbreds, Standardbreds and working Quarter Horses (Yovich et al., 1986; Adams, 1974). In one study, greater incidence of forelimb fractures were found to occur at the lateral side of the left limb, and the medial side of the right limb in horses running counterclockwise (Scott et al., 1979a). Honnas et al. (1988b) noted that many cases of solar margin fractures accompanied foot problems such as laminitis and pedal osteitis. Fractures of the third phalanx are classified according to location and type of fracture (Honnas et al., 1988a; Scott et al., 1979a). Fractures may be articular, non-articular, and solar (◆ fig. 16.22).

Signs of third phalanx fracture include lameness, increased digital pulse, and increased sensitivity of the sole, wall and frog to hammer percussion and hoof testers. The horse may not bear weight on the affected limb. Clinical signs are less obvious in non-articular fractures and the horse may react to the hoof testers only when the area of the fracture is examined (Adams, 1974). Involvement of the extensor process is accompanied by localized swelling at the coronary band (Honnas et al., 1988a); this fracture type may result in the development of buttress foot (Frank, 1953)(page 218). Fractures that do not involve

the DIP joint have a better prognosis (Scott et al., 1979a; Honnas et al., 1988a).

Farriery of Third Phalanx Fractures

Application of a protective horseshoe for treatment of third phalanx fractures is important component of the treatment. Although the hoof forms a rigid case around most of the third phalanx and limits its movement, hoof expansion should be restricted in order to allow a firm bone healing (Scott et al., 1979a). Treatment of most cases of third phalanx fractures includes the application of therapeutic horseshoes and stall confinement. Healing may take six months or longer (Scott et al., 1979; Honnas et al., 1988a; Yovich et al., 1986). Honnas et al. (1988a) indicated that many horses walk with little or unnoticed lameness shortly after the horseshoe is applied. They recommended using a bar shoe with quarter clips and a flat pad for fractures of the body of the third phalanx; the bar shoe and clips limit hoof expansion and reduce shearing forces across the fracture lines, the pad absorbs some shock and protects the painful sole. Pine tar and oakum should be applied between the pad and the sole. The horseshoe is reset every four weeks. The horseshoe should be applied with minimum trauma to the foot by using a light race hammer. The space between the clips and hoof wall can be closed with light hammer blows or by filling it with acrylic resin. Shearing forces on the hoof capsule at resets are minimized by pulling the horseshoe with a crease

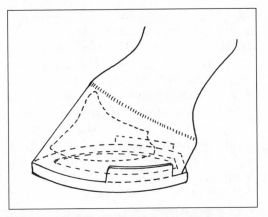

♦ **Fig. 16.23.** Side rims straight-bar shoe for treatment of third phalanx fracture, schematic illustration. The relationship of the horseshoe to the third phalanx is shown. See text for details. (Adapted from Scott E.A. et al. 1979, fig.6.)

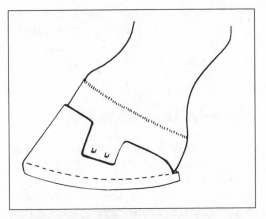

♦ **Fig. 16.24.** Continuous rim horseshoe, schematic illustrations. See text for details. Adapted from Sigafoos R. 1986, fig. 15.

nail puller. Alternatively, the bar shoe can be fitted with side rims placed along the quarters and heels (Scott et al., 1979b) or with a continuous rim horseshoe (Sigafoos, 1986; Moyer and Sigafoos, 1988) (see below). Other types of devices that may be applied include the application of a side rim horseshoe fitted with a heart-bar, or a treatment plate fitted with a solar support pad; both devices provide arch support for the third phalanx and better alignment along the fracture line (Redden in Moyer and Sigafoos, 1988).

Farriery of solar margin fractures includes the application of a wide-web horseshoe and a pad. In addition, the underlying foot disorder should be investigated and treated (Honnas et al., 1988b). Some horses may require surgical debridement of bone fragments. A treatment plate should be applied to cases that undergo extensive debridement. Scott et al., (1979a) recommended that horses returning to racing activity following healing wear protective horseshoes permanently.

STRAIGHT-BAR SHOE AND SIDE RIMS

Scott et al. (1979b) described the application of a *straight-bar shoe with side rims* for treat-

ment of articular and non-articular wing fractures (♦ fig. 16.23). This horseshoe is constructed by welding a 3 mm thick metal bar along the quarter and heel on each side. The height of the rim should be 3 to 4 cm. Following application of the horseshoe, the space between the hoof wall and the rim is filled with acrylic resin.

CONTINUOUS RIM HORSESHOE

Sigafoos (1986) and Moyer and Sigafoos (1988) described the construction and application of a *continuous rim horseshoe* for treatment of third phalanx fractures. The horseshoe is constructed by fitting an egg-bar shoe to the hoof and welding iron sheet metal, 16-gauge thick, around the margins of the horseshoe. The sheet metal should fit the contour of the hoof wall. This forms a metal boot that covers a large section of the hoof wall. The sides of the rim are cut in order to provide space for at least two horseshoe nails on each side. The horseshoe is nailed to the hoof and the space between the rim and hoof wall is filled with acrylic resin (♦ fig. 16.24). The construction of the continuous rim shoe is relatively difficult. Complications that may develop from the application a of continuous rim horseshoe include contracted hoof, bruised heels, hoof wall loss at the quarters and increased lameness; in these cases, the rim at the heels area should be expanded.

 ## NAVICULAR BONE FRACTURES

Navicular bone fractures MAY RESULT FROM direct trauma to the hoof or from complication of navicular disease. Turner and Malone (1997) described a conservative method of treatment of navicular bone fractures in a horse. The affected foot was trimmed and the hoof was shod with a flat horseshoe fitted with four, 3° wedge pads. Elevation of the heel relieved tension from the DDFT and removed pressure from the navicular bone, thus promoted healing. The horse was placed in a stall rest for 60 days. This period was continued with short periods of hand walking. The horseshoe was reset every four weeks, and at each reset, one pad was removed. Once all the pads were removed, the horse was shod with a flat horseshoe.

 ## PEDAL OSTEITIS

Pedal osteitis IS AN INFLAMMATION OF THE THIRD phalanx (osteitis = inflamed bone). The disease may be non-septic or septic (infected). Non-septic pedal osteitis affects primarily the solar margin of the bone. The bone margins become roughened and the vascular channels within it become wider; these changes are seen clearly on radiographs. In addition, the bone may loss minerals. Non-septic pedal osteitis may develop from various insults to the feet (Moyer et al., 1999). Predisposing factors include work on hard roads, chronic laminitis, collapsed heels, flat and thin sole.

Septic pedal osteitis develop when bacteria infect the third phalanx, bacteria may enter the bone through a sub-solar abscess, puncture wound, complicated laminitis or complete hoof capsule loss. A sinus tract or an abscess that communicates with the bone commonly accompanied the disorder; bone infection may involve the solar border or phalangeal process, and may result in pathological fractures (Cauvin and Munroe, 1998).

Farriery of non-septic pedal osteitis includes the application of a wide-web horseshoe and a thick pad; some cases may require protection with an aluminum plate instead of a pad. The solar area of working horses may require permanent protection. Alternatively, a glue-on plastic shoe with a wide web may be applied. The underlying cause of the disorder should be investigated and treated or removed.

Treatment of septic pedal osteitis includes surgical debridement of necrotic bone and bone fragments, and establishment of drainage. A sterile flexible metal probe may aid in detection of infected tracts. In some cases, application of hoof poultice overnight, following hoof trimming, may aid in detection of small draining tracts. Prior to surgery, the hoof should be trimmed, rasped and scrubbed, and a sterile dressing applied overnight (Cauvin and Munroe, 1998). Following surgery, the hoof is fitted with a treatment plate that protects the foot and provides access to the wound. Sterile gauzes, soaked in 5% povidone-iodine solution are packed inside the wound. Treatment may include systemic and topical application of antibiotics. Once the wound granulates, the hoof is fitted with a protective horseshoe, such as a wide-web horseshoe, and a leather pad. Other authors prefer to keep the foot bandaged until the wound is filled with healthy granulation tissue and than apply a treatment plat; once the lesion is completely dry and cornified the hoof may be stabilized by acrylic reconstruction (Cauvin and Munroe, 1998).

 ## SUB-SOLAR ABSCESS

Sub-solar abscess IS A COMMON FOOT DISORDER that may develop from bacterial infection caused by a puncture wound to the sole, septic laminitis (Johnson, 1972), muddy conditions, thrush, gravel, horseshoe nail pricks and keratoma. The condition is also called foot abscess and *suppurative* (pus) *pododermatitis* (podo = a foot in Greek, dermatitis = inflammed dermis). Degenerated regions of white line may be the initiating cause for abscess formation (Josseck et al., 1995). Once a focal point is infected, bacterial growth increases, exudate forms and pressure is built up under the sole (Johnson, 1972). The abscess commonly undermines the sole and expands under the horn in the line of least resistance; tunnels may form along the white line or at the angle of the sole (♦ fig. 16.25; plate 4). The abscess may track backward to the thinnest part of the sole and discharge. Abscesses that develop under the frog tend to track backward to the soft horn-skin junction under the bulbs of the heels and discharge in this area (Holocombe and Giltner, in Pearson et al., 1942; MacGregor, 1998). Sole abscesses may extend under the hoof wall and form a sub-mural abscess (page 151). Abscess development underneath the bars is commonly observed in horses kept on wet pasture. The route of infection in these cases is from small bar cracks exposed to moisture or infected with thrush. Sub-solar abscess has the potential of developing into deep infection of the foot (MacGregor, 1998).

Sole abscess may produce sudden onset of lameness. The affected foot is warmer to the touch and there is increased digital pulse. In earlier cases, the location of the abscess can be detected with hoof testers or hammer percussion. In more advanced cases, there is a generalized pain over the entire solar area. While walking, the horse avoids placing weight on the affected area, and as the case progresses, the horse tends to bear weight only on the tip of the toe (MacGregor, 1998). Drainage of pus at any location, including the white line, coronary band, or bulbs of the heels, indicates possible occurrence of a foot abscess (Scott et al., 1979).

Treatment of Sub-solar Abscess

Treatment of sub-solar abscess includes removal of all undermined horn without disturbing the dermis (Richardson et al., 1986a).

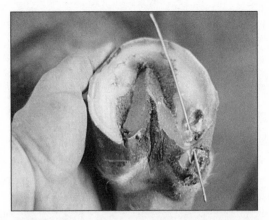

♦ **Fig. 16.25.** Sub-solar abscess with heel bulb involvement in a foal. (Photo by author.)

The site of penetration or the tract of the foreign body is explored, and the entire undermined area is removed carefully with the help of a blunt probe (MacGregor, 1998). Debridement can be carried out while the horse is standing, using regional foot anesthesia (Richardson et al., 1986a).

Prior to debridement, the horseshoe is removed, and each nail is examined for evidence of pus and discharge. The hoof is trimmed and any suspicious area, darkened tissue, or puncture wound is pared out until the abscess is reached. If paring of the hoof does not reveal any lesion, a hoof tester should be used (Johnson, 1972).

Extremely hard hooves that may be difficult to explore should be softened with a poultice overnight. A flexible blunt probe disinfected with alcohol is used to locate undermined areas at the sole. These areas are exposed by carefully trimming the overlying sole with a thin hoof knife. A normal foot does not have hollow spaces beneath the horn. Local abscesses are treated by forming a drainage hole over the abscess with a hoof knife or a loop knife. The drainage hole should be large enough to prevent *dermal prolapse* caused by pressure within the foot that pushes dermal tissue through the hole; the pinched dermis is extremely painful and can make the horse more lame (MacGregor, 1998). A small loop knife or a digging knife is used for debridement of an abscess located

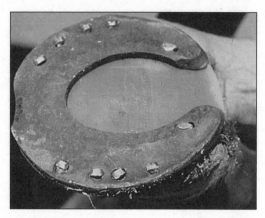

◆ **Fig. 16.26.** Wide-web horseshoe fitted with a flat pad. (Photo by author.)

under the bar. As much bar as possible should be preserved. Following paring of the abscess and establishment of drainage, the foot is soaked in warm Epsom salts solution (Snow, 1984). More sole should be removed if suppuration is still present (Johnson, 1972).

Treatment of the debrided abscess includes poulticing the foot for three to four days and bandaging it with antibiotic ointment (Snow, 1984). A new coat of cells should be evident after 8 to 10 days in most sub-solar abscesses with proper drainage (Fessler, 1989). Superficial abscesses not involving the dermis can be disinfected with 3 percent hydrogen peroxide, and then packed with pine tar and oakum under a foot bandage. As healing progresses, the bandage is replaced with a wide-web horseshoe or a rasp horseshoe fitted with a flat pad (◆ fig. 16.26). Prior to application of the horseshoe, the sole is packed with pine tar and oakum. Warm pine tar can be added between horseshoe resets by pouring it under the pad, twice a week (Johnson, 1972). Deeper lesions involving the dermis can be fitted with a treatment plate (page 158). Once healthy granulation tissue develops, the treatment plate can be replaced with a horseshoe and flat pad.

FLAT PADS

Horseshoe pads are used to protect the solar aspect of the hoof in cases of thin sole,

bruised sole, sole abscesses and wounds. The pad allows the horse to be exercised during the recovery period. Pads may be used to protect the foot against bruising in areas with rigid terrain and from concussion caused by hard ground. The shock absorption properties of pads protect the foot in chronic lameness cases such as navicular disease, ringbone and side bone. *Flat pads* are made from plastic, rubber and leather of various thickness; pad thickness of 3 mm for plastic and 6 mm for leather provide adequate protection to the solar area (see ◆ fig. 16.26). The pad should be hard enough to resist bending. Thick synthetic pads, 10 to 12 mm thick, provide additional protection and better shock absorption. Thick pads may be used to correct differences in limbs height and for making an elevated hoof boot.

In order to prevent accumulation of sand and gravel between the pad and hoof, flat pads should be connected to the horseshoe branches with copper rivets. Prior to the application of the horseshoe, the solar area should be packed with pine tar and covered with a flattened piece of oakum; the pine tar prevents moisture loss and development of thrush and the oakum holds the pine tar and prevents accumulation of debris between the sole and pad. Warm pine tar should be added to the solar area during shoeing intervals in cases where the horse is kept under moist or muddy conditions. Carroll (1989) recommended not using leather pads on horses that are bathed often because leather absorbs and hold water and tends to break down. Balch et al. (1989) indicated that continuous compression and expansion of the pads result in loosening of the horseshoe. Prolonged use of close pads may result in softening and weakening of the hoof. The pad may be cut open to form a *rim pad*. The rim pad protects the solar margins, absorbs shock, and provides better hoof grip. In addition, it permits cleaning of the solar area (page 164).

In cases where more protection to the solar area is required, a 3.0 mm *aluminum plate* can replace the pad. The plate is cut to fit the horseshoe outline, and 3.0 mm diameter holes are drilled equivalent to the horseshoe

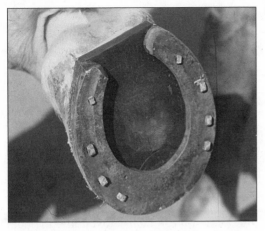

◆ **Fig. 16.27.** Wide-web horseshoes fitted with a wedge pad. (Photo by author.)

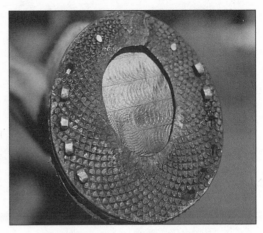

◆ **Fig. 16.28.** Egg-bar rasp horseshoe. Note that the horseshoe nails were placed in the location of healthy hoof wall. (Photo by author.)

nail holes. Prior to application of the plate, the solar area is packed with pine tar and oakum.

WIDE-WEB HORSESHOE

The *wide-web horseshoe* is used in many cases of foot lameness where the horse is footsore. This horseshoe provides excellent protection to the solar area, and permits exercising the horse during the recovery period (◆ fig. 16.27). Foot diseases that may benefit from application of wide-web horseshoes include chronic foot soreness (Moyer, 1990), bruising (Moyer, 1980), dropped sole, pododermatitis, hooves with missing wall section(s), hoof wall cracks, chronic laminitis and pedal osteitis.

Wide-web horseshoes can be forged from various size bar stock, ranging from 6 to 10 mm thickness and 25 to 40 mm in width. The horseshoe weight and width should be proportional to the foot. Wide-web horseshoes may be modified according to the individual case into a bar shoe and rolled toe horseshoe. The horseshoe may be fitted with a plastic or a leather pad.

RASP HORSESHOE

The *rasp horseshoe* is a wide-web horseshoe made from an old shoeing rasp. Forging the horseshoe takes some practice, but produces

a relatively lightweight horseshoe that provides excellent protection to the solar area (◆ fig. 16.28). The rasp is placed in a vise and the handle holder is broken off with a hammer. The rasp is heated to a cherry red and the rough side of the rasp is smoothed by light hammer blows, using a soft hammer. The ends of the bar are heated to yellow white and tapered; then the horseshoe is turned into a regular or bar shoe. In order to prevent its breakage due to its high carbon content, the horseshoe should be allowed to cool in the forge.

SUB-MURAL ABSCESS

Sub-mural abscess or gravel is a common foot abscess that develops under the hoof wall (sub = under, mura = a wall in Latin). The infection may develop from a puncture wound at the white line region, misdriven horseshoe nail, septic laminitis (Johnson, 1972), extending sub-solar abscess, hoof wall crack, thrush, seedy toe (Adams, 1974), and excessive moisture. According to Johnson (1970) and Johnson (1972) sub-mural abscess does not develop from gravel (small stones) migrating up the coronet, but they may be present at the white line when the foot is debrided (Johnson,

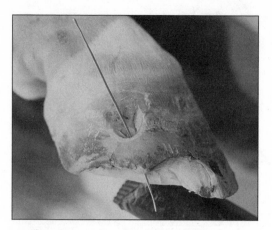

◆ **Fig. 16.29.** Sub-mural abscess following debridement. The metal probe is inserted under a bridge of horn that was left in order to give some support to the hoof wall. (Photo by author.)

1972). Small stones that tend to separate the white line may be an initiating factor in development of gravel by creating a favorable environment for development of thrush. Once an infection begins, suppuration (pus) follows the line of least resistance, between the hoof wall and laminae. If left untreated the infection may reach the coronary band where it erupts and drains (◆ fig. 16.29). Lameness may be moderate to severe, but once the infection erupts at the coronary band, symptoms are relieved. Sub-mural abscess may weaken the quarters of the hoof wall and cause development of "flail" or loose heel (Gubert, 1989).

Henninger and Owen (1986) indicated that *sub-mural crushing* and hemorrhage of the laminae, caused by blunt trauma to the hoof wall, might result in the development of a sterile abscess, which is an abscess without infectious organisms. The abscess may drain at the coronary band.

Examination of the hoof includes inspection for misdriven horseshoe nails, separation and abnormal coloration at the white line, cracks and exudate. Hoof testers should be used to detect tenderness. Hammer percussion of the suspected area will reveal a resonant sound over the hollow wall. Horseshoe nails may cause a circular blackening of the horn next to the white line and adjacent sole.

This finding is usually coincidental. Gravel has to be differentiated from close nail that presses on the sensitive laminae (Johnson, 1972); in the case of close nail, lameness is improved following removal of the nail.

Once a suspected area is found, it should be explored with a sterile blunt probe to determine the direction and depth of the lesion. The undermined area should be completely debrided of thrush, gravel and loose horn. As much hoof wall as possible should be preserved. Debridement of deep areas is established with the use of a digging knife, and in most cases, it can be inserted under the hoof wall without disturbing the dermal laminae. In cases where the hoof wall is very thin, it may be necessary to remove a section of hoof wall that is parallel to the tract. Any loose and undermined heel should be removed in order to allow for new heel growth.

Establishment of proper drainage is important. In cases where the infection has not reached the coronary band, the opening at the bottom side is enlarged with a digging knife. The hoof should be bathed in Epsom salts solution. Alternatively, the exposed area is flushed under pressure with a povidone-iodine solution. A dose syringe is suitable for this purpose. The exposed tract is packed with gauze soaked with povidone-iodine or with pine tar and oakum. In cases where the abscess drains at the coronary band, the bottom opening is enlarged and the undermined wall is flushed under pressure through the opening at the coronet. The foot is kept bandaged and the daily flushing is continued until the infection is controlled (Johnson, 1972).

Farriery of Sub-mural Abscess

Farriery of sub-mural abscess includes the application of a horseshoe and a pad in order to protect the exposed area at the sole. Gubert (1989) recommended the application of a bar shoe to cases with loose heel following removal of the affected wall. Application of a wide-web horseshoe with a drainage hole that allows daily flushing of the wound has been described (O'Grady, 1996). The drainage hole is made by tapping the horseshoe under the location of the drainage tract. The tap is fitted with a stud guard that prevents accumulation of dirt.

Cases with missing sections of hoof wall should be fitted with a bar shoe; the defect in the hoof wall should remain open or protected with a foot bandage until it becomes dry and cornified. The hoof wall may be reconstructed with acrylic repair material. Alternatively, the hoof wall may be reconstructed before healing is complete by establishing a drainage tract under the repair (page 118).

Prevention of gravel is achieved by reducing the exposure of the hoof to moisture, regular application of pine tar, and careful inspection of the white line for small cracks, crumbling horn, separations, and nail holes that may accumulate debris and develop into thrush. These areas should be debrided and treated with pine tar. In cases where the horse is kept shod, these areas should be packed with a hoof pack prior to application of horseshoes.

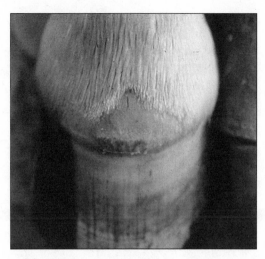

◆ **Fig. 16.30.** Coronitis caused by sub-mural abscess. The skin above the coronary band (clipped area) is red, swollen and tender. (Photo by author.)

CORONITIS

Coronitis IS AN INFLAMMATION OF THE CORONARY band caused by infection, exposure to irritating materials and disease. Coronitis may develop from chronic selenosis (Witte et al., 1993), chronic inflammation caused by fungi (Keller et al., 2000), coronary band wounds, gravel, laminitis and frostbite (◆ fig. 16.30). The inflammatory reaction caused by the application of blistering materials to the coronary band may cause coronitis. Another cause is *vesicular stomatitis*, a viral disease that can affect horses and causes (among other signs) blisters and oozing sores at the coronary band. *Summer sores* lesions characterized by granulation tissue may develop at the coronary band; these lesions, which are caused by the larvae of the stomach worm (Habronema) cause these lesions, which can be quite extensive (Loomis et al., 1975). Coronitis may become complicated by development of abnormal hoof horn and malformed hooves.

Treatment of Coronitis

Treatment of coronitis includes the elimination of the underlying cause, debridement of loose and necrotic tissue, and establishment of drainage. The integrity of the coronary dermis should be maintained. The foot is treated by daily foot soaking in warm water and Epsom salts, followed by the application of antibiotic dressing and a foot bandage.

Farriery of coronitis includes the application of a bar shoe in order to protect and stabilize the foot, especially when a portion of the hoof wall has been removed. The frog may require some form of support in order to prevent third phalanx rotation.

PUNCTURE WOUNDS

PUNCTURE WOUND OF THE FOOT ARE CLASSIFIED into superficial and deep wounds. Superficial wounds include those that penetrate cornified tissue but not the dermis, whereas deep wounds involve deeper structures within the foot, and can result in serious complications (Richardson et al., 1986a). Hence, every case of puncture wound of the foot should be examined carefully and treated as an emergency. Debridement of most foot wounds may be carried out under field conditions by using a regional nerve block. More severe cases may require general anesthesia.

Superficial Puncture Wounds

Superficial puncture wounds are commonly caused by a foreign body, and many cases develop into sub-solar abscesses. Treatment of superficial puncture wounds includes debridement and removal of undermined horn with a sharp hoof knife. In cases where the hoof is extremely hard, it should be softened overnight with a poultice pack in order to facilitate safe debridement. If done carefully, debridement may be performed without using a regional anesthetic. Debridement should be done carefully in order to prevent bleeding and disruption of the dermis. The wound is packed with gauze sponges soaked in povidone-iodine and a foot bandaged is applied; the bandage is changed daily until the wound is dry. The hoof is fitted with a horseshoe and flat pad after packing the solar area with pine tar and oakum. Alternatively, a protective horseshoe may be applied following debridement. Depending on the location of the wound, this could be a wide-web horseshoe, an armor-plated horseshoe that protects the toe region, or a half-bar shoe that protects the heels area. The wound should be treated daily with pine tar.

Deep Puncture Wounds

Deep puncture wounds penetrate the dermis and deeper structures within the foot. The wound may be caused by a sharp foreign body that penetrates any part of the solar area of the foot to various depths. Deep puncture wounds of the foot are classified according to the site of penetration of the foreign body into three regions: sole, frog and collateral sulci, and coronary band (Richardson et al., 1986a). Serious complications can result when the DDFT, navicular bursa or DIP joint are involved. Puncture wounds caused by "picking up" street nails was common in urban working horses (Merillat 1911). Fortunately, it is rare that a nail penetrates deep enough to reach vital structures within the foot. Nail treads are another cause of puncture wounds, they are caused when the horse steps on protruding nails of a loose horseshoe (Merillat, 1911). Police horses may step on sharp objects placed by demonstrators.

PUNCTURE WOUNDS OF THE SOLE

Deep puncture wounds of the sole may involve the sole dermis, third phalanx, navicular bursa and digital cushion. Lameness may be acute and the horse may not bear weight on the foot. The location of the wound in cases where no foreign body is present is determined by trimming the hoof, removal of horn flakes, and systematic application of hoof testers. All areas with discoloration, cracks, fissures and secretions should be explored. Puncture wounds at the bottom of the foot commonly have black discoloration at the entry site (Johnson, 1970; Richardson et al., 1986a). A sterile blunt metal probe is used to determine the depth and direction of suspicious tract(s). Once the puncture wound is located, it should be debrided, and then drainage has to be established. The opening at the outer surface should have at least a 2 cm diameter and the wound edges should be beveled so it does not close before complete healing of the inner part of the wound (Richardson et al., 1986a). Infected dermis can be excised with a scalpel and abnormal bone is removed with a bone curette.

Treatment of the wound includes daily packing with povidone-iodine soaked sterile gauze sponges covered with a foot bandage. Alternatively, the hoof can be fitted with a treatment plate. Once the wound is dry and there are no signs of secretions, the hoof is shod with a horseshoe and a leather pad. Prior to shoeing, the solar area is packed with pine tar and oakum. Warm pine tar is added as required to the sole between shoeing intervals.

PENETRATING WOUNDS OF THE CORONARY BAND

Penetrating wounds of the coronary band area may result from wood splinters, tread wounds caused by horseshoe calks, or from accidental limb contact. The infected wound may result in development of undermined hoof wall below the injury. Injuries to the coronary band have the potential of developing into hoof wall cracks or clefts. The lesion has to be differentiated from sub-mural abscess by careful examination of the sole white line region below it (Richardson et al., 1986a).

Small foreign bodies embedded in the coronary band could be difficult to detect. Therefore, the coronet should be palpated carefully and examined by lifting the hair and examining the skin for signs of pain, redness and swelling (◆ fig. 16.31).

Treatment of coronary band wounds include clipping the hair around the wound, removal of the foreign body if present, and careful debridement of loose horn and necrotic tissue. Undermined hoof wall has to be debrided in order to establish drainage; the hoof wall below the wound is thinned with a hoof rasp and the undermined hoof wall is exposed carefully with a hoof knife or loop knife. Only devitalized tissue and loose horn should be removed. The coronary der-mis should be preserved in order to prevent the development of a permanent hoof wall crack. The wound is flushed with povidone-iodine diluted in saline, under pressure, with the use of a dose syringe. The foot is treated daily with a warm Epsom salts bath, followed by application of antimicrobial dressing and a foot bandage. The hoof wall below the injury should be examined for signs of developing wall crack. Farriery may include the application of a bar shoe in order to stabilize the foot.

PENETRATING WOUNDS OF THE FROG

The pliable nature of the frog makes it prone to puncture wounds. In addition, once a foreign body is removed from the frog, it is difficult to identify the tract. The penetrating object introduces infectious microorganisms that become sealed inside the sole or frog, forming a "closed cavity infection" (Johnson, 1972; Steckel et al., 1989).

Puncture wounds in the frog area may involve the frog dermis, digital cushion, DDFT, navicular bursa and DIP joint. In cases where the wound involves the digital cushion alone, a tapered core of tissue that contains the tract should be removed with a scalpel. Penetrating wounds involving the DDFT should be approached in a similar manner; all necrotic or devitalized tissue should be removed (Richardson et al., 1986a). Following debridement, the wound is treated as described for puncture wounds of the sole. Penetrating wounds of the frog may involve the navicular bursa and lead to development of navicular bursitis (see below).

NAVICULAR BURSITIS

Navicular bursitis IS A SERIOUS INFECTION involving the frog dermis, digital cushion, DDFT and navicular bursa. In some cases, the DIP joint may become involved. Puncture wounds involving the third phalanx, navicular bone or bursa have a poor prognosis (Johnson, 1972). In a retrospective study of 38 hors-

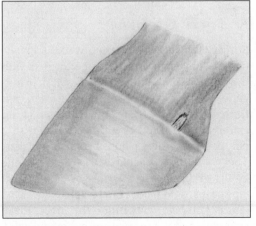

◆ **Fig. 16.31.** Coronary band injury caused by a wood splinter.

es that had navicular bursitis, only 12 horses had a satisfactory outcome, and were used for their intended purpose after recovery (Richardson et al., 1986b). The most common foreign body found in this group was nails. Other foreign bodies included wire, staples, and wood splinters. In 10 cases, no foreign bodies were found. In a different study on a group of 50 horses that had deep puncture wounds at the foot, only 50 percent of the horses with punctured frog fully recovered, whereas 95 percent of the horses with puncture wounds outside the frog became sound (Steckel et al., 1989). The disorder may develop from septic pedal osteitis complicated by pathologic fracture of the palmar/plantar phalangeal process (Cauvin and Munroe, 1998).

Injury to the navicular bursa results when a sharp object penetrates the back 2/3 of the frog. The foreign object penetrates the cornified frog, frog dermis, digital cushion and the deep digital flexor tendon before reaching the navicular bursa. The infection can necrotize the flexor tendon, infect the DIP joint and cause adhesions between the flexor tendon and navicular bone. Involvement of the navicular bursa may lead to inflammation of the deep flexor *tendon sheath* or envelope (Johnson, 1972; Richardson, 1999). Infections of the DIP joint are difficult to treat and the affected horses are often euthanatized (Honnas et al., 1992).

Signs of navicular bursitis include non-weight-bearing lameness and increased digital pulse. The entire foot may be sensitive and warmer than normal. Diagnosis of navicular bursitis includes careful examination of the frog for entry sites, and the use of hoof testers to locate sensitive areas. The hoof should be trimmed before the examination. Once a tract is found, the foot is anesthetized and a sterile flexible blunt probe is carefully inserted into the tract. The probe should not be forced inside the foot. Once the probe is inserted, its protruding side should be bent against the sole in order to prevent accidental penetration if the horse steps on the foot. The foot is radiographed (x-rayed) with the probe inside to determine the depth and direction of the wound (◆ fig. 16.32). Richardson and O'Brien

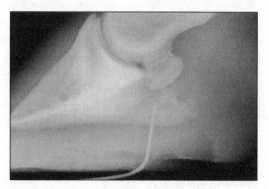

◆ **Fig. 16.32.** Penetrating wound of the frog. Lateral radiograph of the foot shows the position of the metal probe. (Photo by author.)

(1985) indicated that in the first few days following an injury, any damage to the navicular bone might not be visible in radiographs.

Treatment of navicular bursitis requires surgical excision of the affected tissue and treatment of the wound. *Maggot therapy*, with maggots that consume necrotic tissue may be applied (Sherman et al., 2006). Historically, the surgical treatment of navicular bursitis was termed "radical nail prick operation" (Merillat, 1911). A newer treatment technique that includes the use of endoscopy to perform *bursal lavage* of the infected navicular bursae has been described (Wright et al., 1999). The technique is less invasive and have better post-operative healing.

Nail Prick Operation

Surgery for deep penetrating wounds involving the navicular bursa are performed with the horse under general anesthesia; field surgeries for this type of injury have been performed (Weisenberg, 1990). Hooves that are extremely hard and dry are softened with a poultice pack for 24 hours prior to surgery. The poultice is covered with nylon and the foot is wrapped with a grain sack or with duct tape strips; a hoof boot can be applied over the entire bandage. Softening the hoof make exploration of the injured site easier and safer. The farrier tools used in the operation should be sterilized in an autoclave.

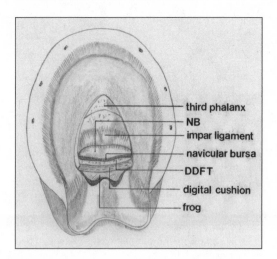

◆ **Fig. 16.33.** The anatomy of the navicular bursae and associated structures. (Adapted from Merillate A.L.1911, fig. 239. Some terms have been changed to modern terms.)

DDFT = Deep digital flexor tendon, NB = Navicular bone.

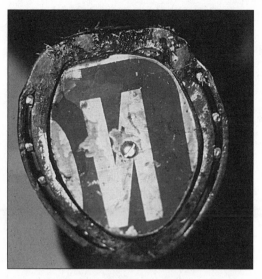

◆ **Fig. 16.34.** One-bolt treatment plate. (Photo by author.)

The foot is prepared for aseptic surgery and a tourniquet is placed on the limb. Exposure of vital structures is carried out by resecting part of the frog and continuing through the frog dermis, digital cushion, flexor tendon, into the navicular bursa (◆ fig. 16.33). Following exposure of the navicular bursa, contaminated, devitalized tissue is removed (Fessler, 1971a), necrotic parts of the navicular bone are excised by curettement. Any discolored or frayed tendon is carefully removed; excessive incision of the flexor tendon may lead to its complete tear. During debridement, extreme care has to be taken to avoid penetrating the impar ligament, which forms a seal between the navicular bursa and DIP joint (Honnas et al., 1988d; Gibson et al., 1990). An infected impar ligament indicates that the DIP joint may also be infected (Richardson et al., 1986b).

Following surgery, the surgical site is packed with sterile gauzes soaked in povidone-iodine, and a foot bandage is applied with extra cotton packed against the sole to control bleeding. Alternatively, the hoof can be fitted with a treatment plate immediately following surgery. Hemorrhage is controlled by tightening the plate against packed bandage material (◆ fig. 16.34). The tourniquet, which may be covered under bandage material, should be removed.

Large quantities of secretions from the wound may be produced one to two weeks following surgery. The foot bandage and sole pack should be changed once or twice a day until secretions stop. A treatment plate can be applied to the hoof several days after the surgery. The plate saves bandage material and permits hand walking the horse. Once the wound is filled with healthy granulation tissue, the hoof is shod with a wide-web horseshoe and leather pad. The solar area should be packed with pine tar and oakum. Warm pine tar can be added to the sole during shoeing intervals as needed.

FOOT BANDAGE

The *foot bandage* is used to protect the foot following foot injuries and debridement procedures involving different areas. The foot bandage can be used to control bleeding following surgical procedures of the solar area (◆ fig. 16.35). A thick plastic bag should be

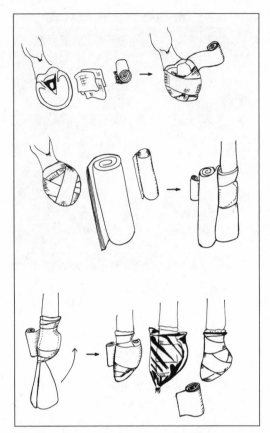

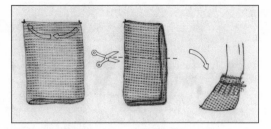

◆ **Fig. 16.36.** Plastic grain sack used to protect a foot bandage. A pocket (hood) is made in the sack by placing one corner into the other. The sack is cut to the desired length and is placed over the bandaged foot. Duct tape, elastic adhesive tape or plastic hay bale rope is used to secure the sack in place. The tape or rope should be loose enough to allow placement of one finger between the sack and digit.

◆ **Fig. 16.35.** Application of foot bandage following debridement of the sole. The wound is packed with sterile gauze sponges soaked in povidone-iodine solution; a sterile gauze roll holds the gauze sponges in place. A sheet cotton roll is wrapped around the foot with rolled brown gauze. Half of the cotton sheet should be left to protrude beyond the foot. This part is folded against the sole and wrapped firmly with the same rolled gauze. A thick plastic bag is placed over the foot and the foot is wrapped with elastic adhesive tape. (Reprinted by permission from Richardson, G.L., et al. 1986, fig. 5. Illustrations modified to text.)

bandaging, the operator should be able to place at least one finger between the bandage and bulbs of the heels. Once the wound begins to granulate, the foot bandage is replaced with a treatment plate or a horseshoe and a pad.

TREATMENT PLATE

The *treatment plate* is a combination of a horseshoe and a plate fitted to the bottom of the horseshoe. The plate protects the solar area, prevents accumulation of manure and urine, saves bandage material, and permits hand walking the horse during the healing period. The treatment plate is applied to the hoof following surgical debridement of foot disorders such as infected third phalanx (Baird et al., 1990), navicular bursitis, puncture wounds (Asmus, 1940; Richardson et al., 1986a), sole abscesses and canker. The treatment plate may be used to provide solar support in cases of solar prolapse (Eustace, 1989b). The treatment plate can be modified and connected to the hoof with screws (Redden 1986b) (page 140).

placed over the bandage in order to prevent passage of moisture or urine into the wound (Richardson et al., 1986a). Further protection is achieved by covering the foot bandage with duct tape strips, a plastic grain sack or a large hoof boot (◆ fig. 16.36). In order to prevent obstruction of circulation, the foot bandage should not be tightened excessively. Following

Various types of treatment plates can be constructed. A *one-bolt treatment plate* is the simplest type to construct from a keg shoe or a bar shoe (◆ fig. 16.37). The device is constructed from a forged straight-bar shoe that

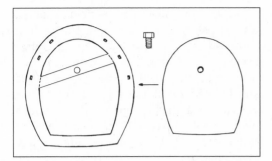

◆ **Fig. 16.37.** One-bolt treatment plate, schematic illustration. See text for details.

is fitted to the hoof. Alternatively, the horseshoe can be made by fitting a keg shoe to the hoof and welding a bar across the horseshoe branches. A diagonal bar, 15 mm wide, is welded across the horseshoe over healthy tissue. The bar should be thinner than the horseshoe in order to accommodate the plate. The bar is welded level with the hoof surface of the horseshoe; the center of the bar is threaded with a 3/8" tap. A plate made from 3 mm sheet metal is cut to fit the inner margins of the horseshoe. A hole is drilled in the plate and used to secure it to the horseshoe with a 3/8" bolt. Klimesh (1997) described the construction of a similar device made with a toe tab. Plated horseshoes used by police cavalry to protect the solar area of the foot from sharp objects can be used as a treatment plate as well. A *four-bolt treatment plate* can be constructed from an open or straight-bar shoe (◆ fig. 16.38). The device is constructed by fitting the hoof with a straight-bar shoe. A metal plate is fitted to the outer margins of the horseshoe. The palmar/plantar part of the plate is left longer and bent at an obtuse angle. The plate is secured to the horseshoe ground surface by four 3/8" bolts bolted into threads made in the horseshoe. The horseshoe nail heads should be level with the ground surface of the horseshoe. The disadvantage of this device is that the bolt's heads may interfere with walking on hard surfaces.

In order to prevent further trauma to the foot, the treatment plate is nailed with a light race hammer. The wound is dressed and wrapped with sterile gauze. The remaining

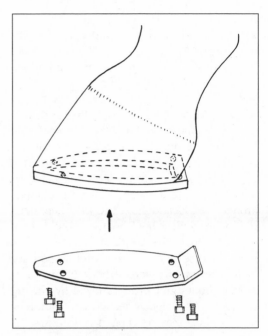

◆ **Fig. 16.38.** Four-bolt treatment plate, schematic illustration. See text for details.

space is packed with sterile gauze and the plate is secured. Securing the plate in this manner following surgery helps to control bleeding.

Following growth of healthy, pinkish granulation tissue, the treatment plate is replaced with a horseshoe and a leather pad. Prior to application of the horseshoe, the sole should be packed with pine tar and oakum. In cases where the sole is flat or tender, a 3 mm thick aluminum plate may be used instead of a pad. Alternatively, the wound may be protected with a wide bar welded across the horseshoe, similarly to armor-plated horseshoe.

HOOF POULTICE

Hoof poultice add moisture into dry hooves and act as an absorbent in the treatment of foot abscesses. Application of poultice prior to debridement procedures of foot abscesses or puncture wounds softens the hoof and permit safer manipulation. Softening the hoof may cause an abscess to break out spontaneously

(O'Grady, 1996), and aid in detection of small sinus tracts related to septic pedal osteitis (Cauvin and Munroe, 1998). The hoof should be trimmed prior to poulticing; when required the poultice is thinned by stirring in water. MacGregor (1998) indicated that poulticing the hoof with hypertonic (high salt content) substances tend to dry the hoof and should be avoided. Generous amounts of poultice are applied over the foot and the foot is wrapped with a strong plastic bag. Elastic adhesive tape or duct tape strips are wrapped around the foot and the entire wrap is protected further with a hoof boot or plastic grain sack. Alternatively, the hoof can be packed with poultice and covered with a poultice boot. The poultice should be kept on for at least 12 hours and then removed by rinsing the foot with water. A second application of new poultice may be applied to foot abscess cases.

A hoof poultice may be used to correct moisture loss from the hoof following trimming or hot horseshoe fitting. Following these procedures, a poultice is applied over the solar area and covered with waxed paper. The hoof is left to absorb moisture while the next hoof is trimmed. Prior to application of horseshoes, the hooves may be rinsed with water or wiped with a towel. The solar area is checked for levelness and the horseshoe is applied. Following the application of horseshoes, the solar area should be dressed with pine tar in order to maintain the moisture within the hoof.

HOOF BOOTS

Hoof boots are used to protect the hoof in cases of foot injuries such as sole abscess, stone bruise and as a replacement for lost horseshoes; in addition, hoof boots are used to protect bandaged feet and to hold poultice material. Hoof boots may be used to protect the solar area against bruising, provide traction on slippery surfaces, and protect the heel bulbs against lacerations when riding over sharp rocks. Various types of commercial hoof boots are available, including a closed rubber boot suitable for poulticing. Alternatively, a *poultice boot* can be constructed from an extra large leather bell-boot by attaching a leather sole to its bottom. When using hoof boots to replace lost horseshoes, the boot should fit snugly. In order to prevent rubbing and chafing at the heel bulbs, the limb should be fitted with a pastern wrap that contains a cotton sheet held by a self-adhering bandage. Hoof boots may be used to provide solar support in laminitis cases; a commercial boot for that purpose is available.

Hoof boots may be modified for various orthopedic treatments. Stokes et al. (1998) described the use of an *elevated hoof boot* to raise the healthy opposite foot in horses with a limb cast. The height of the boot is raised with a wood board cut to fit the boot outline. The board is attached to the boot by flat-head screws (see ◆ fig. 16.58). In cases where a supporting limb laminitis is suspected, an elevated heel boot may be used to reduce tension from the DDFT; the heels are raised by attaching a wedged wooden board (or several wedge pads), cut to fit the boot outline, to the bottom of the boot.

🪚 INJURIES AND DAMAGE CAUSED BY HORSESHOE NAILS

INJURIES BY HORSESHOE NAILS MAY RESULT FROM direct penetration of horseshoe nails into the dermis or by pressure exerted by the nail on the surrounding structures. Damage to the hoof may result from horseshoe nails that split and weaken the hoof wall.

Horseshoe Nails Pricks

Misdriven horseshoe nails that penetrate the dermis causes *horseshoe nails pricks* ("forge pricks") (Merillat 1911). This type of injury is more commonly observed in horses with thin and badly broken or worn hoof wall. In most cases, lameness is noticed immediately after shoeing. Horseshoe nails pricks may develop into sub-solar or sub-mural abscesses.

The offending nail may be located by tapping each clinch with the tip of a small ball-peen hammer to see if the horse is exceptionally sensitive over this area (Milne, 1967). Although any nail can cause the problem, nails that are more palmar/plantar and those that are driven very high are usually the source of pain. Any suspicious nail should be pulled and examined. A moist nail may provide a sign to the site of infection. The horseshoe should be removed and the hoof examined with hoof testers. Suspected nail holes are checked for the presence of infection with a flexible blunt probe. The affected nail hole is enlarged with a digging knife and the wound is flushed with povidone-iodine. The hole is packed with pine tar and oakum and the horseshoe is reset by using the remaining nail holes. Deep and infected wounds require daily flushing. This can be achieved by making a drain in the horseshoe branch. A hole is made where the wound is located; the hole is tapped and fitted with a stud guard that prevents contamination of the wound. The tract provides convenient access for flushing and medicating the wound (O' Grady, 1996). Cases that develop into sole abscesses or sub-mural abscesses should be debrided and treated as described for these conditions. The tetanus vaccination status of the horse should be checked in order to determine if revaccination is required.

Prevention of horseshoe nails pricks can be achieved by using small size, slim horseshoe nails. Forged horseshoes made with proper horseshoe nail pitch and positions are by far more suitable than keg shoes are, and can reduce the incidence of horseshoe nails injuries. The last nail holes should be placed dorsal to the widest portion of the horseshoe. Punching five nail holes on each side of the horseshoe permits alternate nail placement at each shoeing interval, which reduces stress from the hoof wall. Driving three nails on each side is usually adequate. Application of glue-on shoes can eliminate the problem of horseshoe nails pricks and close nails, but does not solve the problem of horses with poor hoof conformation.

Close Nail

Close nail ("pressure quick") is caused by horseshoe nails that are driven too close to sensitive tissue (Johnson, 1972). The condition is more common in hooves with thin wall or in hooves where the horseshoe nail is driven too high. Lameness caused by a close nail commonly develops a few days following shoeing. The horse become sound as soon as the nail is removed (Johnson, 1972). Treatment of close nail includes removal of the offending nail and observing the horse. In cases where lameness develops, the condition should be treated as described for horseshoe nail pricks.

Wall Splits

Wall splits are small cracks in the hoof wall caused by horseshoe nails that are driven into thin, dry and weak hoof wall (◆ fig 16.39). The condition is common in horses that are being shod often. Splits may develop in healthy horn with thick hoof wall if the nail is positioned in the outer part of the hoof wall and not in the inner softer part (Geyer, 1999). Large splits may result from horseshoe nails that are driven into nail holes that are too large. In most cases, wall splits are superficial and are only a cosmetic problem. In some cases, the splits may form a route for development of thrush or may weaken the hoof wall and cause broken sections at the quarters.

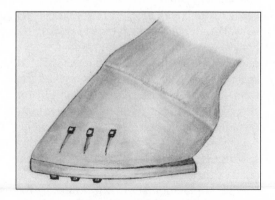

◆ **Fig. 16.39.** Hoof wall splits caused by large horseshoe nails.

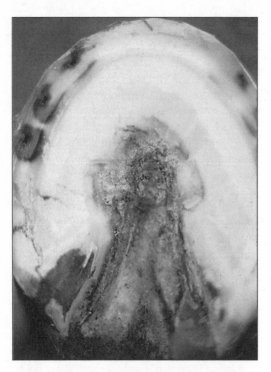

◆ **Fig. 16.40.** Dark spots located around areas of horseshoe nails placement. (Photo by author.)

Treatment of wall splits includes removal of the horseshoes with crease nail pullers, trimming the loose horn, debridement of thrush and application of pine tar over the affected area. Horses with weak hooves may be placed in a pasture and allowed to grow new hoof. In cases that require horseshoes, the hooves should be shod with light horseshoes, using small size, slim-type horseshoe nails. Forging the horseshoes and placing the horseshoe nails according to the hoof conformation can reduce the incidence of wall splits. In cases where the hoof is dry and free from thrush, it can be fitted with a glue-on shoe. This permits new hoof growth without the affect of horseshoe nails. In cases where the heels are too low, they should be raised by holding the horseshoe at an angle while the resin is curing (Craig and Craig, 2004). Prolonged supplementation with biotin may improve the quality of the hoof horn in some cases. Treatment of splits for cosmetic reasons can be done by sealing them with acrylic

resin. Hooves with weak horn tend to splits at the distal margins of the hoof wall of barefooted horses; rounding the margins of the bearing surface of the wall when the hooves are trimmed may prevent development of splits.

Dark Spots

Dark spots are circular spots that are observed at the wall-white line area. The spots are associated with horseshoe nails and commonly develop several weeks after shoeing. It appears that dark spots may be caused by a reaction to horseshoe nails or from leaching from them (◆ fig. 16.40). No data was found on possible causes for these spots.

🖈 SUB-SOLAR BRUISING

Sub-solar bruising IS A COMMON FOOT condition caused by abnormal pressure on the solar dermis that leads to the rupture of small blood vessels, resulting in sub-solar hemorrhages. The blood pigment becomes embedded in the horn. As the horn grows, the sole over the affected area become reddish. Sub-solar bruising may result from a single traumatic event or by continuous insults to the hoof (◆ fig. 16.41).

Predisposing factors for bruised sole include work on rough or rocky ground (Balch et al., 1995b), small horseshoes, loose horseshoes, tucked heel, toe grabs, heel calks, flat sole, long toe and under-run heels (Moyer, 1988a), excessive hoof wear, over-trimming (Moyer, 1981) and improper foot balance (Moyer and Anderson, 1975a). Sub-solar bruising may result from excessive pressure against the sole in cases where the sole was not concaved or the horseshoe was not seated out. The frog may become bruised from stepping on a stone during high speed (Holocombe and Giltner, in Pearson et al., 1942). Chronic sub-solar bruising may exist for an extended period and is often difficult to correct; the horse may be lame or show a reduced performance (Moyer, 1988a). Excessive pressure on the sole may result from snow balling

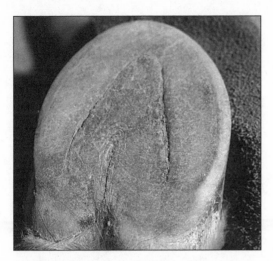

◆ **Fig. 16.41.** Sub-solar bruising. The entire sole is worn and reddish from prolonged walking on asphalt. (Photo by author.)

(see below). The most common site of chronic bruising occurs at the angle of the sole (Moyer, 1979); bruising at this site is termed corn (page 165).

Bruises may be noted during routine hoof trimming as red discolored areas at the sole or frog. In early cases, there is no discoloration and the only signs may be altered gait and reaction to hoof testers; more than one foot may be involved. Bruises of the bulbs of the heels and frog may develop in horses ridden on rocky terrain. A crescent-shaped bruise equivalent to the margins of the third phalanx may be observed in horses with flatfoot, chronic laminitis and pedal osteitis. The bruise develops from abnormal pressure between the third phalanx and sole dermis. The area is sensitive to hoof testers.

Bruises at locations other than the sole may be caused by an external blow to the hoof wall. A trauma to the coronary band often results in reddening of the horn below the site of injury. Hemorrhage at a localized area of the laminae may appear as a red discoloration at the white line below the injury. These signs may appear several weeks or months after the trauma. Pollitt (1995) described a condition caused by *concussive bruising* of the coronet that may be related to abnormal shearing forces at the coronary band. He proposed that the condition might be caused by abnormal distal-proximal pressure on the hoof wall with development of red, hemorrhagic bands parallel to the coronet (see plate 14). The condition was observed in horses with upright pastern and broken back foot axis.

SNOW BALLING

Balling up of snow becomes a problem when the ice begun to warm up and pack the sole; this predisposes the horse to slippage and injuries (Wiseman, 1968). In addition, the horse bears its weight directly over the solar area, which may become bruised (Ards, 2006). Snow balling can be prevented by keeping the horse barefoot, rounding the inner margins of the horseshoe, or using a horseshoe and pad (Wiseman, 1968). Full snowball pads and rim snowball pads are available commercially. Frequent application of vegetable oil over the solar area help prevent the buildup of snowballs (Ards, 2006).

Farriery of Sub-solar Bruising

Farriery of sub-solar bruising includes trimming the hoof, concaving the sole margins and application of a protective horseshoe that is well seated out. The bruise should not be explored unless it has moist secretions or it is undermined. The type of horseshoes used depends on the extent and location of the lesion, presence of lameness and the type of work performed by the horse. Horseshoes that are used include a plain horseshoe, reversed horseshoe, horseshoe and pad or a rim pad, wide-web horseshoe (Moyer, 1981), bar shoe (Moyer, 1988a) and armor-plated horseshoe (Thomas, 1998). A horseshoe and molded pad may be used in horses with thin sole. Moyer (1981) recommended using a plastic rim pad with 0.25″ thickness, for racing Standardbreds. Sole pressure is reduced by concaving the pad with a hot hoof knife. A straight-bar shoe or an egg-bar shoe may be applied to cases where the bulbs of the heels are bruised.

Prevention of sole bruises includes concaving the sole margins with the hoof knife in order to prevent sole pressure. The hoof surface of the horseshoe should be seated out to prevent direct pressure between the horseshoe and sole (Moyer, 1981; Moyer, 1988a). These measures may not provide adequate protection to the feet of horses that receive abnormal loads during landing, such as jumpers and hunters. These horses may be protected by leaving the hoof wall slightly longer or fitting the horseshoe with a rim pad (Balch et al., 1995b).

ARMOR-PLATED HORSESHOE

The *armor-plated horseshoe* is a horseshoe with a plate welded across the toe of the horseshoe; the horseshoe protects the sole from bruising (Thomas, 1998) and following healing of a wound (◆ fig. 16.42). The armor-plated horseshoe may be used instead of a wide-web horseshoe.

The horseshoe is made from a keg horseshoe or forged from bar stock. Following fitting of the horseshoe to the hoof, a 3.0 mm thick metal plate is shaped to fit the inner toe section of the horseshoe. The plate is welded level with the ground surface of the horseshoe. This allows access to the wound for daily treatment with pine tar.

RIM PAD

The *rim pad* is an open flat pad or wedge pad that fits along the web of the horseshoe. The rim pad is made by cutting the inner section of a full pad after connecting it to the horseshoe. The rim pad provides better hoof grip compared to the close pad; it absorbs concussion and allows picking the sole. Rim pads are used in cases of thin sole, bruised sole, solar prolapse and sore palmar/plantar hoof (◆ fig. 16.43).

Horses with flat or thin sole can be fitted regularly with a rim pad in order to prevent bruising. The pad is cut so it protrudes 2 to 3 cm wider than the horseshoe inner margin. A thick synthetic pad should be used in cases where the frog or bulbs of the heels are sensi-

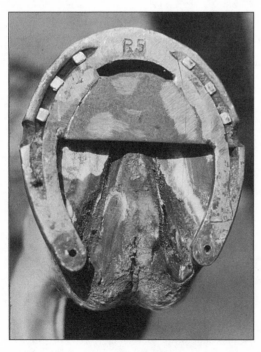

◆ **Fig. 16.42.** Armor-plated shoe. (Photo by author.)

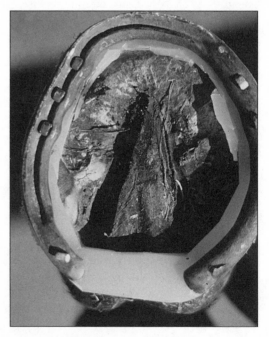

◆ **Fig. 16.43.** Rim pad. The pad also provides some protection to the plantar area. (Photo by author.)

tive. An opening can be made at the center of the pad; the remaining section provides good protection to the palmar/plantar area of the foot. Eustace and Caldwell (1989b) recommended using a rim pad fitted to a heart-bar shoe in order to raise the foot and relieve pressure from the sole in cases of solar prolapse.

HORSESHOE AND MOLDED PAD

The *horseshoe and molded pad* are used for prevention of sole bruising in horses with thin and sensitive soles, and for protection of the heel bulbs. The molded pad is made from a full plastic pad that is heated and pressed against the sole until it molds into the shape of the solar surface. The advantage of the molded pad is that it provides a better grip with the ground compared to a flat pad (◆ fig. 16.44). Prior to using this technique, it should be practiced under the supervision of experienced farrier.

Application of the molded pad is done on level cement or rubber floor. A 5 kg pile of white sand is placed next to the affected limb. The horseshoe is fitted to the hoof, and a soft synthetic pad is connected to the horseshoe with copper rivets. The pad is cut along the horseshoe outline, except at the palmar/plantar area, were a 4.0 cm extension is left. The horseshoe is then nailed to the hoof, the limb is held up and the pad is heated evenly with a hot air blower for 10 seconds (originally the pad was heated for two to three seconds with hot iron rod heated to black heat). The foot is placed immediately on the pile of sand and the opposite limb is lifted and held up for 30 seconds. As the weight of the horse presses the pad, it molds into the shape of the solar area. The pad is cut around the heel bulbs and warm pine tar is poured between the pad and sole.

 CORNS

A *corn* IS A SUB-SOLAR BRUISE THAT DEVELOPS AT the angle of the sole (Butzow, 1961). This site is also called *"seat of the corn"* (◆ fig. 16.45; plate 1). Corns develop as a result of excessive pressure against the angle of the sole. The lesion may be dry, moist or suppurated (containing pus). Corns are more common at the medial side of the hoof (Miller and Robertson, 1943). Causes of corns include small horseshoes, short horseshoe branches, tucking the medial branch of the horseshoe to prevent it

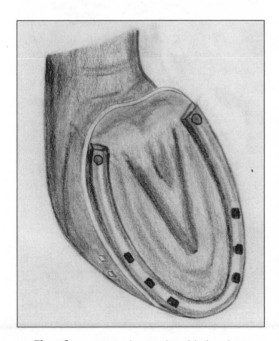

◆ **Fig. 16.44.** Horseshoe and molded pad. Note that the pad covers some of the heel bulbs. See text for details.

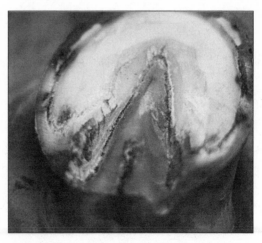

◆ **Fig. 16.45.** Corns, dry form. The corns developed at both angles of the sole (darker areas). (Photo by author.)

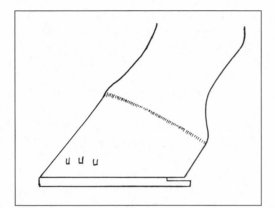

◆ **Fig. 16.46.** Stepping the horseshoe for removal of pressure from the heels, schematic illustration. (Adapted from Miller and Robertson (1943), fig. 195.)

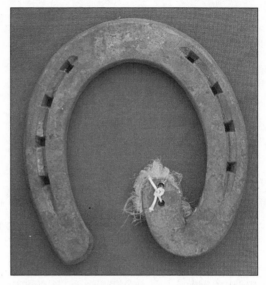

◆ **Fig. 16.47.** Half-bar shoe. In this horseshoe, two holes were drilled in the bar and were used to tie a string of oakum soaked with pine tar. (Photo by author.)

from being pulled, (Balch et al., 1998b; Moyer, 1980), and shoeing "tight" with minimal room for heel expansion followed by growth of the quarters and heels beyond the horseshoe (Balch et al., 1998b). Repetitive pressure against the angle of the sole leads to rupturing of small blood vessels at the sole dermis. As new horn grows, the area becomes discolored with red pigment. The corn may be sensitive to hoof testers, but in most cases, the horse is not lame.

Farriery of Corns

Farriery of corns includes the removal of direct pressure from the affected area and application of a protective horseshoe. Suppurative corns should be explored and debrided prior to application of the horseshoe. Dry corns should be trimmed slightly by concaving the angle of the sole prior to application of the horseshoe. In cases where the palmar/plantar area is sensitive, the horseshoe branch at the heels area may be lowered (stepped) in order to remove direct pressure from the heels (Miller and Robertson, 1943) (◆ fig. 16.46). The types of horseshoes that may be used for protection of corns include plain horseshoe, horseshoe and pad, wide-

web horseshoe, half-bar shoe, double half-bar shoe and a bar shoe. Martinelli and Ferrie (1998) recommended using three-quarter bar shoes to relieve direct pressure from corns. McCunn (1951) recommended using a three-quarter horseshoe. The last two horseshoe types may not be appropriate for horses that work on rocky surfaces. Rather, a wide-web plain horseshoe, well seated out at the affected heel area should be used (Miller and Robertson, 1943).

Prevention of corns includes lowering the surface of the angle of the sole prior to application of horseshoes, fitting the horseshoe full, and shoeing the horse at the proper shoeing intervals.

HALF-BAR SHOE AND DOUBLE HALF-BAR SHOE

The *half-bar shoe* is a horseshoe with one branch turned inward and forward. This horseshoe is used in the treatment of quarter cracks and corns. The *double-half bar shoe* is the same horseshoe but with both branches turned, and it is used in cases of bilateral corns (Rick, 1907). Russell (1882) described a similar horseshoe used for *tender feet*. The horseshoe can be made from a keg horseshoe or forged from bar stock. The angle and length of the turned branch is determined by the location of the lesion, which may be in the angle of the sole, bars, frog sulci or frog (◆ fig. 16.47). The bar(s) should be slightly flattened at the ground surface.

THREE-QUARTER-BAR SHOE

The *three-quarter-bar shoe* is a straight-bar shoe with an open section at one branch. This horseshoe is used to remove direct pressure from the corn area and quarter cracks. This type of horseshoe is more stable than the three-quarter horseshoe and protects the palmar/plantar area of the hoof as well (Martinelli and Ferrie, 1998) (see ◆ fig. 13.10e).

THREE-QUARTER HORSESHOE

The *three-quarter horseshoe* is a horseshoe with a short branch on one side. This horseshoe is used to relieve pressure from the quarters and heels in cases of quarter cracks (Russell, 1878), heel cracks, corns and avulsions

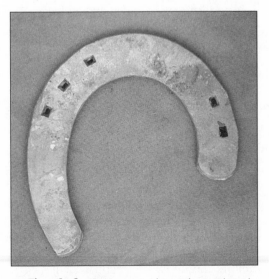

◆ **Fig. 16.48.** Three-quarter horseshoe. (Photo by author)

injuries (◆ fig. 16.48). The horseshoe should not be used in horses that work or are kept outdoors in rocky environments.

 ## NAVICULAR DISEASE

Navicular disease is a foot disorder characterized by decreased performance, gait alteration and lameness. The disease is caused by degenerative changes in the navicular bone and is a major cause of chronic forelimb lameness in horses (Colles, 1982; Black, 1992). Navicular disease is common in Quarter Horses (Graham in DeWitt, 1970), and in high performance horses such as racing, barrel and jumping horses. Young horses and horses that have not been worked can be affected (Diehl and Ueltschi, 1981). In one study, horses between 4 and 17 years of age were affected (Østblom et al., 1984a).

Colahan (1994b) recommended using the term "navicular syndrome" to describe disorders with similar signs as navicular disease; these lameness conditions are characterized by *chronic heel pain*, such as can be observed in cases of under-run heels or sheared heels. More recently, Rijkenhuizen (2006) recommended the use of the term *palmar foot syndrome* to describe a variety of pathological lesions that may be identified in horses with palmar foot pain; such lesions may involve the navicular bone, DDFT, navicular bursa and other structures.

Wright (1993) investigated the clinical features of navicular disease in 118 cases. Most of the horses examined were poor to moderate quality athletes. The development of the disease in these horses may have been related to conformation and management factors. Williams (2001) proposed that some cases might develop as a result of inherent abnormal gait pattern. Factors involved in the development of the disease include conformational abnormalities (Østblom et al., 1982) and genetic predisposition (Rooney, 1974a). Many cases of navicular disease are related to poor hoof conformation, poor trimming (Turner, 1986a) and shoeing practices (Colles, 1982;

Turner, 1986a, Turner 1986b). High ratio of body weight to foot size is a common problem associated with navicular disease, especially in Quarter Horses (Beeman, 1985). The use of horses for athletic activities that are unnatural to their biomechanical structure could be a major contributing factor for development of the disease.

Development of Navicular Disease

Navicular disease may develop as a result of one or a combination of the following predisposing factors: long-toe low heels (broken back foot axis) (Østblom et. al.1982; Østblom 1984a; Moyer, 1979; Leach, 1983a; Rooney, 1974a), narrow feet, contracted heels, underrun heels, asymmetric feet, short shoes, uneven weight distribution (Østblom et al. 1984), unbalanced hooves (Østblom, 1984), small feet (Beeman, 1985), hard ground (Rooney, 1974a), straight pasterns, and toe grabs (Forssell, 1943). Horses with collapsed heels are susceptible to navicular disease due to the increased load on the navicular bone from the DDFT (Wright, 1993b). These factors may lead to development of the disease by increasing fetlock dorsiflextion, increasing breakover time, and increasing concussion forces within the foot.

During locomotion there is a delay in breakover time in feet with broken back foot axis; consequently, the fetlock become overdorsiflexed during the final phase of breakover. This leads to sustained forces of compression against the flexor surface of the bone (Pool et al., 1989), and to abnormal friction and vibration between the DDFT and navicular bone (Rooney, 1974a). Other factors that can cause similar effects include those that prevent cutting into the ground. These may include horseshoes, hard ground, toe grabs and calks. Another predisposing factor is lack of palmar support that may occur with short horseshoes or beveled-heel horseshoes.

As the disease progresses, the flexor surface of the navicular bone may become eroded, and adhesions between the bone and tendon may develop. In some cases, the bone may fracture (Baxter et al., 1995). The palmar area of the foot becomes painful and the horse begins to land toe first, the stride become shorter and stiff, and the horse may stumble; lameness is commonly more pronounced the day after working with pointing of the affected foot (Leach, 1986a). Wilson et al. (2001) indicated that the changes in landing patterns are accompanied by increased compressive forces on the navicular bone early in the stance phase, and this can complicate the condition further. The alteration in the landing pattern causes an increased wear at the toe wall and increased growth of the heels. The decreased weight placement on the palmar aspect of the foot interferes with normal hoof expansion, and as a result, the heels begun to contract. Hoof contraction results in upright quarters and heels that amplify concussive forces and worsen the condition. The disease is frequently accompanied by a small, narrow, atrophied frog with thrush at the central sulcus (Anderson, 1992).

Horses with navicular disease respond to hoof testers applied to the back third of the frog. Lameness is typically mild to moderate and is more pronounced when the horse is trotted in circles (Wright, 1993). X-ray examination is part of the diagnostic procedure of navicular disease. In order to obtain proper radiographs, the horseshoes are removed, the sole and frog are trimmed and all flakes and crevices are removed. Prior to radiography, the frog sulci are packed with Play-Doh that prevents the appearance of artifacts on the X-ray film. The hoof wall is not trimmed unless requested by the owner/trainer and the horseshoes are replaced using the old nail holes.

Prevention of Navicular Disease

The various methods used for treatment of navicular disease do not resolve the pathological changes of the disease (Wright, 1993). In a recent review, Rijkenhuizen (2006) indicated that *prevention* is probably the key for controlling the disease. Prevention of navicular disease should include proper selection of horses, careful monitoring of workload, maintenance of optimal fit and weight, and proper hoof care management. The higher incidence of the disease in certain breeds of horses is highly suggestive of a genetic component, thus selective breeding for horses with better quality feet should be a primary goal, and should include the introduction of horses with superior hoof quality. In Holland, a breeding selection program implemented by the Dutch Warmblood Studbook resulted in reduction of the incidence of the disease (van den Belt et al., 2003). Horse owners should be aware of the relationship between type of activity and development of navicular disease, and the poor prognosis of this disease.

Proper foot management should include trimming and shoeing the horse at the proper intervals and careful balancing of the feet. Horses with stumpy pasterns may benefit from increased hoof angle that creates a broken forward foot axis, which increases the springing action to the fetlock. Horses with small hooves can be shod with thick pads or with plastic glue-on shoes that increase the functional size of the hoof and reduce concussion. Development of long-toe low-heels conformation during the shoeing interval can be minimized by shortening the shoeing interval and by increasing the hoof angle slightly when the hooves are trimmed.

Farriery of Navicular Disease

Farriery of navicular disease is aimed at reducing abnormal forces between the navicular bone and the flexor tendon, and reducing concussion. The underlying cause of the disease should be investigated and treated when possible. Farriery principles of navicular disease include balancing the feet, raising the heels, and providing palmar support to the foot. Cases of navicular disease accompanied with long-toe low-heels should be trimmed to establish proper foot axis. Raising the heels reduces the tension from the DDFT; therefore, less pressure is applied against the navicular bone (Moyer, 1981; Willemen, 1999). Increasing palmar support distributes the concussion forces over a larger area and protects the foot. This effect can be enhanced with the use of a cushioning pad.

Turner (1986) indicated that increasing the hoof angle by 2° to 4° might not have an effect on the flexor tendon in horses with normal hoof angle. Østblom (1984) and Østblom et al. (1984) indicated that raising the heels increases the load on the palmar area of the foot and the heels are rarely built up. Horn production may be stimulated by feed supplement consisting of a mixture of sulfurated amino acids, minerals and biotin (Østblom et al., 1984).

Changing the hoof angle in chronic cases that develop short toe and high heels may be difficult, as lowering the heels increases the tension in the flexor tendon and places excessive pressure on the navicular bone. In these cases, the heels should be trimmed and then raised again with a horseshoe and wedge pad; this prevents excessive tension in the DDFT, provides a larger hoof contact area, and encourages expansion of the hoof. Cases that are accompanied by thrush and infected frog should be debrided and treated with pine tar.

Horseshoes used for treatment of navicular disease include plain horseshoe and wedge pad, wedged horseshoe, bar shoe, rolled-toe shoe and rocker-toe shoe. Application of a half-round horseshoe with a squared toe and wedge pad can improve the gait of the horse (see ◆ fig. 16.55). The wedge pad reduces tension from the DDFT and absorbs some of the concussion that is transmitted to the navicular bone, whereas the half-round horseshoe and square toe reduce the hoof lever arm and ease breaking over. An opening may be made in the center of the pad; a connecting bar, 5.0 cm wide should be left in the pad to protect the palmar aspect of the foot. Gnegy (2003) indicated that pads prevent hoof wall expansion and inhibit the function of the hoof capsule. He recommended raising the heels by welding 10 mm heel lifts at the ground surface of the horseshoe branches.

Other types of horseshoes used in the treatment of navicular disease include aluminum wedged horseshoe (Anderson 1989), aluminum wedged egg-bar shoe, navicular egg-bar shoe (Miller 1994), and a horseshoe fitted with a bar-wedge pad (Moyer 1981). Moyer (1983) recommended the use of a

horseshoe with rolled toe, whereas in Standardbreds that are shod with relatively thin
horseshoes, he recommended squaring the
toe. Schoonover et al. (2005) showed that
horses fitted with aluminum wide-web
wedged horseshoes began to use the affected
limbs significantly better 14 days following
shoeing; the horseshoes were fitted full, and
the heels were extended in order to provide
palmar support. More horseshoe types that
have been described include egg-bar shoe
(Adams 1974; Østblom, 1984; Østblom et al.
1984), egg-bar shoe with elevated heels (Layton, 1965) and glue-on shoe (Moyer, 1980). A
heart-bar shoe may be used in cases where
additional protection to the frog area is
required. Østblom et al. (1984) described the
application of egg-bar shoes on a group of
horses diagnosed with navicular disease. The
heels were not raised and the horseshoes
were made with a rolled toe, toe clip, and
three nail holes on each side. The last nail
hole was placed dorsal to the widest part of
the horseshoe. The horseshoe was fitted full
and with adequate palmar support. The application of the horseshoe resulted in some
relief of pain and the expansion of previously
contracted hooves. Dyson and Marks (2003)
recommended that horses with profound
pathologic changes in the navicular bone be
shod with a bar-shoe with the breakover point
set under the toe. The hoof angle should be
increased until the DDFT becomes less tense
than both the SDFT and SL; the amount of
tension is determined while the opposite leg
is held up. Regardless of the type of horseshoes used, an adaptation period of two to
three weeks may be required before pain
relief is achieved (Schoonover et al., 2005).

WEDGE PADS

Wedge pads are made from plastic or rubber
and are available in 2° and 3°. The wedge pad
is commonly used to increase the hoof angle.
In addition, the wedge pad reduces concussion, increases palmar/plantar support, protects the heel region and relieves tension
from the flexor tendons and suspensory ligament (◆ fig. 16.49). The wedge pad is com-

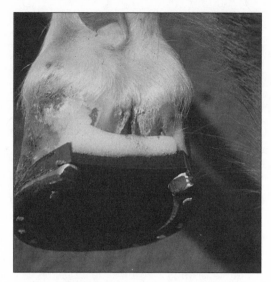

◆ **Fig. 16.49.** Wedge pad. A rectangular piece of
sponge was used instead of oakum. (Photo by
author.)

monly used in the treatment of navicular disease. Turner and Malone (1997) described the
application of wedge pads in the treatment of
navicular bone fractures. Wedge pads may
also be used in chronic laminitis, long-toe
low-heel, under-run heels and clubfoot. In
certain cases, the hoof angle may be lowered
and then raised again with a wedge pad.
Other applications of wedge pads include
shoeing the healthy opposite limb in order to
prevent supporting limb complications, and
raising the heel in pastern subluxation of the
hind limb. Wedge pads may be combined
with the application of a lower limb splint in
order to relieve tension from the suspensory
apparatus.

The height of the hoof can be modified by
shifting the position of the pad forward or
backward. Thicker pads absorb shock more
efficiently and are more suitable for navicular
disease cases. The wedge pad may be used to
correct medial–lateral imbalance caused by
excessive wear at one side of the bearing surface. In this case, the pad is held on the hoof
with the horseshoe over it, and the pad is
rotated until the desired position is obtained.
The pad is connected to the horseshoe and is
cut around the horseshoe outline.

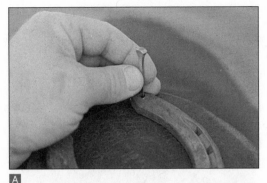

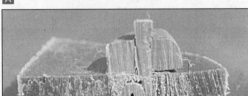

◆ **Fig. 16.50.** Connecting a wedge pad to the horseshoe. A. A 4 mm hole is drilled at the ends of the horseshoe branches. The horseshoe is placed against the pad over the anvil surface. A horseshoe nail held with the tapered side toward the outside of the horseshoe is driven into the pad with a rapid stroke of the hammer. B. Cross section of the horseshoe and pad show how the horseshoe nail recoils on itself (when it hits the anvil) and becomes firmly attached to the pad.

In order to prevent collapse of the pad and accumulation of sand and gravel between the sole and pad, firm attachment between the horseshoe and pad is important. This is achieved by using horseshoe nails to connect the pad (◆ fig. 16.50). Prior to application of the horseshoe, the solar area is packed with pine tar and oakum. Alternatively, the center of the pad may be cut open to permit cleaning the sole.

ROLLED-TOE HORSESHOE

The *rolled-toe horseshoe* is a horseshoe with a round profile at the toe-ground surface, similar to the naturally worn horseshoe. This profile provides less stress, and more natural breakover (Blombach, 1994; Martinelli and Ferrie, 1998) (◆ fig. 16.51).

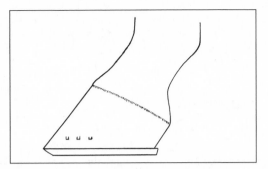

◆ **Fig. 16.51.** Rolled-toe horseshoe, side view, schematic illustration.

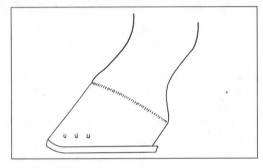

◆ **Fig. 16.52.** Rocker-toe horseshoe, side view, schematic illustration.

Rolled-toe horseshoes are used in cases of navicular disease to ease breakover (Moyer, 1990). This horseshoe may be applied to horses with orthopedic disorders above the foot in order to make the horse more comfortable.

ROCKER-TOE HORSESHOE

The *rocker-toe horseshoe* has a toe-ground surface with a rounded profile similar to the rolled-toe horseshoe but the toe is turned upward (◆ fig. 16.52). The horseshoe allows the foot to breakover with smoother action (Koepisch, 1998b). The rocker-toe horseshoe is used in cases of navicular disease, chronic laminitis, and stumbling. The rocker-toe promotes easier breakover by shortening the hoof lever arm. The horseshoe may be applied to hooves with missing toe wall by using side clips to stabilize the hoof (Helms et al., 1994).

A good fit between the hoof and horseshoe curvature should be achieved by careful trimming of the toe wall. Inappropriate fitting of the horseshoe or its application to horses with thin sole could result in bruised sole and lameness.

HALF-ROUND HORSESHOE

The *half-round horseshoe* is used mostly on the forelimbs. The horseshoe can be forged from round bar stock on a swedge block. The round profile of this horseshoe is similar to that of a worn horseshoe, which allows the limb a more natural motion and reduces fatigue caused by delay in breakover (Sparks, 1970). Hill and Klimesh (1989) indicated that the half-round horseshoe allows the horse's foot to break over easily in any direction.

The horseshoe is commercially available in web sizes of ½", 5/8" and ¾". The weight of the half-round horseshoe is about 20 percent less than that of a regular horseshoe with similar web and thickness.

The half-round horseshoe is commonly used on the forelimbs of Standardbred race-horses, and in horses with accidental limb contact problems. The horseshoe is suitable for various types of lameness problems such as navicular disease, collateral ligament desmitis and orthopedic disorders above the foot (page 240), and it is an excellent horseshoe for healthy horses as well (◆ fig. 16.53). The half-round horseshoe is commonly used with a wedge pad for treatment of navicular disease. Light half-round horseshoes are suitable for foals and for horses with thin hoof wall. The horseshoe can be attached with relatively small horseshoe nails; clips can be added to the horseshoe by welding 15 mm square sections of iron, 3 mm thick, at the desired location, and rounding the ends of the clips with a grinder. Modifications of the half-round horseshoe include squaring the toe, reversing the horseshoe, forming a bar shoe, and a tip shoe.

WEDGED EGG–BAR SHOE

The *wedged egg-bar shoe* is an egg-bar shoe that is wedged from the heel toward the toe. The horseshoe is used to lift the heels and provide

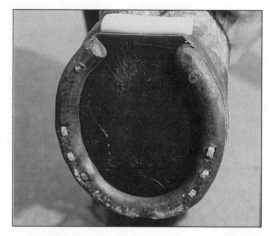

◆ **Fig. 16.53.** Half-round horseshoe and a wedge pad. (Photo by author.)

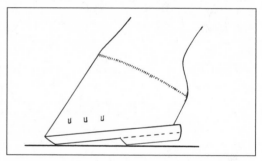

◆ **Fig. 16.54.** Navicular egg-bar shoe, side view, schematic illustration.

palmar/plantar support (Martinalli and Ferrie, 1998). Wedged egg-bar shoes are used in cases of long-toe low- heels, under-run heels and navicular disease. A 3° wedged aluminum horseshoe is commercially available.

NAVICULAR EGG-BAR SHOE

The *navicular egg-bar shoe* was described by Miller (1994) as a "rolled toe horseshoe fitted with elongated calks" (◆ fig. 16.54). Historically, application of the horseshoe to horses with navicular disease resulted in improvement, or retarding of the usual progress of the disease, but the exact function of the horseshoe is not clear. An aluminum navicular egg-bar shoe is commercially available.

ACCIDENTAL LIMBS CONTACT

FOOT AND LIMB INJURIES CAUSED BY *accidental limbs contact* are common. Accidental limbs contact with the fore hoof striking the hind limb of the same side is observed in Standardbred trotters. The hoof may contact the hind leg at various levels; contact at the level of the coronary band is termed *scalping*, and it is common at the toe area (Simpson, 1968). Accidental contact of the hind hoof against the forelimb of the same side is observed during trot, and it is termed *overreaching*. Overreaching may result in injuries to the bulbs of the heels and medial aspect of the coronary band, as well as resulting in lost horseshoes (Shively, 1982). *Forging* is similar to overreaching but the contact is lower with hind hoof contacting the solar area of the foreleg (Simpson, 1968; Shively, 1982); both conditions are commonly observed in horses with long legs and a short back. Accidental limb contact of the hind hoof against the foreleg of the opposite side is observed in Standardbred pacers and is termed *cross firing*. Cross firing may result in injuries to the medial aspect of the coronary band (Simpson, 1968). *Interference* describes the striking of a limb by the opposite hoof (Shively, 1982), and it is observed more commonly in horses with toeing-out conformation. Trauma to the palmar area of the cannon bone, caused by interference, can lead to development of *splints* or small bony protrusions adjacent to the splint bones.

Accidental limb contact may result in bruising and lacerations of the coronary band and bulbs of the heels, and injuries to higher structures such as the sesamoid bones and flexor tendons. Moyer (1983) indicated that coronary band injuries are common in Standardbred horses. The underlying cause that leads to abnormal limb contact should be carefully investigated and corrected if possible. Various types of horseshoes and horseshoe adjuncts are commonly used in an attempt to correct accidental limb contact. These methods do not correct all problems and some may even strain the limb.

Prevention of Accidental Limb Contact

The basic principles for correction of accidental limb contact in trotting horses include increasing the motion of the forelegs and slowing the hind legs. The technique (Simpson, 1968) includes shoeing the fore hooves with half-round horseshoes and the hind hooves with full swedged horseshoes. Swedged horseshoes produce more friction with the ground and strain the limb. Another method includes shoeing the fore hooves with half-round horseshoes and the hind hooves with square-toed horseshoes. In addition, the hoof angle in the hind hooves is lowered by 2° to 3° to slow the breakover time. The horseshoes are set back in order to reduce the possibility of the forelegs being hit by the metal horseshoe. Some horses can be fitted with plain horseshoes on the hind limbs. Horses that continue to overreach may be shod with tip shoes or spooned-heels horseshoes in the fore hooves, and fitted with protective boots.

Prevention of interference injuries includes hot rasping the medial aspect of the horseshoe in order to under set it; this prevent the metal from contacting the opposite limb. In addition the limbs should be protected with appropriate boots such as bell boots, rubber scalpers, and shin boots (Simpson, 1968; O'Brien, 1968).

The use of horseshoe adjuncts in order to prevent accidental limb contact should be avoided. These modifications increase friction and jarring on the foot, which places abnormal strain on the limb.

SQUARE-TOED HORSESHOE

The *square-toed horseshoe* is a horseshoe with a toe that has been straightened perpendicular to the long axis of the horseshoe. The toe may be squared over the anvil's horn or with a squaring block; nearly every type of horseshoe can be squared (Klimesh, 1997) (◆ fig. 16.55). The squared toe encourages the foot to breakover at the center of the foot. This horseshoe is used in horses with limb deviations such as toeing-out in order to encourage

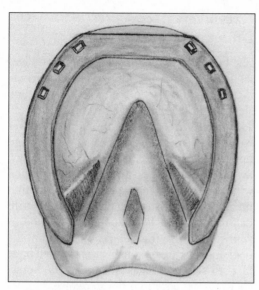

◆ **Fig. 16.55.** Square-toed horseshoe, solar view. The toe wall hangs over the horseshoe.

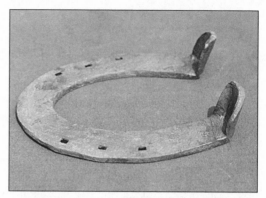

◆ **Fig. 16.56.** Spooned-heels horseshoe. (Photo by author.)

straight limb motion. In addition, the horseshoe is used on the hind limb in order to prevent damage to the front feet caused by overreaching (Klimesh, 1997; Blombach, 1994). The forelimbs may be fitted with a square toe horseshoe in cases of chronic laminitis and navicular disease in order to reduce the hoof lever arm; a similar effect may be achieved with a reversed horseshoe. For treatment of navicular disease, the horseshoe may be fitted with a wedge pad. In cases of chronic laminitis, a space between the toe wall and the hoof surface of the horseshoe should be made in order to relieve pressure from the toe wall and sole.

SPOONED-HEELS HORSESHOE

The *spooned-heels horseshoe* is a horseshoe with long branches bent to fit the angle of the heel. The branches are bent against the tip of the anvil's horn into a "spoon" shape. This horseshoe reduces the change of the front horseshoes being *sprung*, or lost, by overreaching (Adams, 1974) (◆ fig.16.56).

The spooned-heels horseshoe is sometimes used in cases of *shoe boil* to reduce irritation to the elbow.

PROTECTIVE BOOTS

Various types of *protective boots* are available for protection of the foot and limb. O'Brien (1968) described the application of *grab boots* and *bell boots* for protection against overreaching injuries and pulling of horseshoes. He recommended the application of *rubber scalpers* to pacers that crossfire.

The bell boot provides protection to the coronary band and bulbs of the heels; these boots are commonly used in Standardbred horses, jumpers, hunters and in Western agility sports. Bell boots should be fitted to horses that are being transported in order to prevent injuries caused by the horse treading on itself. Heavy leather bell boots should be used on horses shod with horseshoes fitted with studs, such as police horses. Preferably, horseshoe studs should be removed and the holes fitted with stud guards. *Shipping boots* that provide protection to the lower limb are also available. Splints can be prevented by keeping the horse barefoot when possible, shortening and filing smooth the horseshoe branches', avoiding the use of caulks and studs, and application of *splint boots* over the cannon bones area.

 FOOT LACERATIONS

Foot lacerations ARE COMMONLY CAUSED BY WIRE cuts, protruding metal objects and accidental

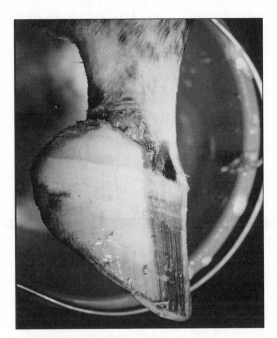

◆ **Fig. 16.57.** Deep foot laceration. (Photo by author.)

limb contact; the injury commonly involves the bulbs of the heels and the coronary band, but deeper structures may be involved. Laceration injuries to the coronary band may result in hoof wall defect and development of quittor (Miller and Robertson, 1943). Injuries to the coronary band may be caused by horseshoe studs, heel calks, toe grabs, barbed wires or wood splinters. Stepping with one leg on the opposite foot is called *tread*. Tread injuries may result during transportation of horses, and can be very extensive if the horseshoes are fitted with horseshoe studs. These injuries are frequently found on the dorsal or medial aspects of the hind feet (Miller and Robertson, 1943). Heel bulb laceration may result from walking on sharp stones. Another cause includes excessive use of hobbles (Back, 1959).

Foot lacerations may involve the coronary dermis, as well as deeper structures, including the lateral cartilages, digital cushion, collateral ligaments, tendons, blood vessels and nerves (Fessler, 1989) (◆ fig. 16.57). Foot lacerations may be accompanied by severe hemorrhage and lameness. Neglecting to treat these injuries can result in excessive granulation tissue in the foot region that interferes with healing (Fessler, 1971a). Damage to the coronary dermis could result in development of chronic hoof wall defect (Booth and Knottenbelt, 1999). Lacerations at the heel bulb area typically heal without complications unless the DIP joint is involved (Janicek et al., 2005).

Treatment of hoof wall lacerations includes trimming the hoof to minimize shearing forces on the hoof capsule, clipping, and aseptic preparation of the digit. The loose section should be stepped in order to remove direct ground pressure from it. The wound is carefully debrided and all loose and undermined horn is removed; this may include the entire section that is loose, but the coronary dermis should be preserved. Whenever possible, the wound margins should be aligned precisely and sutured; sutures should not penetrate the coronary dermis as this may interfere with healing. Careful apposition of the wound margins is important in order to minimize the development of hoof wall defect (Fessler, 1971a). Following suturing, the foot is immobilized with a distal limb cast (Booth and Knottenbelt, 1999; Dabareiner et al., 2004). Mild cases may be fitted with a foot bandage. Dabareiner et al. (2004) indicated that immobilization of the foot in a cast for treatment of heel bulb laceration is an effective method, and may have better cosmetic outcome compared to bandaging alone.

Healing of coronary band lacerations may be followed by development of superficial or deep permanent hoof wall crack. Farriery of these cases depends on the type and location of the crack and the horse's workload (page 179).

Prevention of foot lacerations is extremely important. Major damage to the foot can be prevented by keeping horses in a safe environment, application of protective boots during riding, removal of horseshoe studs during transportation and application of heavy *shipping boots*. The use of horseshoe adjuncts such as toe grabs, studs and trailers should be avoided.

Distal Limb Cast

A *distal limb cast* (foot cast) may be applied to the foot following surgical procedures on foot lacerations (Fessler, 1971b; Steckel and Fessler, 1983; Blackford et al., 1994), quittor, and reconstructive surgery (Booth and Knottenbelt, 1999). The cast immobilizes and protects the foot, reduces healing time and improves the functional and cosmetic outcome of the injury (Bramlage et al., 1991; Booth and Knottenbelt, 1999; Smith, 1993; Dabareiner et al., 2004). The distal cast encases the hoof and extends to the level of the proximal pastern.

Booth and Knottenbelt (1999) described the application of a distal limb cast in the recumbent horse. They recommended the use of a cast made from a resin-impregnated fiberglass tape combined with padding foam. Prior to application of the cast, the hoof is trimmed, and two holes, 2 to 3 mm in diameter are drilled through the distal toe wall. Strong metal wire is inserted into the holes and is connected to a handle that is used to pull the digit into full extension while the cast is being applied. A distal limb cast may be applied to a standing horse; the cast is applied with the limb elevated off the ground. In order to improve fitting and prevent cast sores, the limb should be placed on the ground prior to curing of the fiberglass so the horse will bear weight on it (Dabareiner et al., 2004).

A walking bar may be incorporated in the palmar/plantar aspect of the cast in order to protect it when the horse is hand walked. The bar can be made from 5 x 25 mm iron bar stock bent into a rectangle with one open side. The height of the opposite limb should be raised to the same level as the casted limb; a horseshoe, a horseshoe and thick flat pad, or a frog support pad may be used for that (Booth and Knottenbelt, 1999). Another method for raising the opposite limb includes

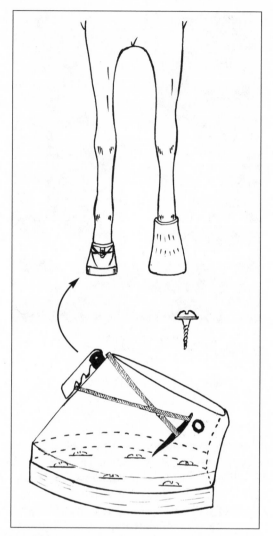

◆ **Fig. 16.58.** Elevated hoof boot, schematic illustrations. A wooden board cut to fit the outline of the boot is connected to the bottom of the boot with round head wood screws.
(After Stokes M. et al. 1998.)

the use of an elevated boot (Stokes et al., 1998) (◆ fig. 16.58).

The cast is removed with an oscillating cutter saw by making a cut on each side of it. In some cases, the two cut halves may be used as a splint by reapplying them to the foot with elastic adhesive tape (Booth and Knottenbelt, 1999).

🐾 HOOF WALL AVULSIONS

Hoof wall avulsions OR CORONARY BAND avulsions are caused by severe laceration injuries that involve the pastern and hoof wall, or by tearing of hoof wall section from the distal end. In both cases, a section of hoof wall becomes loose or detached. Hoof wall avulsions may result from wire cuts and protruding objects. Tearing of the hoof wall may result from overgrown hooves, excessive moisture that weakens the horn, quarter cracks, and false quarter (◆ fig. 16.59). Strong impact against uneven ground or a stone can result in hoof wall avulsion, most commonly at the quarters area. Hoof wall avulsions involving the distal part of the hoof may be superficial and cause no lameness. In more severe cases, the injured hoof wall may remain loosely attached to the laminae or hang from coronary band. The horse becomes acutely lame and there may be a profound bleeding. Hoof wall avulsions involving the coronary band may damage the coronary dermis and disrupt germinal cells; this may result in development of hoof wall crack, or less often, in a horn spur (Markel et al., 1987; Fessler, 1971a) (see below).

Treatment of hoof wall avulsions includes trimming the hoof, and stepping the bearing surface of the hoof wall at the avulsed section in order to remove pressure from it. Once this is done, the degree of damage is assessed. The limb is clipped and aseptically prepared from the fetlock distally (Fessler, 1989). Necrotic or contaminated tissue is removed, and undermined horn and tissue recesses, which might serve to hide foreign bodies and trap exudative material, are debrided (Fessler, 1971a; Steckel and Fessler, 1983; Fessler, 1989). This may require the removal of the entire section of avulsed hoof wall. The coronary dermis should be left intact. Avulsions injuries that involve the pastern are sutured; no suture material should penetrate the coronary dermis (Fessler, 1971a). The margins of the wound should be aligned precisely (Honnas et al.,

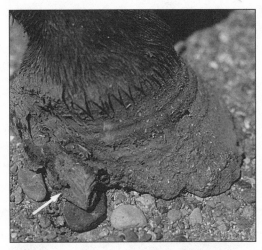

◆ **Fig. 16.59.** Partial hoof wall avulsion at the quarter (arrow) caused by excessive moisture and hoof overgrowth. (Photo by author.)

1988d) in order to maintain parallel hoof wall growth. Misalignment of the wound margins may result in development of permanent hoof wall crack or formation of false quarter. Severe cases should be placed in a distal limb cast. Moderate cases are treated with antibiotic-impregnated dressing applied to the wound surface. Then a pressure bandage that controls bleeding is applied. The bandage is changed daily until secretion decreases and the dermis regenerates. The bandage should be protected with a plastic boot or a waterproof duct tape (Steckel and Fessler, 1983). The hoof may be shod with a protective horseshoe following debridement or several days later.

Farriery of hoof wall avulsion cases includes the application of wide-web egg-bar shoe that provide protection and stability to the foot (◆ fig. 16.60). A z-bar shoe (Gregory, 2004a; Gregory, 2004b) (◆ see fig.13.10d) or a three-quarter horseshoe may be applied to cases with superficial involvement of the quarters or heels area. Following shoeing, the wound should be protected with a foot bandage and the horse kept in a well-bedded stable.

Once the wound is dry and cornified (this may take two to three weeks from the time of the initial injury), the missing hoof wall sec-

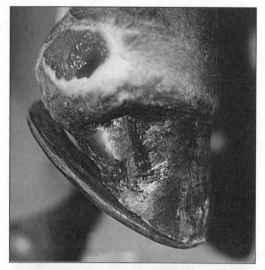

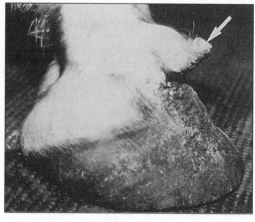

◆ **Fig. 16.61.** Horn spur (arrow). (Reprinted by permission from Coffman et. al.1970, fig.2.)

Horn Spur

A *horn spur* is characterized by abnormal horn growth at the coronary band that commonly grows at a right angle to the hoof wall (◆ fig. 16.61). Horn spur may develop from avulsion injuries that involve the coronary band, followed by disruption to germinal cells that result in abnormal horn growth and scar formation. The lesion is commonly accompanied by permanent hoof wall crack. Markel et al. (1987) described the surgical reconstruction of chronic coronary band avulsion (horn spurs) in three horses. The technique included the removal of fibrous scar tissue in order to provide a bed for replacement of the avulsed segment, suturing the avulsed segment to the hoof wall, and immobilization of the foot.

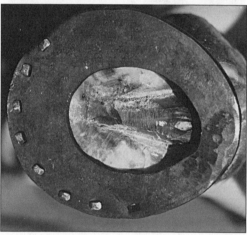

◆ **Fig. 16.60.** Wide-web egg-bar shoe used to protect avulsion injury at the quarter and heel. Lateral and solar view. Note that horseshoe nails were placed at the toe wall. (Photos by author.)

tion can be reconstructed with acrylic repair material. Acrylic remodeling is most helpful for partial avulsions in which the remaining normal hoof contributes to weight bearing (Fessler, 1971a). Preparation of the area for reconstruction includes undercutting the edges of the defect to increase the strength of the repair, and application of fabric material that forms a scaffold for the repair (Moyer, 1981; Moyer and Sigafoos, 1991).

COMPLETE HOOF LOSS

Complete hoof loss MAY RESULT FROM SEVERE laminitis, digital necrosis (a complication following severing of the palmar digital nerves) (Taylor and Vaughan, 1980), chronic selenosis, and foot gangrene (Pollitt, 1995) (◆ fig. 16.62). A firmly attached horseshoe being caught up (snagged) during motion may cause accidental detachment of the hoof.

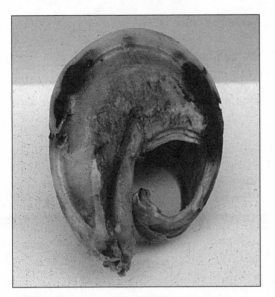

◆ **Fig. 16.62.** Complete hoof loss caused by severe laminitis. (Photo by author.)

Although the hoof has a regenerative capacity, extensive injuries may result in complications such as septic pedal osteitis, abnormal horn growth, and supporting limb laminitis. The new hoof may be malformed and unmatched with the opposite foot (Fessler, 1971a).

Treatment of Hoof Capsule Loss

Emergency treatment of hoof detachment includes wrapping the foot to protect it from further contamination and to control bleeding. A sterile bandage containing povidone-iodine ointment should be applied over the lesion and covered with a heavy foot bandage. Under field conditions, the lesion may be covered with pure pine tar and bandage material.

Treatment of hoof detachment includes debridement and removal of loose and infected tissue. The lesion is covered with sterile gauze soaked in povidone-iodine solution and a foot bandage is applied. The bandage is changed daily and an antibiotic dressing is applied; once the lesion becomes cornified and there are no secretions, the interval of bandaging can be increased. It may take 8 to 12 months for healing to be completed. During this period, the horse should be kept in a well-bedded stable and placed periodically in a sling. The opposite limb should be fitted with a frog support pad or a heart-bar shoe; all limbs should be kept in support bandages.

The prognosis for cases caused by laminitis is poor due to lack of circulation and accompanying necrosis. Some cases of laminitis are treated by complete resection of the hoof. These cases require constant nursing care until the new hoof grows (Chapman and Platt, 1994). Hooves affected by chronic selenosis are displaced from beneath by growth of new horn (Raisebeck, 2000).

HOOF CAPSULE CRACKS

Hoof capsule cracks ARE A COMMON FOOT disorder that can result in lameness and disuse of the horse. Cracks may develop at various parts on the hoof capsule, including the wall, bars and sole. Hoof wall cracks are classified according to the location of the crack into *toe, quarter* and *heel cracks.* The position of the crack is classify as *distal crack* for cracks related to the margins of the hoof wall, and *proximal cracks* for cracks related the coronary band; both types are *incomplete wall cracks,* whereas a crack that extends throughout the entire length of the hoof wall is a *complete wall crack.* Hoof wall cracks that involve the outer layer of horn are called *superficial cracks,* whereas *deep cracks* extend to the dermis. *Bar cracks* are cracks that develop across the bars, and they may be superficial or deep. Other types of hoof capsule cracks include sole cracks, clefts, splits, and cracks caused by chronic selenosis.

Hoof wall cracks may result from a disease or injury to the foot that weakens the hoof wall, poor hoof conformation, environmental factors and abnormal forces placed on the hoof capsule. Predisposing factors for hoof wall cracks are numerous and include injury to the coronary dermis (Johnson, 1972; Merillate, 1911; Evanse et al., 1966), brittle horn, contracted hooves and conformation faults (Merillat, 1911), sheared heels (Blackford et al.,

1991), distortion of the coronary band (Snow and Birdsall, 1990), laminitis (Moyer and Sigafoos, 1993), lack of elasticity to the horn, weak hooves, overloading part of the hoof, nailing too far back, uneven foot and long toe (Evans et al., 1966), accidental limb contact (Johnson, 1972), thrush, abscess migration, under-run heels and thin hoof wall. In addition, an excessively wet or dry environment may result in development of hoof wall cracks. Wounds and lacerations that disrupt the normal keratinization process at the coronary band commonly cause hoof wall cracks originating from the coronary band. Some hoof wall cracks may develop from abnormal shear forces in this area.

Hoof wall cracks located near the solar margins of the hoof wall are commonly the result of poor hoof care, excessive hoof length, improper trimming and shoeing, and hooves that are disproportionately small. Imbalance may create abnormal impact and concussion that can lead to hoof wall failure (Blackford et al., 1991).

Rooney (1974a) indicated that the forces placed on the hoof wall tend to follow the orientation of the horn tubules and this predisposes the hoof wall to vertical cracks. Suchorski-Tremblay et al. (2001) indicated that the possible role of shear stress in crack formation has not been investigated. "Once a crack begins to develop, the potential for further extension and separation of the defect is present because of hoof wall instability" (Stashak, 1989). Existing hoof wall cracks form an ideal site for development of thrush and gravel.

Healing of coronary band laceration is similar to healing of skin wounds and includes migration of epithelial cells from the coronary dermis from both sides of the wound; chronic infection and excessive motion interfere with this process and may result in permanent hoof wall crack (Steckel and Fessler, 1983; Fessler 1971a). Not all permanent cracks and defects cause functional impairment (Fessler, 1971a). The degree of lameness associated with a crack ranges from nonexistent to severe pain (Blackford et al., 1991; Moyer and Sigafoos, 1993). Pain may result from movement of the loose portion of the wall, inflammation and/or infection, but most hoof wall cracks are not painful (Moyer, 1980; Moyer, 1983).

The approach to treatment of hoof wall cracks depends on the type, location and depth of the crack, and the amount and type of work done by the horse. The underlying cause(s) that led to the development of the crack has to be investigated, and conditions such as under-run heel, sheared heels, wall separation, and proximal deviation of the coronary band have to be addressed (Sigafoos, 1995). Depending upon the length and location of the crack, it may take 5 to 10 months for a crack to "grow out" (Lungwitz, 1966).

Farriery Principles for Hoof Wall Cracks

The treatment approach of hoof wall cracks includes investigation of the underlying cause(s), relief of shearing forces within the hoof capsule and balancing the foot. Farriery principles includes removal of direct ground pressure from the crack by trimming the bearing surface of the wall and application of a protective horseshoe; farriery may be combined with hoof wall repair. Superficial cracks may be treated by correcting the foot imbalance, application of egg-bar shoe, and reduced workload as the only treatment (Moyer, 1980). Extensive, infected and painful cracks require more stability than a bar-shoe alone (Moyer, 1980; Moyer, 1981). In these cases, horseshoeing is combined with the application of hoof wall repair material that stabilizes and protects the hoof; the resin becomes a functional part of the hoof wall that bears weight. Failure to relieve the forces that led to the development of the crack in the first place may result in repair failure (O'Grady in Stephens, 2003).

Techniques used in hoof wall repair include debridement of the lesion, undercutting the hoof wall, lacing techniques, application of acrylic resins and synthetic fabrics, establishment of drainage, and application of protective horseshoes (see below).

Additional treatment methods described in the literature include the use of adjustable tension bands to stabilize toe and quarter cracks using an open stainless steel hose clamp held by screws across the crack (Blackford, 1991), older techniques for immobilizing hoof wall cracks include the use of horseshoe nails, brass plates or clamps placed across the cracks, and burning a transverse groove at the upper end of the crack in order to stop the spread of the crack (Merillat, 1911). These techniques usually fails to stop the formation of a complete crack (Evans et al., 1966). The use of most of these techniques has been discontinued with the development of hoof repair resins.

DEBRIDEMENT

The full depth of the crack should be debrided and opened with a hoof knife or with a hand-held motorized burr fitted with a cutting bit (Jenny et al., 1965; Moyer and Sigafoos, 1991). O'Grady (2001) recommended using a tungsten-carbide bit for exploring cracks (◆ fig. 16.63). Large cracks with undermined hoof wall may be debrided by thinning the hoof wall across the crack with a shoeing rasp, followed by exploration of the crack with a hoof knife or loop knife. Small cracks may be debrided with a narrow-bladed hoof knife or with a digging knife.

Areas affected with thrush or sub-mural abscess should be probed and debrided until healthy horn is exposed. The crack should be debrided carefully in order to prevent bleeding. Debridement of deep hoof wall cracks requires the application of regional foot anesthesia and a tourniquet. The repair should be delayed in cases that are bleeding or have infected tissue until the wound become completely dry and cornified. In selected cases, a resin may be applied by forming a drainage tract for the lesion (page 183).

UNDERCUTTING THE HOOF WALL

Undercutting the hoof wall is done following debridement of the crack in preparation for resin application. This technique includes the removal of horn beneath the defect margin in order to forms a shelf or *buttress*. This shelf holds the resin and increases the strength of the repair (Jenny et al., 1965; Evans et al., 1966) (◆ Fig. 16.64). Depending on the thickness of the hoof wall, undercutting may be performed with the end of a hoof knife blade, a loop knife, or with a motorized burr fitted with appropriate bit size. The depth of the undercut area should be 3 to 5 mm for the average size hoof. Hoof wall thickness at the heel area may not be sufficient for this procedure.

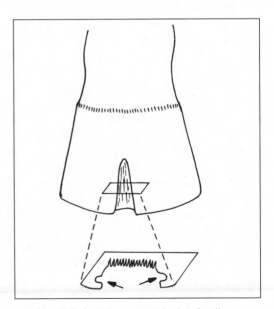

◆ **Fig. 16.64.** Undercutting the hoof wall, schematic illustration. A transverse section of a toe crack showing the undercut area (arrows).

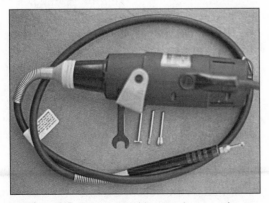

◆ **Fig. 16.63.** Motorized burr and various bits used for debridement. (Photo by author.)

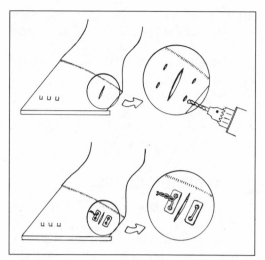

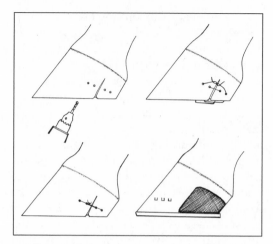

◆ **Fig. 16.65.** Stabilizing technique for incomplete proximal heel crack, schematic illustration. See text for details. (Reprinted by permission from Moyer, W. 1988, fig.2. Illustrations modified to text.)

◆ **Fig. 16.66.** Lacing technique for stabilizing a quarter crack, schematic illustration. See text for details. (Reprinted by permission from Moyer, W. and Sigafoos, R. 1991, fig. 1. Illustrations modified to text.)

LACING TECHNIQUES

Various methods of *lacing techniques* used to stabilize the hoof wall crack have been described (Moyer, 1983; Moyer and Sigafoos, 1993; Moyer and Sigafoos, 1991; Jenny et al., 1965; Evans et al., 1966; O'Grady, 2001). Lacing reduces motion and forms a scaffold for the repair material (Jenny et al., 1965; O'Grady, 2001). Moyer (1983) indicated that the procedure is important when dealing with painful, unstable and extensive cracks. Moyer (1983) described a method for stabilizing incomplete proximal heel cracks with the use of brace plates and stainless steel wire (◆ fig. 16.65). Following debridement, two holes, 2 to 3 cm apart, are drilled in the hoof wall on each side of the defect, beginning 1.5 to 2 cm from the edge and directed toward the margins of the defect. The holes are made with a 2 mm drill bit. Two rectangular brace plates with equivalent holes are placed on each side of the crack and wired together with stainless steel wire. Moyer and Sigafoos (1993) indicated that this technique is particularly important when dealing with racehorses competing on hard, fast surfaces. A similar technique was described by O'Grady (2001) and included the use of stainless steel wire and steel tabs.

Complete quarter cracks and quarter cracks with hoof wall loss may be stabilized with a synthetic multifiber material such as umbilical tape laced through predrilled holes made in the hoof wall (Moyer, 1983, Moyer and Sigafoos, 1993; Moyer and Sigafoos, 1991; Evans et al., 1966) (◆ fig. 16.66). Following debridement, two holes, 2 cm apart, are drilled in the hoof wall on each side of the defect, beginning from the bearing surface of the hoof wall toward the midregion of the defect. The holes should exit the hoof wall 2 cm and 3 cm from the crack margins. The holes are made with a 2 mm drill bit. A string of umbilical tape is placed through the holes as illustrated and the string is tightened. During the lacing procedure, the limb should be held so it bears no weight (Evans et al., 1966). The defect is repaired with 2 to 3 layers of composite and the hoof is shod with a bar shoe (see hoof capsule repair, chapter 14).

WEBBING MATERIAL

The use of *webbing material* in hoof wall repair involves the incorporation of synthetic fabrics with the acrylic repair material. The combined acrylic and webbing material adds significant strength to the repair, particularly to extensive cracks and associated hoof wall loss (Moyer, 1983). The type of fabric selected for the repair is important (Sigafoos, 1995; O'Grady, 2001b) (see composite lay-up, chapter 14).

DRAINAGE

Repair of hoof wall defects prior to cornification of the wound is possible if good *drainage* is established. Drainage allows for flushing and medicating the wound, and permits early return to work. Techniques for incorporating a drainage tract with repair of hoof wall cracks have been described (Moyer and Sigafoos, 1993; Sigafoos, 1995; O'Grady, 2001). One technique includes the application of fabric lacing, suitable for hooves with thin wall (Sigafoos, 1995) (see establishment of drainage, chapter 14).

Toe Cracks

Toe cracks may develop at the distal, proximal or along the entire length of the toe wall. The crack may be superficial or deep.

DISTAL TOE CRACKS

Predisposing factors for *distal toe cracks* include dry, brittle feet, overgrown hoof wall and trauma (Henninger and Owen, 1986). Thrush and white line disease weakens the bearing surface of the toe wall. Toe cracks are commonly caused by excessively long hooves that increase leverage on the toe wall. Initially a split appears at the toe margins; the split continues to separate and expose the white line to manure and debris, which creates an ideal environment for thrush (◆ fig. 16.67). The hoof wall is weakened further and the split continues to separate. A section of hoof wall may break loose. In some cases, the entire length of the toe wall may split. Merillate (1911) indicated that draft horses tend to develop toe cracks, especially in the hind feet, and the exact cause of these cracks is unknown. Distal toe cracks also tend to develop in pastured Thoroughbred mares kept barefoot.

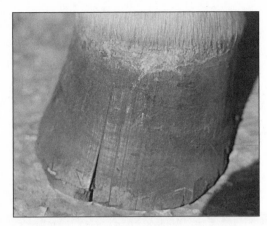

◆ **Fig. 16.67.** Distal superficial toe crack. (Photo by author.)

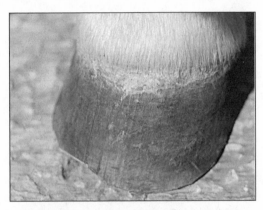

◆ **Fig. 16.68.** Distal superficial toe crack. The same case shown in the previous figure following trimming, direct pressure from the toe wall was removed by trimming an arched section at the distal toe. (Photo by author.)

Farriery of distal toe cracks includes trimming and balancing the hooves, debridement of thrush, white line disease and infection if present, removal of direct pressure from the toe wall, and stabilizing the hoof with a protective horseshoe.

Toe cracks caused by a long toe, as observed sometimes in pastured mares and yearlings, can be treated by trimming alone. The bearing surface of the toe wall should be cut to remove direct pressure from the toe wall in cases where the crack is still present following trimming; this can be achieved by cutting an arched section with half-round hoof nippers or with a hoof knife (◆ fig. 16.68). Working horses are trimmed similarly

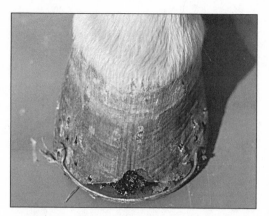

◆ **Fig. 16.69.** Application of horseshoe and side clips following debridement of superficial toe crack. (Photo by author.)

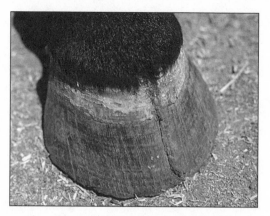

◆ **Fig. 16.70.** Complete superficial permanent toe crack that developed from a coronary band injury. (Photo by author.)

and the hoof is fitted with a regular horseshoe or a bar shoe. The horseshoe is made with two side clips positioned on each side of the crack (◆ fig. 16.69). The clips reduce hoof wall expansion during weight bearing and stabilize the crack.

Cases of deep distal toe cracks are treated by trimming the hoof and preparing it for shoeing. The crack is thoroughly debrided, all loose horn and infected tissue are removed, and the hoof is fitted with a bar shoe and side clips placed alongside the defect. Following cornification of the wound, the toe wall may be reconstructed with a hoof repair material.

PROXIMAL TOE CRACKS

Proximal toe cracks commonly develop as a result of injury to the coronary dermis. Depending on the extent of injury, the crack may be superficial or deep; the crack may extend with hoof wall growth and develop into a complete toe crack.

Farriery of superficial cracks includes the application of protective horseshoes. The crack may be laced and repaired with acrylic resin and fabric material. Once the crack approaches the hoof-bearing surface, pressure on the toe wall is reduced by cutting an arched section at the bearing surface of the toe wall as described for distal toe cracks.

Since proximal toe crack can develop into a complete permanent toe crack, prevention

of its occurrence is important. Following foot lacerations or avulsion injuries, the coronary band should be aligned carefully in order to maintain the normal direction of horn growth.

COMPLETE TOE CRACKS

Most cases of *complete toe crack* develop as a result of injury to the coronary dermis. Depending on the extent of injury, the crack may grow out or develop into a permanent superficial or deep complete toe crack (◆ fig. 16.70). Complete toe crack may result in pain caused by instability of the hoof capsule. The toe wall may open when the hoof is lifted and close when the hoof bears weight (O'Grady in Stephens, 2003).

Farriery of superficial complete toe cracks depends on the amount of load placed on the hoof. Pastured horses may be treated by trimming and removal of pressure from the bearing surface of the toe wall. An arched section is cut at the distal toe as described for distal toe cracks. In cases where the crack tends to split proximally or the horse is being worked, the hoof should be fitted with a plain horseshoe or a bar shoe with side clips placed close to the crack. The toe wall area may be reinforced with acrylic repair material combined with webbing material. Wildenstein (2004) indicated that repairing toe cracks should be done while the hoof is non-weight bearing.

This allows curing of the adhesive without movement at the crack and consequent failure. Deep complete toe cracks should be debrided and treated as a wound. Following cornification of the lesion, the defect margin is undercut and the toe wall is reconstructed. The repair may be reinforced with umbilical tape as described by Moyer and Sigafoos (1993) for repair of quarter cracks with hoof wall loss (page 182). Two to three layers of webbing material should be incorporated with the resin, and the hoof is fitted with a bar shoe and side clips.

Krpan and Crawley (1986) described a method for crack repair using sheet-metal screws placed along the sides of the defect. The screws are laced with stainless-steel wire and acrylic repair material is applied over the area; the hoof is shod with a bar shoe with side clips. Possible complications for this procedure include over-tightening the wires and penetrating the sensitive laminae with the screws.

Quarter Cracks

Quarter cracks are the most common type of hoof capsule cracks. During motion, the thin-walled quarters are placed under compressive, shearing and tearing forces, thus making this region susceptible to development of cracks. Hoof deformation with concurrent restriction of the horseshoe nails (McClinchey, 2004) may be a predisposing factor. Susceptibility to quarter crack development increases in horses with weak hoof, abnormal hoof conformation and imbalanced feet. The medial quarter is prone to crack development since it has a more upright wall and it receives higher concussion during impact (Henninger and Owen, 1986). In Standardbred racehorses, most of the incomplete quarter cracks are located in the medial quarter (Moyer, 1988c). Quarter cracks may develop from injuries caused by accidental limb contact. Stabilization of the quarters area is an important part of treatment as well as the application of straight-bar or egg-bar shoes (◆ fig. 16.71).

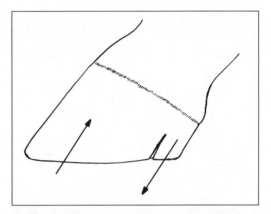

◆ **Fig. 16.71.** Quarter crack instability. Loading the hoof results in considerable movement at the hoof wall, with shearing forces (arrows) developing along the two sides of the crack.

DISTAL QUARTER CRACKS

Distal quarter cracks may be superficial or deep and may develop into a complete quarter crack if left untreated. The crack is exposed to dirt and manure and may be undermined with thrush that weakens the quarter wall further. Predisposing factors for distal quarter cracks include small hooves, poor quality hooves, long hooves, improper medial-lateral balance, excessive moisture, widening of the white line, white line disease, thin-walled hoof, under-run heels, contracted heels and sheared heels.

Distal quarter cracks may develop by a short horseshoe branch fitted close, and by leaving one heel of the hoof too high; both conditions are occasionally observed on the medial side of the same hoof. The pressure placed by the horseshoe branch on the quarter wall is sufficient to result in failure of the horn and development of a crack.

Farriery of distal quarter cracks depends on the extent of the crack and degree of activity performed by the horse. Pastured horses with superficial distal quarter cracks are trimmed, and pressure is removed from the bearing surface of the affected quarter by cutting an arched section at the distal quarter wall (◆ fig. 16.72A). The white line should be debrided and packed with pine tar. A three-quarter horseshoe may be applied to horses

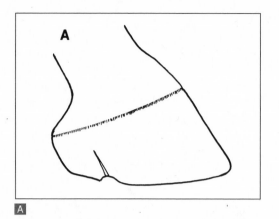

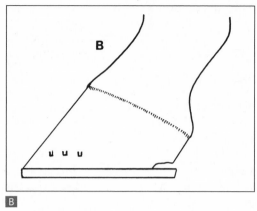

◆ **Fig. 16.72.** Relieving pressure from a distal quarter crack, schematic illustrations. A. Cutting an arched section at the bearing surface of the quarter. B. Stepping the heel and application of protective horseshoe. (Part A adapted from Russell W. 1882, fig. 26; part B adapted from *The Horseshoer* (1966), fig. 78.)

that are not working. Cracks that continue to split are trimmed as described above and the hoof is shod with a bar shoe. Horses with small feet may better tolerate a light half-round bar shoe. Deep distal quarter cracks should be debrided completely, treated as a wound until the area is dry, and cornified; the hoof wall is repaired with a composite and the hoof is shod with a straight-bar shoe or an egg-bar shoe. Application of light horseshoes such as training plates is possible, but may result in failure of the repair under strenuous work. In order to permit normal hoof expansion, the repair material should not be allowed to adhere to the horseshoe. Cases that are accompanied by flail heel should be treated by stepping the affected heel in order to remove direct pressure from it, and application of a bar shoe (*The Horseshoer*, 1966) (◆ fig. 16.72B). Alternatively, the horseshoe branch under the affected heel can be stepped (see ◆ fig. 16.46).

PROXIMAL QUARTER CRACKS

Proximal quarter cracks may be superficial or deep. The crack may develop from laceration injury to the coronary dermis, or from abnormal shearing, compressive or tearing forces placed at the palmar/plantar area of the foot. These cracks may appear initially as hairline

cracks that are difficult to detect (page 189). Causes of lacerations to the coronary band include fence wire cuts, accidental limb contact, or treading with a horseshoe fitted with studs. In cases where the injury to the coronary dermis is accompanied by scar formation, the crack may develop into a complete superficial or deep quarter crack. Proximal quarter cracks may be accompanied by pain and lameness. In some cases, the heel area palmar/plantar to the crack may be loose and painful when palpated. Proximal quarter cracks caused by mechanical failure are commonly accompanied by abnormal hoof conformation such as under-run heels, sheared heels and contracted heels. Quarter cracks are more common in thin-walled hooves and small feet.

Farriery of proximal quarter cracks includes trimming and balancing the hoof, and complete debridement of the crack. The underlying cause(s) should be investigated and treated. Debridement may be carried out with a hoof knife, loop knife or with a motorized burr fitted with a small bit. Superficial proximal cracks should be repaired with acrylic resin. The strength of the repair can be enhanced by burring horizontal notches along the sides of the defect similar to a stepladder pattern, and incorporating a fabric patch into the resin (Moyer and Sigafoos,

1993) (see ◆ fig. 16.74). Alternatively, the crack can be repaired with brace plates and stainless steel wire combined with resin (Moyer and Sigafoos, 1993) (see lacing techniques, page 182). Deep proximal quarter cracks that become infected should be debrided completely. The repair should be delayed until the area is dry and cornified, unless a drainage tract is incorporated into the repair. The hoof is fitted with a bar horseshoe that protects and stabilizes the hoof. Farriery may be modified according to the underlying problem. This may include increasing the base area in under-run heels cases, or relieving the displaced heel in cases of sheared heels.

Some cases may develop a new crack several days after the repair, next to the repaired crack. The new crack may appear initially as a spot of blood or hairline crack at the coronary band. This complication may result from abnormal shear forces that develop under weak repair, excessive loads or both. In this case, the horseshoe and resin should be removed and the underlying cause investigated and corrected prior to application of the new repair. In some cases, the addition of moisture to the hoof capsule by poulticing the foot overnight may prevent the development of new cracks.

Marks et al., (1971) described the application of a horseshoe and pad for unloading the palmar/plantar area of the hoof in order to minimize the shearing forces placed on the crack. They indicated that this method is particularly useful in cases where the heel is not stable and can be moved sideways easily (◆ fig. 16.73).

COMPLETE QUARTER CRACKS

Complete quarter cracks may develop from a distal or proximal quarter crack that extends throughout the entire length of the quarter wall. The crack may be superficial or deep; deep cracks may become infected and/or undermined. The hoof wall section palmar or plantar to the crack may be unstable and painful. Predisposing factors for complete quarter cracks are similar to those for incomplete quarter cracks.

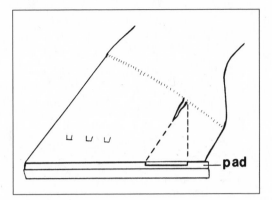

◆ **Fig. 16.73.** Relieving proximal quarter crack, schematic illustration. The "base of support" of the crack is determined by drawing two imaginary lines (broken lines), one from the proximal end of the crack to the ground, and the other by "extending" the line of the crack; this area is relieved by stepping the pad. (Reprinted by permission from Mark, D. et al. 1971, fig. 5. Illustration modified to text.)

Farriery of complete quarter cracks depends on the extent of the crack and type of work done by the horse. Treatment of pastured horses with superficial complete quarter cracks includes hoof trimming, and removal of pressure from the distal margin of the crack by cutting an arched section at the bearing surface of the quarter wall as described for distal quarter cracks (see ◆ fig. 16.72A). The white line should be inspected for presence of white line disease and thrush and debrided accordingly. In cases where the crack is unstable, the hoof should be fitted with a protective horseshoe. This may include a plain horseshoe, three-quarter horseshoe, z-bar shoe or a bar shoe. Evans et al. (1966) recommended cutting away the bearing surface under the crack to form a step that minimizes motion, and supporting the quarters and heels with a bar shoe. Egg-bar shoes provide excellent protection and stability to the hoof. Horses that are being worked should be treated according to the technique described by Moyer and Sigafoos (1993). This includes the complete debridement of the crack with a motorized burr (a hoof knife or a loop knife may be used instead). The quarters and heels areas are sanded and several notches in a

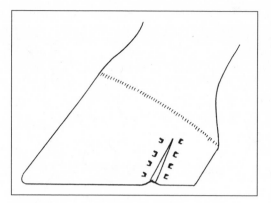

◆ **Fig. 16.74.** Stepladder notches placed along the defect to increase the strength of acrylic repairs, schematic illustration. (Adapted from Moyer W. and Sigafoos D.R. 1993, p. 11, fig 4.)

stepladder pattern are made along the sides of the defect; the notches increase the adherence strength of the resin (◆ fig. 16.74). The defect is repaired with application of two layers of acrylic resin combined with fabric material. Alternatively, reinforcement of the repair may be executed by lacing (Moyer and Sigafoos, 1991) or brass plate (Moyer, 1988) techniques.

Complete quarter cracks that involve the dermis should be debrided completely and treated as a wound until the defect becomes dry and cornified. Infected cracks may be associated with large undermined areas that extend under the hoof wall. These areas should be debrided until healthy horn is reached. The extent of the undermined area is determined with a flexible blunt metal probe. Prior to debridement, the hoof wall over the affected area can be thinned with a hoof rasp. Alternatively, half-round hoof nippers or a motorized burr may be used. Bleeding may have to be controlled by application of a tourniquet. Following debridement, the hoof is fitted with a wide-web bar shoe (◆ fig. 16.75). Quarter cracks with hoof wall loss that are dry and cornified may be repaired by stabilizing the defect with umbilical tape and resin combined with a fabric patch; in cases where the crack is infected, the repair should be delayed or a drainage tract should be established beneath the repair (Moyer and Sigafoos, 1993). Permanent quarter cracks

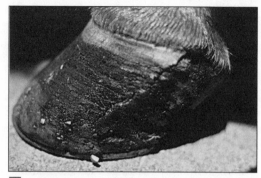

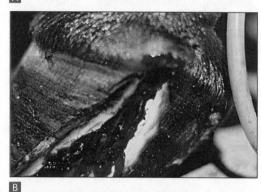

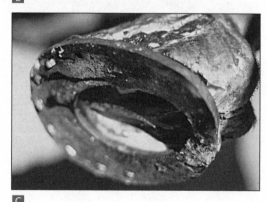

◆ **Fig. 16.75.** Complete deep quarter crack. A. Prior to debridement. B. Following debridement. C. Application of widie-web egg-bar shoe that protects the foot. (Photos by author).

require regular farriery care and periodic hoof repair.

Additional method for repair of complete quarter cracks includes the application of a fiberglass patch and screws combined with a bar shoe (Butler, 1976).

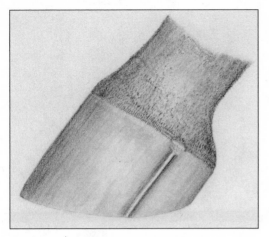

◆ **Fig. 16.76.** False quarter.

FALSE QUARTER

According to Percivall (1855), a *false quarter* is a gap in the hoof wall located at the side of the wall; the gap results from injury to the coronary dermis and it is covered by soft horn secreted by the sensitive laminae. Butler (in Stephens, 2003) indicated that a false quarter is not a crack but a defect in the hoof wall (◆ fig. 16.76). Defects in the quarter area may develop as a result of misaligned coronary dermis following laceration or avulsion injuries to the foot. The misaligned section, which grows against the main hoof, results in the development of false quarter. Another predisposing factor includes under-run heels.

False quarter predisposes the hoof to development of quarter cracks and avulsion injuries, which may result from stepping on a stone at high speed or making sharp turns. Percivall (1855) recommended using a bar shoe and removing direct pressure from the hoof wall at the distal margins of the defect.

Heel Cracks

A *heel crack* is a vertical crack similar to a quarter crack. Proximal superficial heel cracks are treated according to the method described by Moyer and Sigafoos (1993), using a brass plate and stainless steel wire, and acrylic material combined with a fabric patch. The hoof is fitted with a straight or egg-bar shoe.

Carroll (1989) recommended the application of a half-mushroom shoe for treatment of heel cracks. Deep heel cracks should be debrided and treated as a wound until the defect is dry and cornified. Some heel cracks are accompanied by loose heel, and in some cases, the crack may be horizontal. Farriery of these cases includes removal of the affected heel in order to relieve the affected area, and application of a bar-shoe that protects the heel area and permits new horn growth. A z-bar shoe or a mushroom shoe may be applied to horses that do not work on rocky areas. These horseshoes have less chance of being pulled compared to the bar shoe. Heel cracks may develop in horses with under run heels, these cases should be shod as described for this condition (page 209).

Hairline Cracks

Hairline cracks are small fissures that develop below the coronary band as a result of abnormal shearing forces in the hoof wall. The fissure may bleed and can be painful. The hoof wall beneath the fissure may become undermined and the fissure may develop into a hoof wall crack. Predisposing factors include thin hoof wall, under-run heels, proximal deviation of the coronary band and dry hoof wall.

Treatment of hairline cracks includes the removal of underlying cause that lead to abnormal shearing forces. The extent of the fissure should be examined and the undermined wall should be debrided. The hoof should be placed in a poultice pack for 24 hours prior to application of horseshoes. This adds moisture to the horn and relieves shear forces (Snow and Birdsall, 1990). The hoof may be fitted with a regular horseshoe or bar shoe. Thin-walled hooves may be shod with glue-on shoes in order to reduce concussion.

Bar Cracks

Bar cracks appear as narrow fissures across the bar. This type of crack may be difficult to locate and may cause lameness (Moyer, 1980). Bar cracks may extend into the sole; the crack

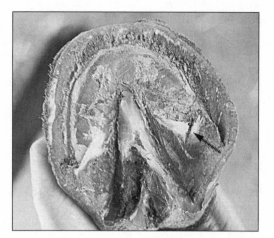

◆ **Fig. 16.77.** Bar crack (arrow). (Photo by author.)

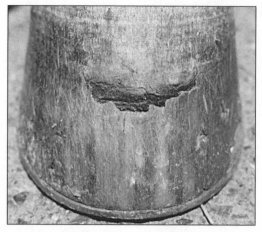

◆ **Fig. 16.78.** Toe cleft. (Photo by author.)

forms an ideal environment for thrush and a route for sole abscess (◆ fig. 16.77).

Treatment of bar cracks includes careful debridement of the undermined bar; as much horn as possible should be preserved. The exposed crack is packed with pine and oakum and the hoof is fitted with a half-bar shoe that covers the affected area. Alternatively, a plain horseshoe and flat pad can be applied.

Sole Cracks

Most cracks that appear in the sole result from normal exfoliation of the sole. These cracks may contain debris and thrush, but in most cases they are superficial and insignificant. *Sole cracks* may result from stepping on a sharp object or from extension of bar cracks. Treatment of sole cracks includes careful debridement of the lesion, application of pine tar, and when required, shoeing the hoof with a protective horseshoe and pad.

Clefts

Clefts or cross cracks appear as a transverse defect in the hoof wall. These cracks are caused by previous injury to the coronary band such as by trauma or sub-mural abscess that drained through the coronary band (Johnson, 1972) (◆ fig. 16.78). Clefts may develop following sever frostbite injuries to

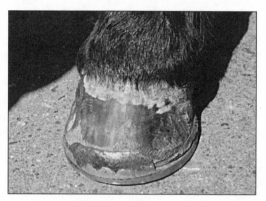

◆ **Fig. 16.79.** Toe rim horseshoe. The rim was welded at the toe area of the horseshoe in order to protect the distal margins of the toe wall. (Photo by author.)

the coronary band (Holocombe and Giltner, in Pearson et al., 1942). Horizontal cracks may develop at the heels by abnormal pressure placed on that region; pressure may result from sharp turns at high speed or from a short horseshoe branch.

Most clefts are insignificant and grow downward with the hoof wall. Clefts that are dry and cornified can be left intact, or filled with a resin for cosmetic reasons. In wet areas, the cleft should be treated daily with pine tar. Under muddy or dirty conditions, the cleft can become infected with thrush that could develop into sub-mural abscess.

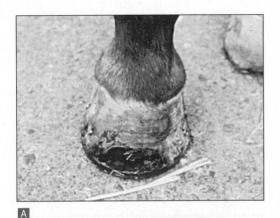
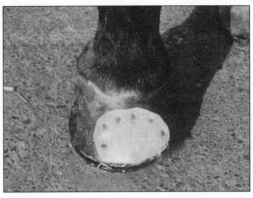

◆ **Fig. 16.80.** Plastic patch. A. The toe wall following debridement of sub-mural abscess and application of protective horseshoe. B. Placement of plastic patch held with several wood screws. (Photos by author.)

Infected clefts should be debrided and packed with pine tar and oakum. A plastic patch may be applied over the defect (see below). Once the cleft reaches the distal margins, the hoof wall distal to it may break. Prior to that, the hoof-bearing surface under the cleft can be stepped in order to relieve pressure from that area. The space that is formed is treated periodically with pine tar and oakum and the hoof is shod with a regular horseshoe or bar shoe. Alternatively, the toe area can be protected with a *toe rim horseshoe* (◆ fig. 16.79).

PLASTIC PATCH

A *plastic patch* is used in the treatment of hoof wall defects such as clefts or debrided sub-mural abscess. The patch protects the affected area and maintains medications within the defect. The patch is cut from a 3 mm thick, soft plastic sheet, and is connected to the hoof with 3 mm diameter wood screws placed at the sides (◆ fig. 16.80). Prior to application of the patch, the defect in the wall is packed with pine tar and oakum.

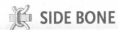 SIDE BONE

Side bone IS A PROGRESSIVE *calcification* (bone formation) of the lateral cartilages. In some

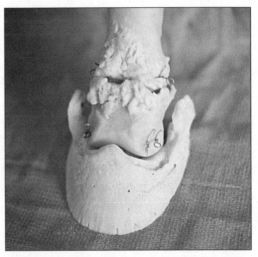

◆ **Fig. 16.81.** Side bone. This specimen has extensive side bone formation on both sides of the third phalanx, and a high ringbone. (Photo by author.)

cases, a considerable amount of cartilage may be converted into bone (Bradley and Grahame, 1946) (◆ fig. 16.81). Non-ossified lateral cartilages readily yield to pressure. This flexibility is lost when it begun to ossify (Butzow, 1961); consequently, the ossified cartilages interfere with normal expansion and contraction of the hoof at the quarters and heels (McCunn, 1951), shock absorption is affected, and the hoof may develop contracted heels. The new bone may fracture and cause lameness (Pollitt, 1995).

Calcification of cartilage may be symmetrical on both sides of the foot or more extensive on one side. A study on the occurrence of side bone in 450 horses showed that most of the horses were affected on the lateral aspect of the foot, 95 percent of side bone was found in heavy draft horses and 16 percent in Warmblood horses. The side bone was not a source of lameness (Verschooten and Van Waerebeek (1994). Development of side bone is a common aging process, and it may result in lameness (Sisson and Grossman, 1953; Butzow, 1961), although obscure locomotion problems are more common than true lameness (Ruohoniemi et al., 2004). Side bone is common in horses such as hunters and jumpers that are subjected to abnormal concussion forces.

Farriery of side bone includes the application of a horseshoe fitted with a thick pad that reduces concussion. The pad can be cut at the center to permit cleaning of the sole. Alteration of the medial-lateral balance should be avoided as it may cause lameness. Dry hooves should be hydrated periodically with a hoof poultice, followed by application of pine tar to the solar area.

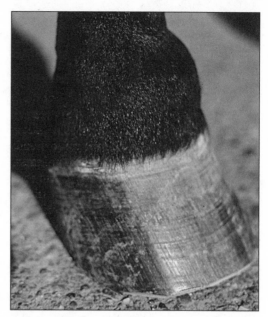

◆ **Fig. 16.82.** **High ringbone.** Deposition of new bone resulted in bulging of the pastern area. (Photo by author.)

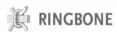 RINGBONE

Ringbone IS CHARACTERIZED BY DEPOSITION OF new bone over the digital bones and joints. Depending on the location of bone deposition, ringbone is classified as *non-articular* or *articular*. A ringbone near the DIP joint is termed *low ringbone*, whereas ringbone near the PIP joint is termed *high ringbone* (see ◆ fig. 16.81). Another form of ringbone that involves the extensor process is called buttress foot (page 218).

Predisposing factors for ringbone include toeing-out or toeing-in foot conformation (Adams, 1974) as well as chronic imbalance (Dyson, 1988) and abnormal concussion. Butzow (1961) indicated that when one side of the

hoof wall is lower than the opposite side, the collateral ligaments on the low side become abnormally strained, and this may initiate the process of bone deposition. As the process of ossification progresses, hoof conformation becomes modified, the heels increases in length as a result of reduced wear, and the pastern appears more upright and bulging (◆ fig. 16.82). The gait may be altered by mechanical interference to normal digit function or pain (McCunn, 1951). Non-articular ringbone causes lameness until the adjacent joint becomes fused and lameness subsides (Frank, 1953).

Farriery of ringbone includes trimming the hoof without alterations in hoof angle; hence, the hoof angle that is favored by the horse should be maintained. Alteration in the medial-lateral plan should be avoided since it may cause lameness. In cases where the horse is working, the hooves can be shod with a horseshoe and a thick pad in order to reduce concussion.

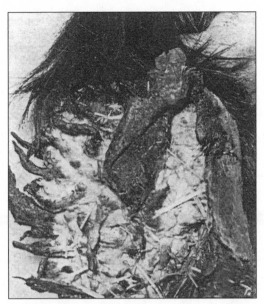

◆ **Fig. 16.83.** Severe canker. Note the growth of disorganized finger-like projections of horn tissue. (Reprinted by permission from Prescott, C.W. 1970, fig. 2.)

CANKER

Canker OR NECROTIC PODODERMATITIS IS A disease of the foot characterized by chronic overgrowth of horn tissue accompanied by fetid odor. The disease is more common in temperate regions (Wilson et al., 1985) and it affects primarily the hind feet (◆ fig. 16.83). Poor foot hygiene and neglected hooves predispose the hoof to the disease (Prescott, 1970). Horses stabled in filthy, urine soaked bedding (Prescott, 1970; Johnson, 1972) or pastured in marshy areas (Johnson, 1972) may develop canker. Historically, canker was a common disease in the hind feet of draft horses (Wilson et al., 1985). The exact cause of the canker is still under investigation. Nagamine et al. (2005) isolated *spirochaete* bacteria from lesions in three horses. Jongbloets et al. (2005) described one case of canker that may have developed as a result of an immune reaction.

The disease begins at the frog and slowly spreads to the adjacent sole and hoof wall (Wilson et al., 1989; Johnson, 1972; O'Connor,

1960). The sole and frog become covered with grayish-white papillae or finger like projections that may reach a length of 5 to 6 cm and a diameter of 0.5 cm. Grey purulent material with a foul odor forms between the papillae. Lameness may not be present unless the case is advanced (Johnson, 1972). In severe cases, the hoof wall may separate from the laminae (Prescott, 1970).

Treatment of canker includes debridement of abnormal tissue and application of systemic and topical medications. Wilson et al. (1989) indicated that radical surgical debridement disrupts deep structures, and recommended minor surgical debridement as the treatment management of canker; this includes the removal of only grossly abnormal tissue and preserving germinal epithelium. Topical application of irritating agents should be avoided. O'Grady and Madison (2004) described two methods for treatment of canker. The first method includes the use of cautery (heat therapy). The second method includes the use of hoof knife and cryotherapy (cold therapy). They recommended that all abnormal tissue should be removed until normal dermis is reached. The affected area is treated with topical medication and a foot bandage is applied, followed by daily application of topical medication.

Farriery of canker includes the application of a treatment plate to cases with enough hoof wall strength. The device protects the diseased foot, gives access for medication, saves bandage material and allows hand walking the horse. The treatment plate should be as light as possible. This may be achieved with an aluminum bar-shoe fitted with an aluminum plate.

KERATOMA

Keratoma IS A BENIGN TUMOR OF THE HOOF THAT develops at the inner surface of the hoof wall or sole (Lloyd et al., 1988). The tumor is firm and smooth and has an oval or conical shape; it may extend a short distance from its origin or extend along the entire length of the inner

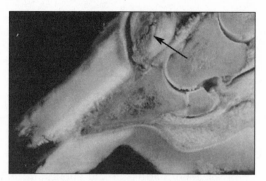

◆ **Fig. 16.84.** Keratoma, longitudinal section through the foot (arrow). This tumor developed as a cylindrical mass between the skin and third phalanx, most tumors are located between the hoof wall and third phalanx. (Reprinted by permission from Hamir, A.N. et al., 1992, fig. 1.)

hoof wall (Frank, 1953). One case report described a tumor located at the coronary band (Hamir et al., 1992) (◆ fig. 16.84). The cause of keratoma is unknown but it may arise in response to hoof infection (Lloyd et al., 1988) or trauma (Kunze, 1986; Lloyd et al., 1988). The tumor may press the surrounding area and cause bulging and deformity of the hoof wall with distortion of the laminae and the third phalanx (Lloyd et al., 1988). The pressure exerted by the tumor on sensitive structures cause lameness. Localized deviation of the white line and draining tracts may develop by a tumor that approaches the bearing surface of the hoof wall (Henninger and Owen, 1986; Pickersgill, 2000).

Treatment of keratoma includes surgical resection of the tumor and application of a protective horseshoe that stabilizes the foot. Bosch et al. (2004) indicated that surgically treated horses have better outcomes compared to conservative treatment. The surgical approach depends on the site and extent of the tumor. Wagner and Balch (1986) and Lloyd et al. (1988) recommended performing a wall strip procedure for tumors extending from the coronary band to the sole (page 195). Local tumors situated under the hoof wall may be treated similarly unless the tumor is located near the white line. In that case, the tumor is resected through the wall-sole junc-

tion. Alternatively, local tumors may be removed through an opening made in the hoof wall. Honnas (1998) described the use of Galt trephine to access keratomas situated in the sole or wall area (see ◆ fig. 16.88). Boys Smith et al. (2006) indicated that cases that underwent partial hoof wall resection had less postoperative complications than those that underwent complete resection, but overall recovery in all cases was very good. Sole keratomas are resected through the sole. A margin of healthy-appearing tissue from around the tumor should be excised with minimal disruption of normal germinal epithelium (Lloyd et al., 1988). Following resection of the tumor, the wound is packed with sterile gauze sponges soaked with povidone-iodine and the foot is bandaged.

Miscellaneous Tumors of the Foot

Foot tumors in the horse are rare (Berry et al., 1991). Reports on tumors other than keratoma include case reports of *malignant melanoma* of the foot (Honnas et al., 1990; Kunze et al., 1986; Floyd, 2003); *carcinoma* in the hoof wall (Berry et al., 1991); *hemangioma* (a benign tumor of blood vessels) in the distal phalanx (Gelatt et al., 1996), and *mast cell tumor* of the third phalanx (Ritmeester et al., 1997).

Farriery of Keratoma

Farriery of keratoma that involve the solar white line area includes the application of a treatment plate (O'Grady and Horne, 2001). Cases involving the hoof wall should be fitted with a bar shoe and side clips (Lloyd et al. 1988; Honnas et al., 1988d). A heart-bar shoe and side clips may be used in cases with extensive toe wall loss (Pickersgill, 2000). In addition, the hoof may have to be stabilized with a steel plate placed across the defect (Pollitt and Daradka, 2004; Pickersgill, 2000) (◆ fig. 16.85). Boys Smith et al. (2006) described the application of a regular horseshoe and side clips placed at the widest part of the horseshoe. Some cases were shod with a heart-bar shoe fitted with a treatment plate.

The horseshoe can be applied immediately following surgical removal of the tumor (Wagner and Balch, 1986), or it may be applied after formation of granulation tissue (Lloyd et al., 1988 ;). Following cornification, the defect in the hoof wall may be reconstructed with acrylic resin (Boys Smith et al., 2006).

Helms et al. (1994) provided a detailed description on toe wall reconstruction in a mare with toe wall keratoma. Forty-eight hours after surgery, the hoof was fitted with a rocker-toe shoe and side clips; the horseshoe was reset at monthly intervals. Following complete cornification of the laminar bed, the area was ground. The remaining hoof wall was sanded and the entire hoof was cleaned with acetone. The defect in the hoof wall was reconstructed with hoof repair material, reinforced with 3 layers of polyethylene fabric in alternating layers of resin and fabric, covered with a wrap. The foot was wrapped with elastic adhesive tape and the composite was allowed to harden for 10 minutes. Following curing the entire hoof was covered with resin combined with a double layer of resin-impregnated fabric. The mare was confine in a stall for 12 hours until the resin was completely hard.

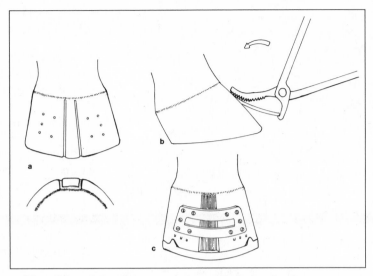

◆ **Fig. 16.85.** Full wall strip procedure at the toe wall, schematic illustration. Two parallel grooves are made along the entire length of the hoof wall; the strips are connected at the white line (a). The strip is grasped with modified alligator forceps and pulled (b). A stabilizing plate is applied and the hoof is shod (c). See text for details.
Adapted from Pollitt and Daradka 2004, fig.1.

Wall Strip Procedure

The *wall strip procedure* may be used in the treatment of keratoma, laminitis, white line disease, gravel and partial hoof wall avulsion. The procedure is commonly done in surgical removal of keratoma. The strip may include the entire length of the hoof wall or part of it.

Preparation for a wall strip procedure includes hoof trimming, clipping the hair from the lower half of the pastern, and covering the hoof for 24 hours with gauzes soaked in alcohol under a foot bandage.

Pollitt and Daradka (2004) described a procedure for a full-length toe wall strip, used in laminitis research. They indicated that this procedure allows clean separation of the hoof wall horn with minimal damage to the dermis. This procedure with some modifications is described below.

Prior to the wall strip procedure, the hoof is trimmed for shoeing, and a wide-web bar shoe with side clips is fitted to the hoof. A *stabilizing plate* is shaped to fit the curvature of the hoof wall at the affected area. The plate is made from 5 mm x 30 mm bar stock of mild steel (◆ fig. 16.85). Several holes, 3.0 mm in diameter are drilled in the plate and used to connect the plate to the hoof with wood screws. The plate is connected to the hoof wall with screws and then removed.

The horse is anesthetized and the foot is prepared for aseptic surgery. Two parallel grooves are made along the entire length of the hoof wall; the grooves should contain the affected area. Grooving should start from the bearing surface of the hoof toward the coronary band; the depth of the cut should not reach the laminar dermis. The coronary band should be approached carefully in order to avoid penetration of the coronary dermis. A third groove that connects the parallel grooves is made at the white line.

Grooving the hoof wall can be done with an oscillating plaster saw, or with a high-speed motorized burr, fitted with 9.5 mm diameter high-speed circular saw. In order to prevent thermal injury, the blade of the saw should be cooled with saline. The groove at the white line can be made with a sterilized loop knife. Once the grooves are completed, the strip should become mobile. At this point, a modified alligator forceps is used to grasp the strip firmly and the strip is peeled upwards. Following debridement of the lesion, the stabilizing plate is applied using the same predrilled holes, and the hoof is shod with the previously fitted horseshoe. Boys Smith et al. (2006) described the application of a perforated metal plate to stabilize the hoof following hoof wall resection; the plate was glued with PMMA.

The wound is covered with sterile gauzes soaked in povidone-iodine and the foot is wrapped with a foot bandage. The lesion is treated until the defect in the hoof wall becomes completely dry and cornified. At that time, the defect in the hoof wall may be repaired with acrylic resin or remain open. The horseshoe should be reset every four weeks until the defect grows out.

Partial length wall strip procedures are sometimes performed in order to remove a distal section of hoof wall. In this case, the upper limits of the parallel grooves are connected with a groove. The hoof may be stabilizing by placing a simple bar across the defect in order to prevent excessive motion (Pickersgill, 2000). Alternatively, the tumor may be removed through a "window" made in the hoof wall with a 2 cm trephine (Boys Smith et al., 2006).

THRUSH

Thrush IS BACTERIAL INFECTION OF THE HOOF characterized by a fetid black discharge that is related to the breakdown of horn (◆ fig. 16.86). The disease involves primarily the central and lateral sulci of the frog. The most common agent isolated from thrush is *Spherophorus necrophorus*, an anaerobic bacterium that thrives in the absence of oxygen (Johnson, 1972). Predisposing factors for thrush include poor sanitation, improper feet care and lack of exercise; the disease appears primarily in stabled horses. The bacteria thrive in small cracks at the hoof wall, in separated white line, and in hooves that are impacted by manure or dirt. Thrush may undermine the sole and white line and form "worm like" channels that predispose the horse to sole abscess and sub-mural abscess. (see ◆ plate 4). Deep thrush tends to develop at the bulbs of the heels in contracted heels and sheared heels cases. These cases commonly have a deep groove at the heel bulbs that is ideal for thrush development (Moyer and Anderson, 1975b). Budras et al. (1998) indicated that greasing the sole and frog can creates an anaerobic environment favorable

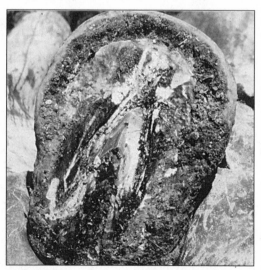

◆ **Fig. 16.86.** Thrush with deeply infected frog. (Photo by author.)

for growth of horn-decaying bacteria and fungi.

Hooves affected with thrush may have frog sulci that are deeper than normal. The foot may be tender and the horse may resent hoof picking (Johnson, 1972). The frog may be completely undermined (Fessler, 1971b). In severe cases, the coronary band may swell and the horse become lame (Johnson, 1972). Complications of thrush include involvement of the frog dermis, inflammation of the digital cushion, and necrotic tendonitis. These cases may look similar to canker (Fessler, 1971b).

Treatment of Thrush

Treatment of thrush include elimination of predisposing factors, trimming the hooves and complete debridement of the affected area; all loose and disintegrated horn should be trimmed, and undermined sole channels should be explored and opened. Mild cases of thrush are treated by topical application of pine tar, one to two times per week. The hooves should be thoroughly picked before treatment. Cases that are more progressive are treated by topical application of povidone-iodine followed by daily application of pine tar.

Farriery of tender feet that are afflicted with thrush includes complete debridement of the affected area and application a horseshoe and leather pad. The solar area should be packed with pine tar and oakum. Farriery of cases accompanied by contracted heels should be modified accordingly (page 208).

Prevention of thrush includes daily hoof picking in order to prevent accumulation of manure and dirt in the hooves (Butzow, 1961), and weekly application of pine tar over the solar area. In order to be effective, this routine should be accompanied by proper sanitation, foot care and exercise. Prevention of thrush in horses that are shod regularly includes debridement of loose horn and powdery areas at the white line and application of a petroleum-and-pine-tar-based hoof pack into recessed areas prior to application of the horseshoe.

PINE TAR

Pine tar is obtained by destructive distillation of wood of the pine family. The material has antimicrobial properties and is used to treat chronic skin disease in humans. In horses, pine tar is used as a topical medication for prevention and treatment of thrush and hoof abscesses, and for preserving moisture within the hoof horn.

In a study done by Robertson and Hood (1996) on hoof wall sections, the hydration properties of several commercial hoof dressings were compared. The study showed that pine tar has excellent ability to maintain hoof moisture.

Routine use of pine tar includes topical application following hoof trimming. Ideally, the horse should stand on a wet area for 30 to 60 minutes following trimming to allow for absorption of lost moisture, then pine tar is applied over the solar area. This procedure is repeated as required between the trimming intervals. In addition, the solar area should be dressed once a week with pine tar for prevention of thrush. The hooves of horses that are shod with full pads should be packed with pine tar and oakum prior to shoeing; the pine tar prevents the development of thrush and sole abscesses; the oakum maintains the pine tar and prevents accumulation of debris under the sole. Water and sand tend to remove the pine tar; additional pine tar can be poured between the sole and pad every two to three weeks in order to replenish the lost pine tar.

Under excessively wet conditions, the application of pine tar may prevent the development of sole abscesses. Dickson and O'Malley (1987) recommended the application of pine tar in areas with heavy annual rainfall to keep moisture out of the feet.

In emergencies, pine tar dressing may be applied to an injured foot in order to protect it until the horse can receive treatment. The content of a one-liter can (~ one quart) of pure pine tar is poured over a large cotton pad placed next to the limb. The limb is placed at the center of the pad and the pad is folded over the foot and bandaged.

PETROLEUM AND PINE-TAR-BASED HOOF PACKING

Hoof care products containing *petroleum* and pine tar are commonly used as *hoof packing*. The hoof packing material seals crevices and holes in areas that are covered by the horseshoe and prevents the development of thrush. Areas that are treated include crevices caused by white line separation, holes made by thrush, and toe wall separations such as those observed in foals with contracted tendons. A hoof pack may be applied under a pad instead of pine tar.

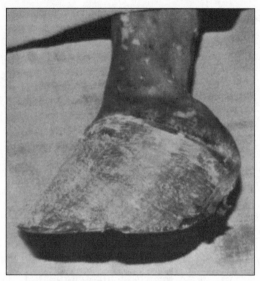

◆ **Fig. 16.87.** Quittor. Several infected tracts can be observed above the coronary band. (Reprinted by permission from Honnas, C.M. et al. 1988d, fig. 5.)

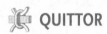 **QUITTOR**

Quittor IS AN INFECTION OF THE LATERAL cartilage characterized by purulent (pus formation) inflammation, necrosis, and development of persistent drainage tracts proximal to the coronary band at the quarters area (◆ fig. 16.87). The disease may develop following laceration injuries or puncture wounds in the coronary band next to the lateral cartilages (Hickman, 1964). Injuries to the coronary band may result from accidental limb contact, wood splinters, accidents or treading on the opposite foot with a horseshoe fitted with studs. The cartilage, which has a limited blood supply, becomes necrotic by spread of infection from the contaminated wound (Johnson, 1972). Historically, the disease was more common in draft horses (Fessler, 1971b); present occurrence of the disease is uncommon.

Treatment of Quittor

Treatment of quittor includes aseptic preparation of the foot and surgical debridement of the lesion. Honnas et al. (1988c) and Honnas et al. (1988d) describe a surgical procedure that includes debridement of the cartilage

through a skin incision made above the coronary band and establishment of drainage by making a drainage hole through the hoof wall, distal to the lesion. The hole can be made with a Galt trephine (Honnas and Moyer, 2000) or with a motorized burr fitted with a high-speed cutting tool (◆ fig. 16.88).

In order to reduce the risk of penetrating the DIP joint during the surgery, the digit should be in held in extension during the operation. To achieve this, two holes are made in the hoof wall, one at each quarter. Strong metal wire is inserted through the holes and attached to a handle, which is used to pull the digit and maintain it in an extended position (Honnas et. al., 1988d).

Following surgical debridement, the lesion is treated by daily flushing with povidone-iodine solution, antibiotic ointment and protective foot bandage. The defect in the hoof wall may be sealed with acrylic resin once the lesion heals and the opening in the hoof wall becomes dry and cornified. The hoof should be fitted with a protective horseshoe if the horse is being worked.

Prevention of quittor includes proper wound care following injuries to the coronary band. The cartilage should be examined care-

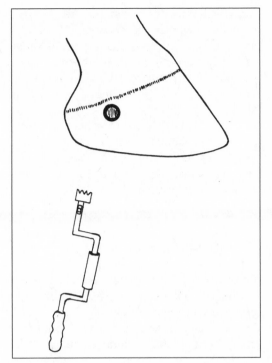

◆ **Fig. 16.88.** Establishment of ventral drainage in the hoof wall with a Galt trephine, schematic illustration. The drainage tract is made by drilling a hole with a 19 mm trephine below the lesion. The same tool is used to expose keratomas.
Reprinted by permission from Honnas, C.M. et al. 1988, fig. 6. Illustration modified to text.

fully and any loose or infected cartilage should be removed during wound debridement (Fessler, 1971b). Other measures include the application of protective boots during transportation, and minimizing the risk of accidental limb contact during work.

🦠 ONYCHOMYCOSIS

Onychomycosis IS A FUNGAL DISEASES OF THE HOOF (onycho = claw or nail; mycosis = fungal disease) caused by a variety of fungi that may invade the hoof horn and surrounding skin. These fungi are keratinopathogenic, which means that they capable of breaking down horn with their enzymes. Keratinopathogenic fungi are found in healthy hooves and dis-

eased hooves. Keller et al. (2000) found a significant correlation between the presence of keratinopathogenic fungus and poor horn quality. Poor horn quality in this study included hooves with horn cracks, white line disease, brittle horn, parakeratosis at the heel bulbs (thickening of the skin due to excessive horn production), laminitic hooves and bruises. Many horses also had swollen coronary bands. No correlation was found between the clinical condition, and bedding or hygiene. In addition, no correlation was found between the incidence of the disease and age, sex and breed. The disease may affect horses that are well-groomed and kept on shavings (Chapman, 1993). Fungi were isolated from hooves affected by white line disease (Kuwano et al., 1996; Kuwano et al., 1998) (see white line disease, page 143).

It is not clear how keratinopathogenic fungi are associated with hoof disorders (Keller et al., 2000). Fungal invasion may be initiated by break down of horn (primary invasion), or the hooves may be invaded through cracks and hoof wall separation that are already exist in poor quality hooves (secondary invasion). This author believes that with so many horses with poor hoof quality (conformation and substance), fungal invasion is secondary in most cases.

HEEL DERMATITIS

Heel dermatitis IS A SKIN DISEASE CAUSED BY A bacterial or fungal infection of the skin above the hoof. The disease may also caused by mites (see below). Areas that are commonly affected include the palmar/plantar aspect of the fetlock, pastern and heels (◆ fig. 16.89). Other names for heel dermatitis include scratches, greasy heel and mud heels. Heel dermatitis commonly develops in horses kept in muddy or swampy environments, and it is more common in horses with white legs markings. The affected skin becomes crusted, scabby and thickened and the horse may become lame (Thomas, 2001).

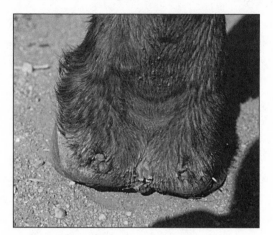

◆ **Fig. 16.89.** Heel dermatitis. Healing of this case is nearly complete, with some scabs and secretions present at the heel bulbs. (Photo by author.)

Treatment of heel dermatitis depends on the cause and severity of the lesion; mild cases may be treated by gentle scrubbing of the affected area with a povidone-iodine scrub followed by complete rinsing of the digit with water. Once the lesion is dry, a topical antifungal or antibacterial ointment is applied. The horse should be kept in a dry and clean environment, and the lesions should be exposed to sunlight. Severe cases of heel dermatitis may require debridement of the lesion and the application of topical and systemic medication. The palmar/plantar area may be protected with an extended-heels horseshoe or with an extended egg-bar shoe until healing is complete (see plate 9).

 FOOT MANGE

Foot mange IS A SKIN DISEASE CAUSED BY THE mite *Chorioptes equi.* The disease commonly affects the palmar/plantar aspect of the pasterns of heavy horse breeds that have long-haired feet; the hind feet are more commonly affected (Cremers, 1985; Hammill, 2005). Other names for foot mange include leg mange, chorioptic mange and heel mange. A thickened skin with scab-like crusts and sores characterizes the lesions caused by this mite. Affected horses are irritated by intense itch-

ing, which cause them to stomp their feet, rub their legs together and chew on the affected areas. Treatment of foot mange includes topical application of mineral oil rubbed deep into the skin on a regular basis. In addition, the horses may require systemic medication against mites (Hammill, 2005).

Application of horseshoes to horses affected by foot mange may be difficult due to painful pasterns. An egg-bar shoe may provide additional protection to the heel bulbs until the lesions are healed.

 CHRONIC SELENOSIS

Chronic selenosis IS A DISEASE THAT IS CAUSED BY prolonged intake of excessive selenium given in the feed or water (Sutton and Butler, 1980). The source of the selenium may be from selenium accumulating plants such as alfalfa (Witte et al., 1993), excessive selenium supplementation (Dewes and Lowe, 1987) or feeds containing high levels of selenium intended for other farm animals. Horses are more susceptible to *selenium poisoning* compared with other types of livestock (Valberg in Corum, 2004). The excessive selenium interferes with keratin production by replacing sulfur in the keratin structure, which leads to abnormal horn production (Reeves et al., 1989). Signs of selenosis that involve the feet include coronitis, sore feet, and development of hoof wall deformities characterized by hoof rings, corrugated hoof surface and horizontal hoof wall cracks. Severe cases may result in complete sloughing of hooves (Witte et al., 1993) (◆ fig. 16.90). These changes may be accompanied by loss of laminar support and rotation of the third phalanx.

Farriery of Chronic Selenosis

Treatment of chronic selenosis includes the removal of the selenium source, hoof trimming and placement of the horse on sandy ground (Raisbeck, 2000). The bearing surface of the affected hooves should be stepped at the toe wall in order to reduce leverage

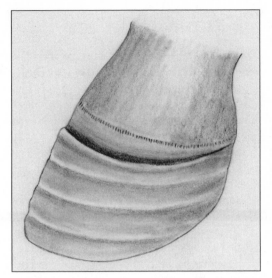

♦ **Fig. 16.90.** Chronic selenosis followed by development of corrugation lines and an horizontal groove at the hoof wall.

from this area. The hooves should be fitted with frog support pads and affected horses should be kept in a well-bedded stable. Some horses may have to be placed periodically in a sling.

Farriery of hooves affected by selenium toxicity includes the application of a heart-bar shoe to support the frog (Raisbeck, 2000). The horseshoe should be applied to cases at risk of rotating the third phalanx. Mild to moderate cases may be fitted with an egg-bar shoe and a flat pad. The solar area should be packed with soft, acrylic material or impression material. The horseshoe should provide palmar/plantar support that allows the horse to shift some weight toward the heels. Alternatively, the hooves may be fitted with glue-on shoes combined with impression material that provides solar support. Glue-on shoes eliminate the use of a hammer, thus reducing the risk of laminar tear. Prior to shoeing, the bearing surface at the toe wall should be dubbed in order to remove direct pressure from the area. No information was found on the reconstruction of affected hooves, but those that are not affected by secondary infec-

tion can be debrided and reconstructed with acrylic resin. Hoof wall reconstruction stabilizes the hoof capsule and reduces the risk of third phalanx rotation. The undermined wall should be removed and the defect margin undercut; several layers of resin-impregnated webbing material should be applied in order to form a strong composite. The hoof should be fitted with a light egg-bar shoe.

 ## SHELLY WALL

Shelly wall OR SHELLY HOOVES ARE CHARACTERIZED by poor quality hoof with horn that is brittle, cracking and flaking (♦ fig. 16.91). The condition is associated with thin hoof wall and exposure to extreme changes in environmental humidity, such as daily movement from dry stall to wet pasture (Marcella and Perry in Stewart-Spears, 2004). Application of nail-on horseshoes may worsen the condition of the hoof. The prevalence of shelly feet in closely related horses suggests that the condition has a hereditary base.

Treatment of shelly feet includes removal of the cause, if known. The condition of the

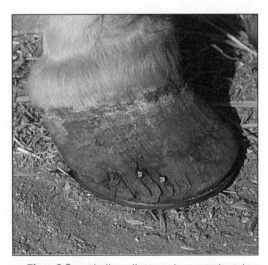

♦ **Fig. 16.89.** Shelly wall. Note the vertical cracks over the hoof wall surface, and the split distal margins at the quarter, mainly near the horseshoe nails. (Photo by author.)

hooves may improve in some cases by a daily supplement of biotin; it may take 6 to 12 months before improvement is noticed. Horses with shelly hooves should be removed from the breeding stock.

 ## SOFT HOOVES

Soft hooves COMMONLY DEVELOP BY PROLONGED exposure of the hooves to moisture. The condition may develop in horses that are being kept in pasture during the night or after unusually heavy rain. The excess moisture predisposes the hooves to development of thrush and abscesses. Shoeing horses with soft hooves is difficult and can be frustrating. The horseshoes tend to become loose, and clinching the horseshoe nail may result in the nail cutting through the hoof wall (Goubaux and Barrier, 1892). The horse may become lame from excessive sole pressure (Calahan in Podoll, 2006).

Prevention of soft hooves includes placement of the horse in a dry stable during periods of prolonged rain, and pasturing the horse only during the daytime in regions with heavy nighttime dew. Horses with the condition should be kept barefoot until the hoof wall becomes hard enough to hold a horseshoes. Horses that are being shod should be fitted with light horseshoes nailed on with slim nails. The position of the nail holes is alternated between shoeing intervals in order to remove strain from the hoof wall. The hooves should be maintained at a longer length and sole pressure should be removed by seating-out the sole (Calahan in Podoll, 2006).

 ## FROSTBITE

Frostbites MAY AFFECT THE FEET OF HORSES exposed to extreme cold, caused by heavy snowfall. The lesions may range from hair loss to skin sloughing and development of ulcers. The area most commonly affected is the coronary band, mainly at the dorsal area. Initially the skin become pale and bloodless, this is followed by redness, heat, pain and swelling. Frostbite may result in development of hoof wall clefts below the injury caused by abnormal horn production. In some cases the frog may be frostbitten and slough off (Holocombe and Giltner, in Pearson et al., 1942).

Treatment of frostbite includes debridment of infected tissue, medication and protection of the affected feet; the horse should be placed in a stable. Farriery of hooves affected by frostbite depend on the type of injury; the sole may be protected with a horseshoe and leather pad; the solar area should be packed with pine tar and oakum. Grown out clefts are trimmed prior to being detached and the hoof is shod with a protective horseshoe (page 190).

 ## THERMAL INJURIES

THERMAL INJURIES MAY RESULT FROM EXPOSURE to fire, excessive heat production during curing of acrylic resins, or when grooving the hoof wall with electric tools. Another important cause is hot shoe fitting; Rick (1907) indicated that this practice can cause sever damage to the hoof, which could result in founder, especially in heavy horses.

Little data is available on the treatment of thermal injuries involving the feet, affected feet should be rinsed immediately with cold water and the horse should be observed for signs of lameness. Slinging the horse in order to relieve pressure from the hooves may be helpful.

Chapter 17

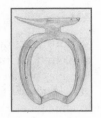

Farriery of Abnormal Foot Conformation

VARIOUS TYPES OF *abnormal foot conformations* are common among horses. These abnormalities may be inherited or developmental in origin. Abnormal foot conformation may affect locomotion and shock absorption patterns of the foot. The condition may be accompanied by asymmetrical hoof wear that results in straining of the stay apparatus, collateral ligaments and digital bones. Farriery of abnormal foot conformation may correct some of the cases and permit the use of such horses. The possible heritability of various conditions should be considered, and affected horses should be removed from the breeding stock.

 ## TOEING–OUT

Toeing–out, OR SPLAYFOOTED CONFORMATION, is characterized by an outward deviation of the foot; the deviation may result from faulty conformation of the entire limb, or deviation at the level of the fetlock or pastern joints (Hermans, 1987) (◆ fig. 17.1). Toeing-out is a very common conformational fault observed in horses; Marks (2000) indicated that the hind limbs in nearly all normal horses rotate outward. This conformation may result in accidental contact with the opposite limb, or *plaiting*, during motion (Shively, 1982b).

During motion, the deviated foot tends to breakover at the medial toe wall. This alteration in hoof and ground interaction affects the normal distribution of ground forces and consequently the shape of the hoof; the medial wall become shorter and steeper (Butzow, 1961; Caldwell, 2001) and the lateral wall become longer, more acute and flared. Chronic cases may develop proximal deviation of the coronary band at the medial hoof wall. The heels may become sheared and contracted (Caldwell, 2001). Excessive wear at the medial aspect of the bearing surface results in increased tension on the medial collateral ligaments, and increased compression on the lateral digital joints (see ◆ fig. 9.7). The uneven distribution of weight across the digit predisposes the horse to ringbone. (For toeing-out in foals, see ◆ page 79.)

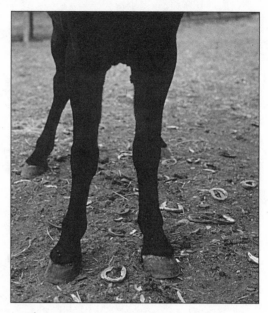

◆ **Fig. 17.1.** Toeing-out conformation. (Photo by author.)

Farriery of Toeing-Out

Farriery of toeing-out conformation depends on the age of the horse. An attempt to correct this conformational fault or improve the appearance of the limbs after closure of the growth plates will strain the digit and cause lameness. Therefore, the practice to lower the lateral side of the hoof in order to straighten the digit is contraindicated in older foals and mature horses. Hooves of yearlings and adult horses should be trimmed with minimal alteration in the medial to lateral plane. The hoof is trimmed so both sides of the hoof are at equal heights. In cases where wear on the medial side is excessive, the hoof may be fitted with a protective horseshoe with the medial branch of the horseshoe fitted full in order to center the foot with the limb axis. Breakover at the center of the foot may be encouraged by application of a square-toed horseshoe. In cases where the medial hoof wall is excessively worn, the horseshoe may be fitted with a wedged shim pad cut from a wedge pad. The pad is attached to the hoof surface of the horseshoe. Alternatively, a side wedge horseshoe may be used to raise the low side.

SIDE WEDGE HORSESHOE

The *side wedge horseshoe* is a horseshoe that is wedged from side to side (Koepisch, 1998a). The horseshoe is used in cases where one side of the hoof is too low. These may include cases of toeing-out, toeing-in, sheared heels (Koepisch, 1998a) and crocked wall. The lateral wedge horseshoe is fitted full on the low side in order to center the foot with the limb axis. Aluminum side wedge horseshoes are commercially available.

 ## TOEING-IN

Toeing-in OR PIGEON-TOED FOOT CONFORMATION is characterized by inward deviation of the foot. The condition is not uncommon and may have a heritable base (♦ fig. 17.2). Some cases of toeing-in may develop from over-correction of toeing-out conformation in foals. Cases of toeing-in may have a deviation at the level of the fetlock joint, and in some, the joint exhibits a pronounced stiffness. During motion, toeing-in results in a "paddling" motion characterized by outward movement of the foot at the beginning of the step, followed by inward movement (Shively, 1982b).

Toeing-in foot conformation increases the pressure on the medial aspect of the digital joints, and increases tension on the lateral collateral ligaments of the digit, which predisposes the horse to lameness. The abnormal stance and the tendency to break over at the lateral aspect of the toe wall results in alteration of the shape of the hoof, which is characterized by excessive wear at the lateral bearing surface of the hoof wall and flaring of the medial toe wall. (For toeing-in foals, see page 80.)

Farriery of Toeing-In

Farriery of toeing-in includes trimming the hoof in order to achieve equal heights on the

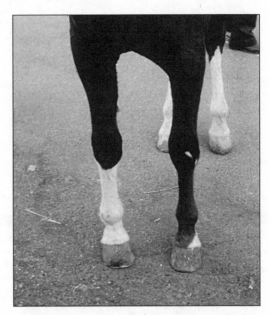

♦ **Fig. 17.2.** Toeing-in conformation. (Photo by author.)

medial and lateral aspects of the hoof. An attempt to correct the condition in mature horses or older foals by lowering the medial side of the hoof wall places abnormal strain on the digit and can result in lameness. Abnormal wear may be prevented with protective horseshoes. In cases accompanied by excessive wear, the horseshoe can be fitted with a wedged shim pad attached to the lateral branch of the horseshoe hoof surface. Alternatively, a side wedge horseshoe may be applied. The horseshoe should be fitted full on the lateral side in order to center the foot with the limb axis.

 ## LONG-TOE LOW-HEELS

Long- toe low-heels IS A VERY COMMON FOOT conformation fault observed in horses (Wright 1993). The condition may result from trimming the heels too low, or it may develop by hoof overgrowth accompanied by excessive wear at the heels. Another cause is weak heels that tend to break and collapse (♦ fig. 17.3).

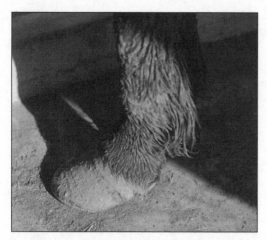

◆ **Fig. 17.3.** Long-toe low-heels foot conformation. (Photo by author.)

Østblom (1984) indicated that the application of conventional horseshoes confine the hoof wear to the heels and causes a low hoof angle toward the end of the shoeing interval. Application of horseshoes that are too small is another predisposing factor (O'Grady, 1995b; Gnegy, 2003). The long toe and short heel forms a broken back-foot axis that predisposes the horse to stay apparatus injuries caused by delay in breakover, and navicular disease caused by increased strain on the DDFT. The condition may be accompanied by contracted heels.

Farriery of Long-Toe Low-Heels

Farriery of long-toe low-heels includes trimming the hoof in order to increase the hoof angle and establish normal foot axis. The condition may be corrected by trimming alone or with the application of horseshoes. The heels may be raised with a horseshoe fitted with a wedge pad or bar wedge pad. Alternatively, a wedged horseshoe or a wedged aluminum egg-bar shoe may be applied. Gnegy (2003) described the application of a horseshoe fitted with heel lifts welded to the ground surface of the horseshoe. Glue-on synthetic shoes may be applied, and in this case, the hoof angle is raised by pressing the horseshoe at the toe

and lifting the heels slightly during the curing process. Horseshoes used for long-toe low-heels should extend backward in order to provide additional palmar/plantar support; it may take several shoeing intervals to correct the condition.

Prevention of Long-Toe Low-Heels

Although the extent of damage to limbs as a result of long-toe low-heels is not clear, it could be significant. Therefore, prevention is important and relatively simple in most cases. The trimming or shoeing interval should be maintained according to the requirements of the individual horse; this interval can be quite variable among horses; the shoeing interval should be decreased with increased activity. The dorso-palmar/plantar balance should be maintained by trimming the heels minimally. The effect of excessive wear at the heels can be minimized by trimming the hoof to increase the hoof angle by 2° to 3°; this will result in a more upright hoof angle toward the next shoeing (Koepisch, 1998a).

CONTRACTED HEELS

Contracted heels OR CONTRACTED HOOVES IN horses is a common foot disorder characterized by narrowing of the hoof, contraction of the heels and atrophy of the frog. The condition is more common in the forelimbs but can develop in any limb. Contracted heels may develop from abnormal foot conformation, extreme hoof length (Stashak, 1987; Adams, 1974), disuse of the limb, horseshoes that don't fit properly, and unsanitary stabling conditions. Hoof contraction may result from environmental factors that remove moisture from the hoof; these include stabling the horse on urine and manure, and the use of hoof dressings and medication that dry the hoof. Disuse of the limb caused by painful conditions, and splinting or casting the limb for a prolonged time commonly result in contraction of the hoof. Stanley (2004) indicated that glue-on metal horseshoes causes con-

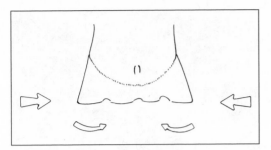

◆ **Fig. 17.4.** Planes of contraction in contracted heels, palmar/plantar view, schematic illustration. Narrowing (straight arrows) and curling (curved arrows) of the quarters and heels result in significant contraction in a short period of time.

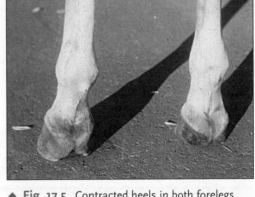

◆ **Fig. 17.5.** Contracted heels in both forelegs. (Photo by author.)

tracted hooves. Whereas, Craig and Craig (2003) showed that application of synthetic glue-on shoes results in expansion of normal hooves. Lungwitz (1966) described two variations of hoof contraction, *proximal hoof contraction* and *contracted sole*, both caused by dryness and too little exercise.

Hoof contraction is more pronounced at the heels due to the yielding nature of the palmar/plantar area of the foot. The planes of contraction include narrowing of the hoof wall, with concurrent inward curling of the quarters and heels toward the center of the foot (◆ fig. 17.4). Anderson (1992) indicated that curved bars are commonly observed in cases of contracted heels. According to Turner (1992), a hoof is classified as contracted if the frog width is less than 67 percent of the frog length. Mansmann (2000) indicated that mismatched feet with a width difference of more than 2 mm might signify a developing problem.

Initially, cases of contracted heels may show reduced performance. The pressure on internal structures caused by the contracting horn may be great enough to cause lameness; this condition was described by Rick (1907) as *hoof bound*. Some cases may be accompanied by increased sole concavity, and the hoof outline may become similar to that of a mule's hoof. Some feet may have *heel bulb contraction* characterized by formation of a deep groove between the bulbs of the heels (see ◆ fig 17.6;

plate 23). Crevices and grooves formed at the frog and bulbs of the heels form an ideal environment for development of thrush. Another complication that is associated with contracted heels is disruption of shock absorption (Rooney, 1974a). As the palmar/plantar aspect of the hoof wall becomes more upright, its ability to expand during weight bearing is reduced. This results in increased impact forces being transmitted to bone and ligaments, which predispose the horse to concussion-related lameness (◆ fig. 17.5).

Many cases of contracted heels have a long-toe low-heels foot conformation accompanied the condition. Measurements taken from a group of horses with long-toe hoof conformation showed a 7 percent decrease in the width of the hoof (measured between the angles of the sole), and 18 percent decrease in the maximum width of the frog (Glade and Salzman, 1985). Contraction may result from change in load alterations in the hoof caused by the low hoof angle and tensed DDFT (Avisar, 1995). Other factors that interfere with normal hoof load include neglected hooves (Layton, 1965) and poor hoof and horseshoe contact.

Contracted heels may develop secondary to lameness disorders such as observed in navicular disease and contracted flexor tendons. In both cases, weight bearing is being shifted toward the toe wall, and as a result, the heels become contracted. A study on navicular disease (Wright, 1993) showed a disparity between the hooves in bilateral cases, with the majority of smaller hooves being in the limbs with the most severe lameness. Sheared heels is another condition that may be accompanied by contracted heels.

Farriery of Contracted Heels

Farriery of contracted heels includes treatment of the underlying cause, hoof trimming, and application of therapeutic horseshoes when required. Lambert (1966) indicated that most of the treatment methods used for contracted heels are aimed at the symptoms and not the causes. The hooves should be trimmed short and balanced; some horses may become sore-footed following trimming, but improve within a few days. Several authors (Emery et al., 1977; Lungwitz, 1966; Stashak, 1987) pointed out that contracted heels and long-toe low-heels commonly occur together. In these cases, the hoof angle should be increased by 3° to 5° following trimming, and the horse should be exercised daily. Horses that tend to develop long-toe low-heels foot conformation should be trimmed every three to four weeks in order to maintain more a uniform hoof angle; some cases show dramatic improvement in the degree of contraction following one trimming (Stashak, 1987; Avisar, 1995).

Following trimming, the hooves should be re-hydrated by placing the horse in a puddle of water for 30 minutes or by applying a poultice pack for 12 hours. Following hydration of the hoof, the solar area is dressed with pine tar. Cases accompanied by heel bulb contraction are treated by packing the groove between the heel bulbs with a string of oakum soaked in pine tar (◆ fig. 17.6). Ideally, the horse should be kept barefoot in a pasture.

Farriery principles of horses with contracted hooves that are being shod include forward placement of horseshoe nails, fitting the horseshoe full, and providing palmar/plantar support. In order to encourage wall expansion, the last nail holes should be positioned

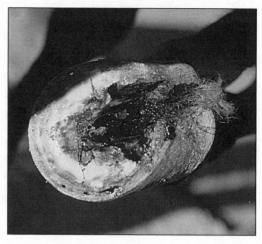

◆ **Fig. 17.6.** Treatment of heel bulb contraction with a string of oakum soaked in pine tar; the oakum is placed in the groove formed at the heel bulbs. (Photo by author.)

forward to the widest part of the hoof. The horseshoe branches should expand gradually from quarters to heels; a base for expansion that is 1/4 of the horseshoe's web should be established at the heels. The horseshoe branches should extended 2 cm palmar/plantar from the point of the heels. Good contact between the hoof and horseshoe is essential for proper hoof wall expansion. The types of horseshoes used for treatment of contracted heels include tip shoes, bar shoes, wide-web horseshoes, and beveled edge horseshoes (The Horseshoer, 1966; Turner, 1992). The tip shoe allows more natural hoof contact with the ground and does not interfere with hoof wall expansion; tip shoes have to be reset every three to four weeks in order to prevent the development of convexed toe. The beveled edge horseshoe encourages expansion of the hoof, but precise fitting of the horseshoe is required for its proper function. The bar shoe provides good expansion surface for the hoof wall in addition to heel support, and it can be beveled.

The application of a wide-web horseshoe combined with acrylic resin was described by

Jenny et al. (1965). This method includes fitting the horseshoe full and reconstructing the slope of the hoof wall at the quarters and heels with resin. Glueing the hoof to the horseshoe surface interferes with hoof wall expansion and should be avoided. Berns (1918) described the long-term effect of contracted heels in a group of horses with clinical signs similar to navicular disease. The horses were trimmed short and shod with horseshoes (with expanding springs) and leather pads. These horses became sound after a period of soreness. The use of expanding springs and spreading devices causes discomfort and is too risky.

BEVELED EDGE HORSESHOE

The *beveled edge horseshoe* is a horseshoe with branches that slope from the inner side of the horseshoe hoof surface toward the outside. The horseshoe is used in cases of contracted heels to encourage outward expansion of the hoof wall. The beveled edge horseshoe is fitted full, with the branches gradually expanding from quarters to heels. The hoof wall that corresponds to the slope of horseshoe should be trimmed precisely until it fits against the horseshoe; this can be achieved with hot shoe fitting and a hoof knife (◆ fig. 17.7). Prior to application of the horseshoe, the hoof should be re-hydrated.

 UNDER-RUN HEELS

Under-run heels IS A FOOT CONFORMATION characterized by weak and collapsed heels that are angled forward (◆ fig. 17.8). Other names for the condition include run-under heels, underslung heels, collapsed heels and sloping heels. The condition is observed primarily in the forelimbs and is common in performance horses (Turner, 1992). The abnormal foot conformation predisposes the horse to chronic heel soreness, musculoskeletal injuries, bruised heels, heel cracks, navicular syndrome (Turner, 1986b) and long-toe low-heels conformation (Moyer, 1981). Predisposing factors for under-run heels include neglected hooves, weak heels and small horseshoes. The high prevalence of under-run heels in Thoroughbreds and Quarter horses (Moyer, 1981; Moyer, 1990) suggests that it may have an hereditary basis; in Japan, the condition is considered a genetic problem (Oikawa and Kasashima, 2002). Under-run heels may be classified as a special case of long-toe low-heels but the latter condition responds to treatment better. Failure to treat the condition early may result in permanent alterations in

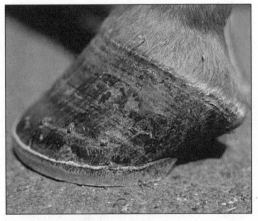

◆ **Fig. 17.8.** Under-run heels. Note the pronounced difference between the toe angle and the heel angle. The lack of support at the palmar area resulted in downward displacement of the coronary band at the heel bulbs. (Photo by author.)

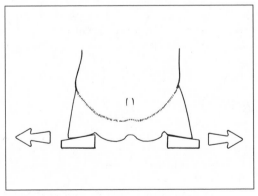

◆ **Fig. 17.7.** Beveled edge horseshoe, palmar/plantar view, schematic illustration. The bevel encourages hoof expansion (arrows).

hoof wall growth that can be very difficult to correct (Moyer, 1981).

Turner (1986b) defined under-run heels as a condition in which the toe angle and the heel angle differ by 5° or more. As a result of this difference, the hoof has smaller base distance and reduced palmar/plantar support. During impact, concussion forces are concentrated over a smaller surface area (Moyer, 1980). In some cases, the horn tubules at the heels begin to bend forward and the heels collapse (Moyer and Sigafoos, 1993; Sigafoos, 1991). The change in the foot axis results in excessive fetlock dorsiflextion and carpus hyperextension during motion (Moyer, 1980).

Under-run heels are associated with musculoskeletal injuries in Thoroughbred racehorses (Balch et al., 2001). The risk for suspensory apparatus failure (SAF) is 6.75 times greater when the toe-heel angle difference is greater than 10° (Kane et al., 1998). In a study on a group of 50 sound performance horses, 52 percent had under-run heels (Turner, 1988). A similar study on horses with navicular disease showed that 77 percent had under-run heels (Turner, 1986b).

Farriery of Under-Run Heels

Farriery principles of under-run heels includes the establishment of proper foot axis, increasing the hoof surface area, and providing palmar/plantar support. Increasing the hoof angle by trimming alone may result in insufficient hoof base distance and palmar/plantar support due to the angulation of the heels. Anderson (1981) and Koepisch (1998a) recommended lowering the heels in order to increase the base distance and then fitting the hoof with an aluminum wedged horseshoe that raises the heels. This method provides more uniform hoof dimension during the shoeing interval (Koepisch, 1998a), and encourages parallel horn growth at the heels with respect to the rest of the hoof wall. The horseshoe should extend backward in order to provide good palmar/plantar support (Moyer, 1981). The risk of a horseshoe being pulled by a hind limb may limit the amount of

support in the forelimbs. Other methods of raising the heels include the application of a horseshoe and wedge pad (Balch et al., 1995b) or bar wedge pad. In order to prevent weakening and collapse of the heels, the shoeing interval should be limited to four weeks.

Horses with quarters and heels that are badly collapsed may be fitted with mushroom horseshoes. This horseshoe removes direct pressure from the bearing surface of these areas and encourages new wall growth. The stem of the mushroom horseshoe should be fitted with a pad that provides a weight-bearing surface for the frog.

Reconstruction of the hoof wall with acrylic resin in under-run heels cases has been described (Moyer 1993 and Sigafoos; Sigafoos, 1991). The procedure is aimed at increasing the thickness of the heels and quarters, raising the palmar/plantar hoof area, and relieving the sole. The technique is difficult and time consuming, although Sigafoos (1991) reported a success rate of 75 percent in 32 treated cases of severe under-run heels.

BAR WEDGE PAD

The *bar wedge pad* or heel lifts is an open wedge pad used to support and increase the height of the heels; the pad is used in cases of under-run heels and long-toe low-heels. The pad is connected to the horseshoe branches with copper rivets (◆ fig. 17.9).

In cases where one heel has to be raised, an *insert pad* or *shim* can be made from a wedge pad or bar wedge pad. The insert pad is connected to the horseshoe with two copper rivets.

WEDGED HORSESHOE

The *wedged horseshoe* is a horseshoe that is tapered from the heels toward the toe (◆ fig. 17.10). This horseshoe is used to increase the hoof angle by raising the palmar/plantar aspect of the foot in cases of weak heels, low heels, under-run heels, navicular disease and suspensory apparatus injuries. The wedged horseshoe may be fitted at 180° in selected

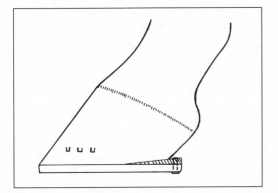

◆ **Fig. 17.9.** Bar wedge pad, side view, schematic illustration. Note that the pad fills the space under the heels and quarters and does not reach the toe.

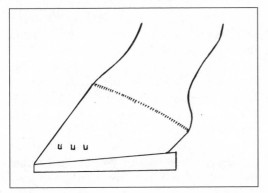

◆ **Fig. 17.10.** Wedged horseshoe, side view, schematic illustration.

cases of chronic laminitis in order to raise the toe wall and reposition the third phalanx. Asmus (1940) described the use of an iron wedge horseshoe with a rolled toe for horses with sore tendons. Koepisch (1998a) indicated that the wedge horseshoe permits more natural motion than a wedge pad does.

The horseshoe may be constructed from aluminum or iron bar stock. A method for calculating the desired angle, heel lift and ground surface length has been described (Sigafoos, 1989). Aluminum wedged horseshoes are commercially available as open or bar shoes, with 2 or 3° slope. The aluminum horseshoe weighs about 1/3 of that of a comparable iron horseshoe; therefore, it is more suitable for therapeutic purposes.

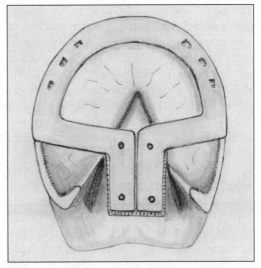

A

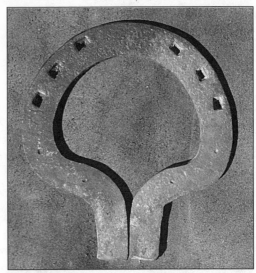

B

◆ **Fig. 17.11.** Mushroom horseshoe. A. Schematic illustration showing the relationship between the hoof and horseshoe, the parallel lines represent padding material. B. Forged horseshoe. (Photo by author.)

MUSHROOM HORSESHOE

The *mushroom horseshoe* is a horseshoe that fits the outline of the toe wall and then continues as a "stem" that is positioned under the frog (◆ fig. 7.11). The horseshoe is used to transfer load from the quarters and heels to the frog in cases of collapsed heels, sheared heels, sore heels, corns, quarter cracks and heel cracks. A *half-mushroom horseshoe* can be applied to cases where only one side is affected (page 213). Schmotzer et al. (1988) described the construction of a mushroom horseshoe made by welding a frog bar to a tip shoe; the horseshoe was fitted with a toe extension and was used in cases of contracted DDFT.

The mushroom horseshoe can be constructed from iron or aluminum bar stock; forging the horseshoe requires practice. In order to relieve the hoof wall, the "stem" should bear some weight (Carroll, 1989). This is achieved by fitting a piece of leather pad to the "stem" of the horseshoe; the pad should be connected with copper rivets. Alternatively, a soft resin may be applied over the "stem" with the use of a mold designed for use in heart-bar shoes.

 ## SHEARED HEELS

Sheared heels IS A CONFORMATIONAL DISTORTION of the foot characterized by proximal deviation of the coronary band at one heel, with increased in height of the same heel (◆ fig. 17.12). Russell (1882) described this conformation as *raised coronet*. Lungwitz (1966) described a similar condition, which he termed *wry foot*, characterized by gradual

bending of the hoof in toeing-out foot conformation, particularly in foals. In this case, the hoof becomes steeper at the inner hoof wall, with slanting at the outer hoof wall, and the inner heel becomes displaced upward.

Predisposing factors for sheared heels include abnormal limb deviation (Caldwell, 2001), chronic lameness that causes the horse to overuse one side of the hoof (Moyer and Anderson, 1975), lowering one side of the hoof in an attempt to correct a limb deviation, and application of a horseshoe with a short branch. Sheared heels develop as a result of excessive ground pressure against one heel caused by imbalance (Moyer and Anderson, 1975b; Finnegan and Rumph, 1991; Lungwitz, 1966; Page et al., 1992). The simultaneous placement of ground forces on one heel and driving forces on the opposite heel leads to development of shearing forces between the heels; consequently, the heel that is subjected to the excessive ground force is being displaced gradually upward together with the coronary band (Moyer and Anderson, 1975; Snow and Birdsall, 1990) (◆ fig. 17.13). In some cases, the heel may be "rolled" under the foot, and the foot axis is no longer cen-

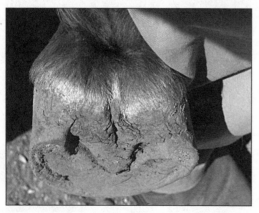

◆ **Fig. 17.12.** Sheared heels, palmar view. Note that one heel is displaced upwards. (Photo by author.)

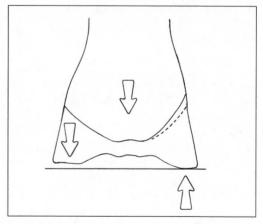

◆ **Fig. 17.13.** Development of sheared heels, palmar/plantar view, schematic illustration. Excessive ground pressure on one heel and driving force on the opposite heel result in upward displacement of the heel and proximal deviation of the coronary band. The dashed line represents the normal position of the coronary band. (Reprinted by permission from Moyer, W. and Anderson, J.P. 1975, fig. 1. Illustration modified to text.)

tered with the limb axis (Moyer and Anderson, 1975). Sheared heels may be accompanied by contraction of one or both heels (Lungwitz, 1966). A deep groove may develop between the heel bulbs, creating a favorable environment for development of deep thrush (Moyer and Anderson, 1975). Sheared heels predispose the horse to chronic heel soreness and lameness; the excessive load on the affected heel may result in hoof cracks and navicular disease. The clinical signs of sheared heels may be identical to those of navicular disease (Moyer and Anderson, 1975; Lungwitz, 1966).

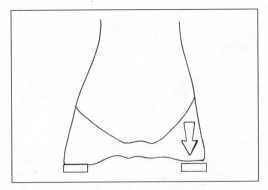

◆ **Fig. 17.14.** Shoeing principles for sheared heels, palmar/plantar view, schematic illustration. The heel and quarter on the proximally displaced side are lowered in order to relieve that side. (Adapted from Moyer W. and Anderson J.P. 1975, fig. 5.)

Farriery of Sheared Heels

The principles of farriery of sheared heels include the application of a therapeutic horseshoe that relieves the displaced heel, supports the foot and protects the heel. The primary cause of the condition should be investigated and corrected.

The hoof is trimmed to establish medial-lateral balance. Prior to shoeing, the hoof should be poulticed for 24 hours. The bearing surface of the heel and quarter of the displaced side is stepped (lowered), and the hoof is shod with a straight-bar or egg-bar shoe (◆ fig. 17.14). This procedure alleviates the discomfort caused by shearing and encourages distal displacement of the affected heel (Moyer and Anderson, 1975). The bar shoe may be stabilized further by welding a short diagonal bar, at the affected side, from the horseshoe branch to the center of the bar. This is particularly useful when a light horseshoe is used. In cases where the heel is "rolled" under the foot, the horseshoe should be centered with the foot axis by fitting it full on that side (Moyer and Anderson, 1975). Excess horn on the flared side should be trimmed.

Carroll (1989) indicated that a half-mushroom horseshoe can be used to relieve the displaced heel by turning the horseshoe branch at the affected side into a "stem." Alternatively, a z-bar shoe may be used for that purpose. Both horseshoes may not provide enough stability in actively working

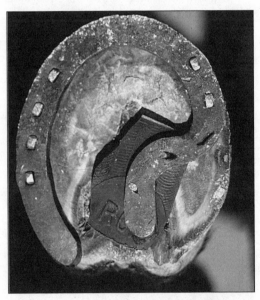

◆ **Fig. 17.15.** Forged half-mushroom horseshoe used to relieve pressure from the heel and quarter area. (Photo by author.)

horses, or enough protection for horses kept on rocky environment.

HALF-MUSHROOM HORSESHOE

The *half-mushroom horseshoe* is a horseshoe with one branch that has been turned into a "stem" positioned under the frog (◆ fig. 17.15). This horseshoe relieves pressure from the bearing surface of the quarter and heel on one side of the hoof. The half-mushroom horseshoe may be used in the treatment of heel and quarter cracks, corns, sheared heels, weak quarters and flail heel. The stem should be fitted with a leather or synthetic pad or soft acrylic resin that supports the frog. The pad is connected to the stem with copper rivets. The half-mushroom horseshoe may be used in horses that tend to pull horseshoes by stepping on the medial branch.

Z-BAR SHOE

The *z-bar shoe* is a modification of the bar shoe, with one branch of the horseshoe placed over the frog (◆ fig. 17.16). The horseshoe is similar to the half-mushroom shoe. The z-bar shoe is used to relieve pressure from one side of the hoof at the quarter and heel. The horseshoe is used in the treatment of quarter cracks, heel cracks, hoof wall avulsions, corns, sore heel, bar cracks and sheared heels (Carroll, 1989; Gregory, 2004a). The part of the horseshoe that is under the frog may be used to support weight; in this case, a triangular shaped leather pad or soft acrylic material should be fitted between the horseshoe and frog. Forging the z-bar horseshoe requires some practice (Gregory, 2004b).

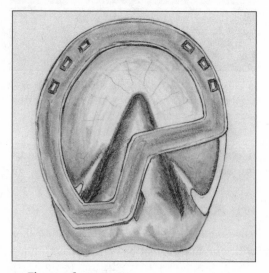

◆ **Fig. 17.16.** Z-bar shoe.

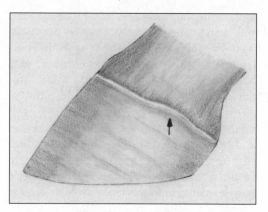

◆ **Fig. 17.17.** Proximal deviation of the coronary band (arrow).

🦯 PROXIMAL DEVIATION OF THE CORONARY BAND

Proximal deviation of the coronary band IS A conformational distortion of the foot characterized by upward displacement of a section of coronary band (◆ fig 17.17). Snow and Birdsall (1990) proposed that proximal deviation results from abnormal shearing forces caused by hoof imbalance. Sigafoos (1995) indicated that the condition might be associated with chronic refractory toe cracks or proximal quarter cracks. Caldwell (2001) noted that displacement of the coronary band might result from toeing-in or toeing-out foot conformation. Moyer and Anderson (1975b) described the displacement of the coronary band in cases of sheared heels. A special case of the condition may include downward displacement of the coronary band at the heel bulbs that is observed in under-run heels, and sloping pasterns (Aldrich, 1997).

Farriery of Proximal Deviation of the Coronary Band

Farriery of proximal deviation of the coronary band includes balancing the hoof and relieving pressure from the affected area. Snow and Birdsall (1990) recommended the addition of moisture to the hoof capsule prior to farriery in order to relieve abnormal shearing forces within the hoof; this includes pulling the horseshoe, trimming the sole and soaking the foot in warm water for 15 minutes. The hoof is fitted with a frog support pad and wrapped with moistened cotton held by an elastic adhesive bandage. The horse is stabled overnight until the hoof assumes its physiologic shape. This procedure is followed by trimming and balancing the foot. The hoof is shod with a bar shoe in order to distribute ground pressure more evenly.

In cases accompanied by a proximal hoof wall crack, shear forces are removed by making a horizontal groove between the crack and the coronary band (Sigafoos, 1995).

⚜ CLUBFOOT

Clubfoot IS A CHRONIC FOOT DISORDER characterized by a hoof with a short toe and high heel that gives the foot a stumpy appearance; the toe wall may be convexed and the white line at the toe is commonly wider than normal. Clubfoot in mature horses may be the result of severe or untreated contracted DDFT as foals, or of injury to the stay apparatus (◆ fig. 17.18). Most cases are observed in one forelimb. Butzow (1961) indicated that the hoof angle in clubfoot is greater than 60° to 65°, and the foot axis is "broken" forward. Depending on the degree of weight carried by the affected foot, the heels may be contracted or wider than normal. The affected hoof is smaller than the opposite hoof and the opposite foot may be wider than normal due to excessive weight bearing; the incidence of slight hoof pair asymmetry is not uncommon and it may reflect mild cases of contracted DDFT that were not treated as foals. These cases are difficult to detect. The differences in conformation between the feet may result in gait alterations that could cause lameness. Clubfoot may be accompanied by permanent stiffness of the DIP joint capsule that seriously impairs the usability of the horse. (For clubfoot in foals, see page 84.)

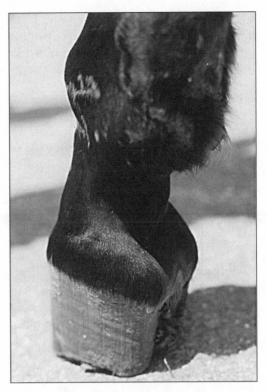

◆ **Fig. 17.18.** Clubfoot. This case developed from injury to the flexor tendons followed by scar tissue formation that limited the use of the limb. (Photo by author.)

Prevention of Clubfoot

The high prevalence of clubfoot in mature horses indicates that the disorder is hereditary in origin. The condition may not be noticeable in horses that underwent desmotomy of the inferior check ligament and appear healthy. Prevention of clubfoot includes the removal of foals and horses that are affected with the disorder from breeding stock (Loving, 1997).

Farriery of Clubfoot

Farriery of clubfoot includes trimming the affected hoof without modifying the hoof angle. Lowering the hoof angle results in abnormal tension in the DDFT, which forces the horse to bear excessive weight on the toe.

This may result in laminar tear with signs similar to road founder. The differences in appearance between the opposite feet may be improved by raising the hoof angle of the normal foot by 2° to 3°. The convex toe is rasped until it is continuous with the proximal toe wall. The hoof should be inspected for presence of thrush at the frog area and for separations at the white line. These areas should be debrided and treated with pine tar.

Horseshoes that are used to protect the foot include a light, plain horseshoe, tip shoe, and half-round horseshoe. Cases that are accompanied by contracted heels should have the heels trimmed low and than raised again with a wedged aluminum horseshoe, or a horseshoe and bar wedge pad; this loads the heels and encourages hoof expansion. The hoof may be poulticed overnight prior to shoeing. Tip shoes should be reset more often as they tend to concentrate pressure at the toe wall. The opposite hoof is commonly shod with a horseshoe that prevents spreading of the hoof wall and maintains the hoof angle.

A surgical procedure in adult horses can improve the condition, although some stiffness to the hoof wall may remain (Wagner et al., 1985b). The surgery involves the resection of the inferior check ligament of the DDFT as is done with foals.

MULE FOOT

Mule foot CONFORMATION IS CHARACTERIZED BY narrow hooves with quarters that are nearly parallel to each other and a steep hoof wall (◆ fig. 17.19). The condition is also called mule heels or narrow foot. Mule foot conformation has reduced ability to absorb shock, consequently the horse becomes predisposed to concussion related lameness and quarter cracks. Loving (1997) indicated that mule foot is more common in Quarter Horses, Arabian, Saddlebred, Tennessee Walking and Fox Trotter horses. Ellis (1998) indicated that a condition of "donkey-like shaped feet" exists in certain Thoroughbred sire lines.

Farriery of mule foot includes the application of light horseshoes such as training

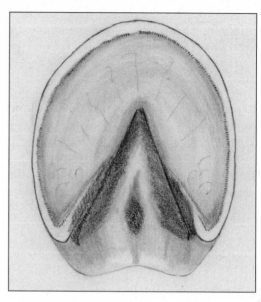

◆ **Fig. 17.19.** Mule Foot.

plates or half-round horseshoes. The horseshoe should be fitted full to permit hoof expansion. The horseshoe may be fitted with a rim pad in order to absorb some concussion.

BEAR FOOT

Bear foot OR "COON FOOT" CONFORMATION IS characterized by a digit with a sloping pastern and upright hoof with "broken forward" foot axis; the toe wall may be concave from proximal to distal direction (Lungwitz, 1966; Shively, 1982a) (◆ fig. 17.20a). Development of bear foot conformation appears to be secondary to change in weight distribution over the foot. The condition is associated with weak suspensory apparatus, long pasterns (Loving, 1997), and it is common in old horses with collapsed suspensory apparatus. The use of horses with this disorder may be limited.

Farriery of bear foot includes the application of an extended heels horseshoes or egg-bar shoe in order to increase palmar/plantar support. Affected limbs may be fitted with a support bandage. Cases accompanied by severe suspensory apparatus collapse may be fitted with fetlock sling shoe. (for example of bear foot see ◆ fig. 18.9).

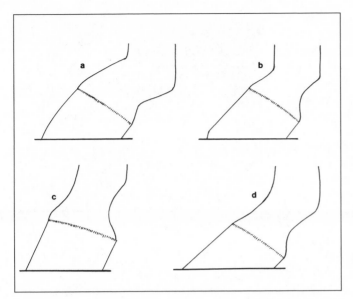

◆ **Fig. 17.20.** Abnormal hoof and digit conformation, schematic illustrations. Bear foot (a), bull-nosed hoof (b), stumpy foot (c), sloping pastern (d). (Adapted from Shively, M. J. 1982a, fig. 4, B-E.)

increases the hoof angle and provides additional palmar/plantar support.

STUMPY FOOT

Stumpy foot CONFORMATION IS characterized by a hoof with a "boxy" appearance accompanied by upright and relatively short pastern (◆ fig. 17.20c). The condition is also called stumpy pastern, upright pastern or upright hoof. Stumpy foot may be similar in appearance to clubfoot, but it appears in all four limbs and the foot axis is not "broken"; the condition is more common in ponies and draft breeds, and their crosses with other horses. Weight bearing in stumpy foot conformation falls on the dorsal aspect of the foot (Aldrich, 1997; Butzow, 1961). Consequently, there is a lack of hoof expansion (Butzow, 1961) and impaired shock absorption. Rooney (1981b) indicated that horses with this type of conformation are predisposed to non-articular ringbone.

Farriery of horses with stumpy foot includes trimming the hoof in order to increase the hoof angle; this flexes the DIP joint and provides some flexibility to the digit. The hoof angle may be raised with the application of a horseshoe and wedge pad. Concussion forces in working horses should be reduced by application of horseshoes fitted with thick pads or with glue-on shoes.

BULL-NOSED HOOF

Bull-nosed hoof IS A HOOF WITH A DUBBED TOE wall (◆ fig. 17.20b). The condition results from setting the horseshoes too far back and rasping the toe wall until the hoof fits the horseshoe (Shively, 1982a). Another practice that results in this conformation is dubbing the toe wall in horses with flat sole, where no sole can be trimmed, in order to make the hoof appear short at the toe wall. Aldrich (1997) indicated that bull-nosed hoof may cause increased ground pressure over the palmar/plantar aspect of the hoof with a consequent decrease in heels angulation.

Dubbing the toe wall in order to shorten the HLA may be done in cases of chronic laminitis, navicular disease and in horses with accidental limb contact problems.

Farriery of bull-nosed hoof conformation includes the application of an extended heels horseshoe that provides palmar/plantar support and allow normal hoof growth. In cases of flat sole, the hoof should be trimmed short and shod with a wedged aluminum horseshoe or horseshoe and wedge pad that

SLOPING PASTERNS

Sloping pasterns CONFORMATION IS characterized by a low hoof angle, weak pasterns, and a foot axis of 45° or less; the foot axis may be "broken" or continued with the pastern axis (◆ fig. 17.20d). The condition is also called low foot, low pastern and sloping hoof. Sloping hoof is accompanied by weak suspensory apparatus, although the ride on these horses may be smoother than usual due to the flexibility of the limb (Shively, 1982a). During motion, the fetlocks may touch the ground and become injured; weight bearing shifts toward the palmar/plantar aspect of the heels, which may expand more than normal. The pastern tends to bend over at the heels, and consequently, the coronary band may become sheared downward (Aldrich, 1997). Horses with excessive sloping of the hooves and pasterns have limited use due to the extreme strain that is placed on the suspensory apparatus.

Farriery of sloping hoof includes the application of an extended heels horseshoe in order to provide palmar/plantar support. The limbs of working horses should be fitted with support bandages or with fetlock support boots.

Prevention of sloping hoof includes the removal of affected foals and horses from breeding stock.

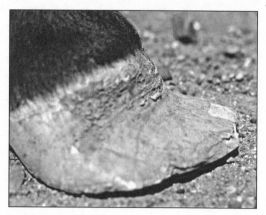

◆ **Fig. 17.21.** Convexed toe. (Photo by author.)

white line should be debrided and treated with pine tar. The hoof is shod with a protective horseshoe. The type of horseshoe used depends on the underlying cause. A wide-web, seated-out horseshoe, or a reversed horseshoe, may be used to remove pressure from the toe wall.

CONVEXED TOE

Convexed toe OR DISHED TOE IS A FOOT conformation characterized by upward bending or curling of the toe wall caused by excessive pressure on the bearing surface of the toe (◆ fig. 17.21). The condition may develop in clubfoot, seedy toe and chronic selenosis, and it is common in foals with contracted DDFT. Convexed toe may develop from hoof overgrowth (Aldrich, 1997). The condition is commonly accompanied by widening of the white line, which may become infected with thrush or white line disease. The excessive pressure on the toe wall may result in development of distal toe cracks, and the foot may become predisposed to development of sole abscess. Severe cases of convexed toe may be accompanied by laminar tear and third phalanx rotation.

Farriery of convexed toe includes treatment of the underlying cause, trimming the foot with minimal changes in the hoof angle, and rasping the toe wall until it becomes continuous with the proximal hoof wall. The

BUTTRESS FOOT

Buttress foot OR PYRAMIDAL DISEASE IS A FOOT conformation characterized by alteration in the shape of the toe wall caused by ossification (deposition of new bone) over the extensor process of the third phalanx (◆ fig. 17.22). Ossification may result from tearing and avulsion of the common digital extensor tendon at its insertion point (Rooney, 1981b) or following fracture of the extensor process (Frank, 1953; McCunn, 1951). Rooney (1981b) indicated that horses with short toe and high heels conformations are predisposed to the condition. The deposition of new bone over the extensor process results in an outward bulging of the coronary band with consequent protrusion of the toe wall that may attain a triangular shape when viewed from the dorsal perspective (Frank, 1953). The normal range of free movement of the foot may be limited (McCunn, 1951) but the horse may walk sound (Frank, 1953).

Farriery of buttress foot cases includes thinning the proximal toe wall to relieve pres-

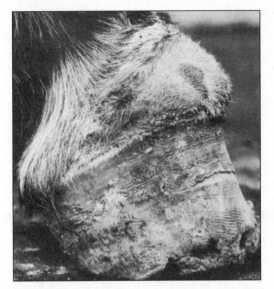

◆ **Fig. 17.22. Buttress foot.** (Reprinted from Frank, E.R. 1953. Veterinary Surgery. Minneapolis, Burgess Publishing Company.)

sure on the sensitive laminae (Frank, 1953), and the application of a horseshoe and thick pad that absorbs some concussion.

🔧 FLARED HOOF

Flared hoof IS CHARACTERIZED BY A HOOF outline that is flared on one side and upright on the opposite side (Lungwitz, 1966). The condition is also called hoof asymmetry, crooked wall and deformed foot. In some cases the hoof may be flared at the toe. The process may begin from a disease that weakens the white line, uneven forces placed on the hoof wall, or both. Flared hoof may develop from thrush, white line disease, chronic laminitis, abnormal hoof conformation, crooked stance caused by chronic lameness (Loving, 1997), faults and neglect of the foot (Lungwitz, 1966), limb deviation (Caldwell, 2001) and imbalance (◆ fig. 17.23). Slight hoof asymmetry with greater slope and wider margins on the lateral side is normal.

The abnormal stance results in flaring away of the hoof wall at the side that receives less pressure, and curling under of the hoof wall at the side that receives more pressure.

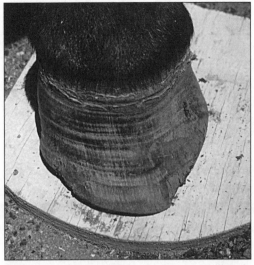

A

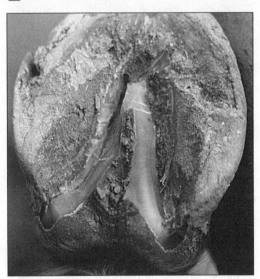

B

◆ **Fig. 17.23. Hoof asymmetry.** A. Asymmetry at the toe wall that developed from standing crooked as a result of chronic injury to the pastern. B. Asymmetry in one quarter caused by flaring. (Photos by author.)

The condition is commonly accompanied by widening or separation of the white line at the flared side and development of thrush in this area. The uneven pressure predisposes the foot to proximal deviation of the coronary band and sheared heels (Moyer and Anderson, 1975b).

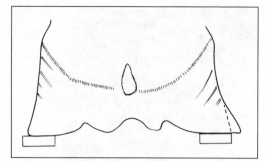

◆ **Fig. 17.24.** Fitting the horseshoe to a hoof with side-to-side asymmetry, palmar/plantar view, schematic illustration. The horseshoe is placed full on the deficit side and close on the flared side in order to center the horseshoe with the limb.

Farriery of Flared Hoof

Farriery of hoof asymmetry includes trimming the hoof level, debridement of separated white line and application of pine tar or hoof pack. The hoof may be shod with a wide-web horseshoe, wide-web bar shoe or a side-support horseshoe. The horseshoe should be fitted full on the deficit side and close on the flared side in order to center the foot axis with the limb (Moyer, 1990) (◆ fig. 17.24). Excess flare should be trimmed. The wide-web horseshoe provides good medial-lateral stability and permits placement of horseshoe nail holes according to the hoof outline. A double crease horseshoe can be used in cases where a light horseshoe is required; the inner crease at the deficit side is used for horseshoe nail placement (see below).

In order to prevent the horseshoes from being pulled by the opposite limb, the space between the horseshoe branch and the hoof wall at the deficit side can be filled with acrylic resin (Jenny et al., 1965). The repair material should not adhere to the horseshoe as this interferes with hoof expansion.

SIDE-SUPPORT HORSESHOE

The *side-support horseshoe* is a horseshoe with one branch that is wider than the other (Koepisch, 1998a). The horseshoe is used to center the hoof with the limb in cases of

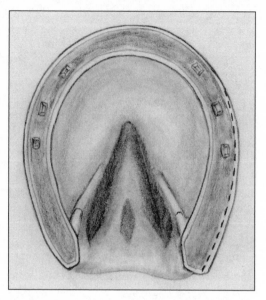

◆ **Fig. 17.25.** Side support horseshoe, palmar/plantar view, schematic illustration. The dashed line represent the hoof outline.

flared hoof and to protect the hoof from excessive wear (◆ fig. 17.25).

The side-support horseshoe can be forged from a wide-web bar stock such as 4.0 cm x 0.6 cm (1½" x ¼"), one branch is drawn to 2/3 the web of the opposite branch. The wide branch is placed at the deficit side and fitted full so it protrudes gradually from the widest part of the quarters toward the heels (Koepisch, 1998a); the horseshoe nail holes are placed closer to the inner side of the branch. This centers the horseshoe with the limb. An aluminum side-support horseshoe is available commercially.

DOUBLE CREASE HORSESHOE

The *double crease horseshoe* is a light horseshoe with an inner and outer crease, with dimensions of 2.2 cm x 0.6 cm (◆ fig. 17.26). The horseshoe is used as a light, wide-web horseshoe or side-support horseshoe; it may be applied to cases of weak hoof wall, missing sections of hoof wall, white line disease, flared hoof and clefts. The double crease permits positioning of the horseshoe nail holes at the outer or inner web at different positions

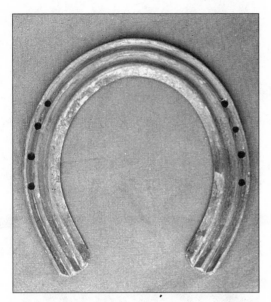

◆ **Fig. 17.26.** Double crease horseshoe. (Photo by author.)

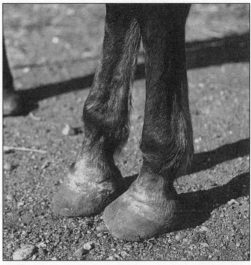

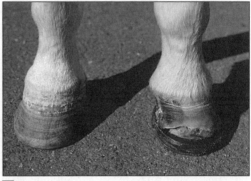

◆ **Fig. 17.27.** Hoof pair asymmetry. A. The fetlock of the right limb is knuckling over and the heels on this hoof tend to grow high. The left hoof, which bears more weight, is flat with low heels. B. Application of a horseshoe and a thick pad to a case with different hoof height. (Photos by author.)

around the hoof wall. In cases that require additional stability, the horseshoe can be forged as a bar shoe. The double crease horseshoe may be applied to weanlings and yearlings with severe foot deviations as a side-support horseshoe.

The horseshoe can be forged from light bar iron stock with the use of a creaser, or with a swedge block. Two creases are made along the entire length of the bar and the horseshoe is turned and shaped with a wooden mallet. The nail holes are made by drilling 3 mm holes at the desired positions. Small size, city-head nails should be used for nailing the horseshoe. The horseshoe may not be available commercially.

HOOF PAIR ASYMMETRY

Hoof pair asymmetry OR MISMATCHED FEET ARE characterized by a pair of fore or hind feet that have different shape, size and hoof angle. Hoof pair asymmetry develops in chronic conditions such as clubfoot or fetlock flexoral deformity (knuckling over). The condition develops from alterations in weight bearing

on the affected limb and excessive weight bearing on the opposite limb. Horses with mismatched feet may stumble during work due to interrupted limb action (◆ fig. 17.27A).

In a study on a group of 50 sound horses, Mansmann et al. (2000) found that 54 percent of the horses had mismatched feet. They indicated that obvious mismatching is suggestive of a previous, current or developing problem; the study defined mismatched feet as feet with hoof angle differences of 2° or higher, and/or with differences in hoof width of 2 mm or more, between left and right feet.

Farriery of hoof pair asymmetry includes matching the feet as much as possible without interfering with their function. This is achieved by fitting the healthy hoof with a horseshoe and wedge pad. Lowering the hoof angle of the affected hoof should be avoided as this will places excessive strain on the stay apparatus.

Mismatched feet may result from one hoof becoming shorter than the opposite hoof, such as following extensive debridement of one foot. In this case, the shorter hoof should be fitted with a horseshoe and a thick flat pad (◆ Fig. 17.27B).

 THIN-WALLED HOOVES

Thin-walled hooves IS A COMMON HOOF conformation fault in horses characterized by inadequate hoof wall thickness, and in most cases by small feet (see below). The condition is observed in Quarter Horses, Thoroughbred, Saddlebred (Loving, 1997) and Warmblood horses (◆ fig. 17.28). Thin-walled hooves have limited shock absorption capability which predispose the horse to concussion-related lameness. Abnormal shear forces that develop in the hoof wall may result in development of hairline cracks and hoof wall cracks. The quarters and heels may collapse, resulting in development of long-toe low-heels. Driving horseshoe nails in hooves with thin wall is difficult, as is maintaining horseshoes in place. Horseshoe nails are easily driven too close to the dermis and the horse may become lame (Hickman, 1964).

Farriery of thin-walled hooves includes the use of light horseshoes and small horseshoe nails. The horseshoe is forged from a light bar stock and the horseshoe nail holes are placed according to the hoof conformation. In order to reduce strain from the hoof wall, six holes are punched on each side of the horseshoe, and three holes are used alternatively at each reset. The strength of shoeing can be increased by welding a toe clip or side

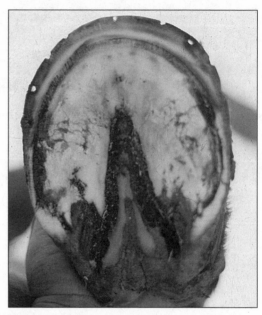

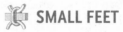 **Fig. 17.28.** Thin hoof wall. (Photo by author.)

clips to the horseshoe. Alternatively, the hooves can be fitted with glue-on shoes.

Horse owners and breeders should be advised to remove horses with thin hoof wall from breeding stock.

 SMALL FEET

Small feet ARE A COMMON FOOT PROBLEM observed in horses. The condition is characterized by disproportion between hoof size and body weight; most cases are accompanied by thin hoof wall (◆ fig. 17.29). Small feet are common in Quarter Horses, Thoroughbred and Saddlebred horses (Loving, 1997). The condition predisposes the horse to concussion related injuries, hoof wall cracks and navicular disease. Turner (1986b) indicated that small feet are a sign for poor prognosis in cases of navicular disease. Loving (1997) indicated that small feet are a heritable condition, and recommended that these horses should not be used as a breeding stock.

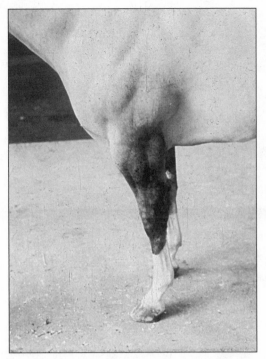

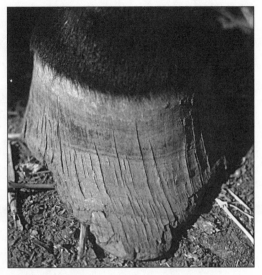

◆ **Fig. 17.30.** Dry hoof accompanied with longitudinal splits in the hoof wall. (Photo by author.)

◆ **Fig. 17.29.** Small feet with disproportionately large body size in a Quarter Horse. (Photo by author.)

Farriery of Small Feet

Farriery of small feet conformation includes the application of a horseshoe that is fitted full all around in order to increase the bearing surface area of the hoof (Turner, 1992). The margins of the horseshoe should be filed smooth to decrease the possibility of the horseshoe being pulled, or injury from accidental limb contact. The horseshoe should be light and the nail holes should be placed according to the conformation of the hoof. The horseshoe may be fitted with toe or side clips. The degree of concussion that is transmitted to the foot can be reduced by fitting the horseshoe with a thick pad or a rim pad. Alternatively, the feet may be fitted with glue-on shoes. The advantage of the glue-on shoe is that it increases the bearing surface area of the hoof significantly, it absorbs shock, and no horseshoe nails are applied.

DRY HOOVES

Dry hooves ARE CHARACTERIZED BY DRY, CRACKED hoof wall, shriveled frog and contracted hoof. The condition affects horses kept in stables and horses that are raised in arid areas or areas with hot summers (Dickson and O'Malley, 1987) (◆ fig. 17.30). Many horses raised in desert areas have hooves that are dry and hard. These hooves are adapted to the environment and have normal conformation.

Causes that lead to moisture loss from the hoof include stabling horses in manure, urine and sand (Butler, 1977a; Dickson and O'Malley, 1987). Butzow (1961) indicated that horses confined to dry stables and corrals have a tendency to develop dry hooves and contracted heels. Dickson and O'Malley (1987) point out that the application of cosmetic hoof paint dries the hoof wall.

Treatment of dry hooves includes the addition of moisture to the hoof capsule and prevention of its loss (Butzow, 1961). The horse should be placed in a clean environment with a ground surfaces low in salt content. Horses raised in sandy paddocks or arid

◆ **Fig. 17.31.** Maintaining hoof moisture. A water puddle attracts a group of horses in an arid area. (Photo by author.)

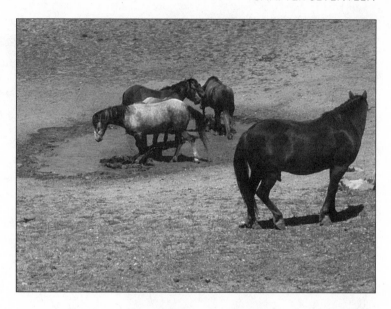

areas can have their feet moistened periodically in a water hole, creek or a footbath (Dickson and O'Malley, 1987). Alternatively, the feet can be washed daily or packed with clay (Butler, 1977a) (◆ fig. 17.31). Following addition of moisture to the hoof, the solar area is covered with pine tar. Butzow (1961) indicated that proper exercise increases circulation and helps maintain proper hoof moisture.

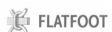 FLATFOOT

Flatfoot IS CHARACTERIZED BY A SOLE THAT IS near level or level with the bearing surface of the hoof wall (◆ fig. 17.32). The condition is also called flat sole, dropped sole, puddle foot and mushroom foot. Flatfoot may develop in chronic laminitis, weak hoof wall, excessive hoof wear or delay in shedding of the sole. It is commonly observed in heavy horses such as draft horses, and it may develop in horses with weak and flaring hoof wall. Flat sole predisposes the horse to sub-solar bruising, sore feet and lameness. The area most prone to bruising is at the dorsal (front) area of the sole (Thomas, 1998). Working horses with flatfoot may become bruised over the solar area even when shod.

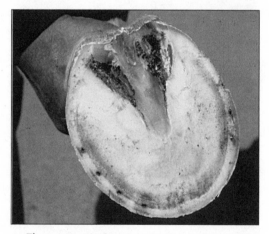

◆ **Fig. 17.32.** Flatfoot. Note the bruised area between the frog and toe. (Photo by author.)

Farriery of Flatfoot

Farriery of horses with flatfoot includes the application of a wide-web horseshoe. The horseshoe should be well seated-out in order to prevent contact between the sole and horseshoe (Martinelli and Ferrie, 1998). Alternatively, the hoof may be shod with a horseshoe and a rim pad, full pad or a molded pad. A full pad may be cut into an open pad, leaving the inner margins of the pad to cover part of the solar area. Thomas (1998) recommended the use of a ¼" neoprene pad. The pad should be cut open in cases where the frog is bulging out. Working horses may be protected with armor-plated horseshoes, provided that the weight of the horseshoes does not interfere with limb function. Alternatively, a wide-web synthetic glue-on shoe can be used; the resin should not be placed over the flat solar area.

In cases where the hoof angle is too low but no sole can be trimmed, the hoof should be shod with a wedged aluminum horseshoe that increases the hoof angle and provides good palmar/plantar support. Alternatively, a horseshoe and wedge pad may be used.

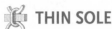 THICK SOLE

Thick sole IS CHARACTERIZED BY A FLAT FOOT with a thick sole (Moyer, 1980; Anderson, 1992). Other names include false sole and retained sole. The condition is caused by a retained sole that fails to shed. Anderson (1992) indicated that thick sole is more common in horses that are stalled on deep bedding with little exercise (◆ fig. 17.33). The retained sole causes the sole to lose its flexibility (Anderson, 1992; Emery et al., 1977) and the ability of the hoof to absorb shock is reduced (Emery et al., 1977). The flat hoof surface interferes with normal hoof and ground interaction.

Farriery of thick sole includes careful trimming of the sole with a hoof knife or half-round hoof nippers. The hooves may be poulticed for 24 hours prior to trimming in order to soften the sole. Prevention of retained sole includes placing the horse in a pasture, preferably in a rocky environment, and increasing the amount of exercise.

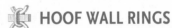 THIN SOLE

Thin sole IS CHARACTERIZED BY A SOLE THAT yields easily to thumb pressure. The condition may result from excessive hoof wear or hoof trimming, and it is observed in hooves that grow slowly. Thin sole is commonly observed in Thoroughbred horses, which have a characteristic thin and concave sole. The condition predisposes to sub-solar bruising and lameness and the horse may be sore-footed following horseshoeing. The feet may be protected with a light horseshoe and a flat pad, rim pad or a molded pad.

HOOF WALL RINGS

Hoof wall rings ARE CAUSED BY INTERMITTENT hoof wall growth with development of alternating ridges and depressions that encircle

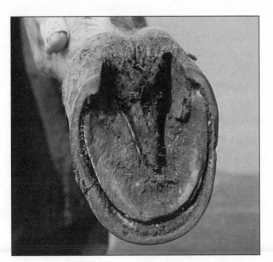

◆ **Fig. 17.33.** Thick sole. In this case, there is a separation at the white line that shows the retained sole. (Photo by author.)

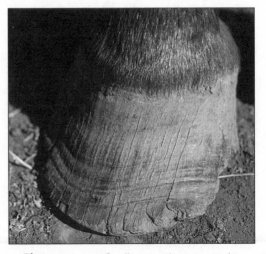

◆ **Fig. 17.34.** Hoof wall rings. The rings on this hoof developed as a result of seasonal diet change. (Photo by author.)

the hoof, parallel to the coronary band (Smythe and Goody, 1967) (◆ fig. 17.34). The condition is also called horizontal rings, fever rings, feed rings and grass rings. Most hoof wall rings are insignificant but have to be differentiated from hoof rings caused by chronic laminitis and chronic selenosis (see below). Hoof rings may develop from a dietary change or systemic illness that causes unequal zones of horn growth (Smithcors, 1961c). Hoof growth is accelerated when horses are turned into spring pastures, which results in grass rings. Horses that are placed outside during the winter may develop circular depressions over the hoof (Smythe and goody, 1967). Rooney (1999) proposed that hoof rings might develop by the action of compressive forces at the outer portion of the hoof wall. Pressure rings may be observed in foals with ALD (see ◆ fig. 11.27).

Abnormal Hoof Wall Rings

Abnormal hoof wall rings commonly develop in horses with chronic laminitis. The *laminitic rings* typically diverge from the toe toward the heels, whereas rings caused by other factors are parallel to the coronary band (see ◆ fig. 16.9; plate 14). This divergence is the result of slower horn growth at the toe relative to the heels (Ritmeester and Ferguson, 1996; Ritmeester et al., 1998). The differences in growth rate leads to development of convexed toe. Smyhte and Goody (1967) indicated that laminitic rings have deeper and wider circular grooves compared to normal rings. Rings caused by chronic selenosis may be corrugated and the hoof wall may develop horizontal hoof wall cracks.

OFFSET PASTERNS

Offset pasterns IS A CONFORMATION FAULT characterized by pasterns that are positioned toward one side of the foot when viewed from the dorsal perspective (◆ fig.17.35). The author observed one case, in the forelimbs of a Quarter Horse gelding. The condition resulted in excessive pressure on the offset side that led to

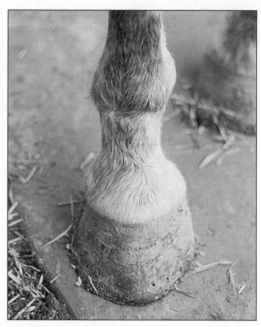

◆ **Fig. 17.35.** Offset pastern. The pastern of the forelimb is positioned toward the lateral aspect of the foot. (Photo by author.)

collapse of the heel on that side. This predisposes the horse to collateral ligament desmitis and joint disease. Offset pasterns resemble toeing-out or toeing-in foot conformation.

Farriery of offset pasterns includes trimming the hoof in order to correct the mediolateral imbalance, and preventing the collapse of the heels. Following trimming, the hoof is shod with a wide-web horseshoe fitted full on the offset side. Alternatively, a lateral support horseshoe may be used. In cases where a gap exists between the horseshoe and heels, the horseshoe should be fitted with a leather shin. Alternatively, the heel may be reconstructed with acrylic resin. A regular hoof-trimming interval of four weeks should be maintained in order to prevent the collapse of the heels in affected limbs.

HABITS THAT EFFECT HOOF SHAPE

Horses may develop *habits* that can affect hoof shape and health; identifying these changes during pre-purchase examination can provide clues about the horse's behavior. Habits that effect hoof shape include resting one hind foot over the opposite foot, pawing, weaving, walking back and forth, and placing the limbs under the chest when lying down (Goubaux and Barrier, 1892). Standing with one hind foot over the other occurs when the horse is in resting position; the coronary band becomes rubbed and bruised, and the hoof wall below it may show signs of wear. In addition, horses fitted with sharp caulks may lacerate the coronary band if they are startled, by treading themselves (Magner, 1980). *Pawing* is a habit that develops in horses confined to a stable with little exercise. The hoof becomes excessively worn at the toe-bearing surface, and if the horse is shod the horseshoe are worn down rapidly. Prevention of pawing includes regular exercising of these horses. *Weaving* is a habit characterized by constant sideway motion of the head and forelimb while the horse stays more or less in the same place. Consequently, the fore hooves wear down at the medial quarters bearing surface; the excessive pressure result in convex hoof wall at this area. Weaving is a habit that is difficult to eliminate, Goubaux and Barrier (1892) recommended placing the horse in cross-ties that prevent side motion of the head. Some horses acquire the habit of walking back and forth in the stable or paddock, which result in excessive wear and bruising of the hooves (see ◆ fig. 16.41). Prevention of this habit includes regular exercising of the horse; the introduction of a companion animal may help in some cases.

Another habit, which does not affect the hooves, but result in *shoe-boil* or inflammation of the elbow is observed in horses that lay down with the forelimbs placed under the chest, with the horseshoe branches pressing the elbows. Prevention of shoe-boil include shortening the horseshoe branches or application of spooned heels horseshoe (see ◆ fig. 16.56). Alternatively, the foot can be fitted with *sausage boot* placed around the lower pastern, the boot is made from a padded leather or rubber ring that prevent direct pressure on the elbow (Lyon, 1934) (◆ fig. 17.36). Keeping the horse barefoot when practical, solve this problem.

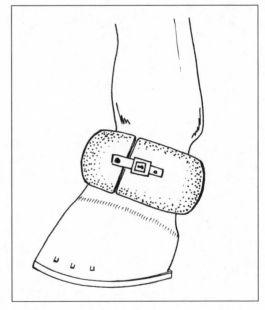

◆ **Fig. 17.36.** Sausage boot.

Chapter 18

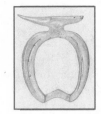

Farriery of Tendon and Ligament Injuries

TENDONITIS OF THE DIGITAL FLEXOR TENDONS

Tendonitis IS AN INFLAMMATION IN A TENDON caused by excessive strain that leads to tearing of fibers within the tendon; consequently, the tendon become inflamed and painful. Most cases of acute tendonitis result in acute lameness that appears during or immediately after exercise. The structures commonly involved include the superficial digital flexor tendon (SDFT) and deep digital flexor tendon (DDFT). Tendonitis is more common in the forelimbs, and it is common in racehorses. Healing time for tendon injuries is prolonged, resulting in significant economic losses. Repeated insults on the SDFT may lead to development of *bowed tendon* or chronic tendonitis that can seriously limit the usefulness of the horse (◆ fig. 18.1). Another form of tendonitis results from infection caused by microorganisms following injury to the limb.

Predisposing factors for tendonitis of the digital flexor tendons include long-toe low-

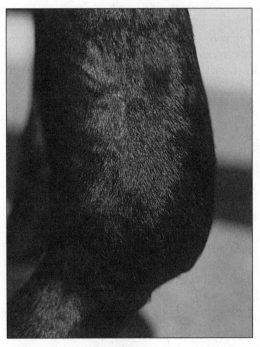

◆ **Fig. 18.1. Bowed tendon.** This condition developed from chronic SDFT tendonitis accompanied by scarring and thickening of the tendon. Note the "bow" shape at the palmar aspect of the metacarpus. (Photo by author.)

heels, under-run heels, soft tracks (Oikawa and Kasashima, 2002), lack of fitness, fatigue, hard ground, short horseshoes, traction devices and sloping pasterns. These factors increase breakover time and fetlock dorsiflextion, which lead to development of abnormal tension in the SDFT, DDFT and their corresponding check ligaments, the suspensory ligament (SL) and sesamoidean ligaments.

The treatment approach to acutely lame horses with tendonitis depends on the structures involved. Raising the heels reduces strain from the DDFT but not from the SDFT (Thompson, 1998; Meershoek et al., 2002) or the SL (Thompson 1998). Meershoek et al. (2002) indicated that application of a heel wedge in SDFT tendonitis cases increases the forces on the tendon and may exacerbate the existing lesion. Therefore, tension from the SDFT and SL should be reduced by raising the heels and flexing the fetlock joint simultaneously; this may be achieved with the application of a lower limb splint or a board splint. Tension from the DDFT is reduced by raising the heels with wedge pads or a Patten shoe; the heels should be raised until relief of tension can be felt when the tendon is manipulated sideways with the hand (Dyson and Marks, 2003). In all cases, the affected limb and the opposite healthy limb should be wrapped with support bandages. Prior to being transported to a medical facility, the limbs of cases of non-weight bearing lameness should be wrapped with a well-padded support bandage and immobilized with a lower-limb splint or a board splint. Smith et al, (2002) described the use of a *tendon support boot* designed to support the fetlock joint during exercise; the boot may be applied to cases of flexor tendon or suspensory ligament injuries.

Prevention of Tendonitis

Because tendons and ligaments have poor healing capacity, the prevention of tendon injuries is extremely important. Studies that correlate poor balance and stay apparatus

injuries in horses are lacking or anecdotal in origin. The reason for that may be the difficulty in carrying out field research of this type. One source (Gee, 2006) described lower incidences of bowed tendons and suspensory ligament injuries in Walking Horses attributed to improved shoeing practices. Nevertheless, the incidence of tendonitis may be significantly lowered by proper hoof care management that includes maintaining short shoeing intervals, balancing the feet, applying horseshoes that are proportional to the hooves, avoiding the use of traction devices, and providing adequate palmar/plantar support. Raising the hoof angle by 2° to 3° in order to compensate for a decrease in hoof angle toward the end of the shoeing interval can reduce tension from the stay apparatus. Oikawa and Kasashima (2002) indicated that application of egg-bar shoes following correction of hoof irregularities stabilizes the hoof and reduces strain from the SDFT. Application of support bandages or tendon support boots during exercise may prevent some injuries. In addition, the level and type of activity, and the degree of fitness of the horse are important factors that have to be considered by horse trainers and owners.

Farriery of Tendonitis of the Flexor Tendons

The farriery methods used in the treatment of tendonitis of the flexor tendons depend on the structures involved and severity of the injury. In all cases, the old horseshoe should be pulled and the hoof trimmed in order to raise the heels maximally. Horseshoes may be used as a base for attachment for various adjuncts such as pads, splints or combinations of these.

Mild cases of DDFT tendonitis are treated by raising the heels with an aluminum wedge horseshoe or a horseshoe and wedge pad, combined with a support bandage. The horseshoe branches should extend backward in order to provide additional palmar/plantar support. Moderate cases of DDFT tendonitis are treated by immobilizing the lower limb

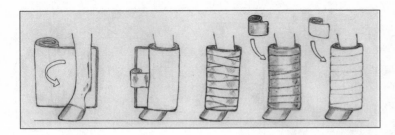

◆ **Fig. 18.2.** Steps in application of a support bandage to a left forelimb. See text for details.

with a horseshoe-splint combination that raises the heels and supports the lower limb. Severe cases of DDFT tendonitis are treated by immobilizing the limb with a *lower limb cast*, with the foot maintained in slight flexion. A walking bar may be incorporated into the cast in order to protect it when the horse is hand walked.

Mild cases of SDFT tendonitis are treated by raising the heels and maintaining the fetlock joint in a slightly flexed position; this may be achieved with a horseshoe and wedge pad combined with a support bandage or with a tendon support boot. Moderate cases of SDFT tendonitis are treated with a horseshoe-splint combination fitted with raised heels; the splint should maintain the fetlock in a flexed position. Severe cases of SDFT tendonitis are treated by immobilizing the limb with a lower limb cast with the foot and fetlock maintained in flexed position.

SUPPORT BANDAGE

The *support bandage* is used in the treatment of stay apparatus injuries and on healthy limbs for prevention of supporting limb complications (◆ fig. 18.2). The support bandage forms a thick cylinder that supports the fetlock joint and prevents excessive fetlock dorsiflextion during weight bearing, which reduces tension from the flexor tendons, check ligaments and suspensory ligament. The bandage should cover the coronary band and reach the proximal cannon bone. The use of appropriate wrapping materials is important. The risk of *bandage bows* is reduced when a whole roll of cotton wool is applied, with uniform pressure. In cases accompanied by an open wound, a primary layer consisting of a non-adhesive wound dressing is applied and held in place by orthopedic felt.

Keegan et al. (1992) indicated that soft bandage support of the fetlock may not be effective in treatment of injuries or for support of the opposite limb in non-weight- bearing lameness, but it may be beneficial for reduction and prevention of limb edema, and assist in circulation of the limb.

The wrapping materials for the support bandage include:

- Thick cotton roll, 12" wide.

- Open-weave stretch bandage.

- Self-adhesive bandage.

- 4" elastic adhesive tape.

A thick cotton roll is wrapped uniformly around the distal limb. The cotton is held in place with an open-weave stretch bandage applied in a spiral fashion. Wrapping begins from the mid-cannon up to the carpus/tarsus, then down to the foot and up to the mid-cannon. A self-adhesive bandage is applied over the stretch bandage in a similar fashion, and the cotton layer is tightened further. A final wrap with elastic adhesive tape is applied; this wrap holds the bandage material together and provides additional support.

LOWER LIMB SPLINT

The *lower limb splint* is designed to immobilize the distal limb and allow the transport of the horse to a medical facility (◆ fig. 18.3). The device is applied to cases with injuries to the stay apparatus or fractures involving the distal limb; these cases include tendonitis of the flexor tendons and suspensory apparatus fail-

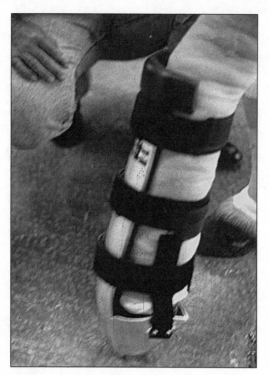

◆ **Fig. 18.3.** A commercial lower limb splint. (Photo by author.)

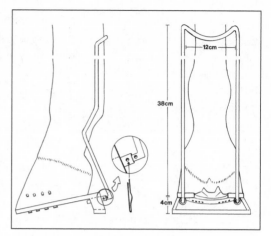

◆ **Fig. 18.4.** Construction of a horseshoe-splint combination, schematic illustrations. See text for details.

ure. The lower limb splint fits over the dorsal aspect of the lower limb and maintains the fetlock in a flexed position. The device is attached to the limb with Velcro straps; the bottom part of the splint can be fitted over a horseshoe in most cases. One complication that may occur with the application of the device is development of pressure sores (Snyder et al. 1986). This complication can be prevented by application of a well-padded transport bandage over the distal limb, and by daily inspection of the limb. The lower limb splint is commercially available.

HORSESHOE-SPLINT COMBINATION

The *horseshoe-splint combination* is a device used to support the fetlock, relieve tension from the suspensory apparatus and immobilize the distal limb. The device is applied to cases of tendonitis and laceration injuries involving the SDFT and DDFT, and traumatic rupture of the SL. The splint consists of

padded metal frame connected to a horseshoe. A properly fitted splint forms a sling that supports the palmar/plantar aspect of the distal limb while maintaining the fetlock joint in a flexed position. The device should distribute equal weight along the palmar/plantar aspect of the lower limb in order to prevent pressure sores. Prior to application of the splint, open wounds are treated and dressed with an appropriate antibiotic ointment covered with a bandage, and the limb is wrapped with a well-padded support bandage. The splint can be removed for inspection and treatment of injuries

The horseshoe-splint combination is constructed from iron, or stainless steel rods. The diameter of the rod should be 10 mm for iron and 8 mm for stainless steel (◆ fig. 18.4). The splint is shaped by placing the rod in a leg vise; the rod is heated at the bending points with an oxyacetylene torch and bent into the desired angles. The splint is shaped to fit the palmar/plantar contour of the distal limb; this outline can be traced from a radiograph. The splint should be wider than the limb. The average distance between the splint branches is 12 cm and the total height is 38 cm. The upper end of the splint should be 10 cm below the carpus/tarsus in order to permit flexion; this end is also angulated so it clears the limb about 3 to 4 cm. These figures should be

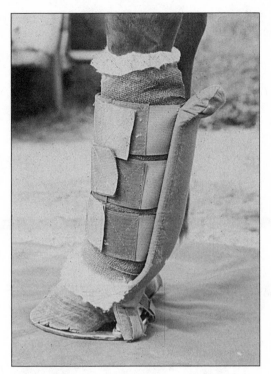

◆ **Fig. 18.5.** Horseshoe-splint combination. The splint was fitted with a padded sleeve and Velcro straps. (Photo by author.)

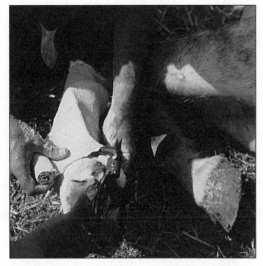

◆ **Fig. 18.6.** Incorporating a splint with plaster cast in a case of flexor tendon injury. (Photo by author.)

adjusted according to the size of the limb. In order to prevent pressure sores, the splint should be fitted with a padded sleeve along its entire length. The sleeve is fitted with three Velcro straps or with leather straps with buckles. The horseshoe branches should extend 4 cm from the heels in order to form a base for splint attachment. One method for splint attachment includes welding a metal pipe, 2 to 3 cm in length on each branch. The pipes should be parallel to each other. The inner diameter of the pipes should be equal to the diameter of the splint. The ends of the splint are bent until they fit smoothly into the pipes. A 3 mm hole is drilled through the pipe and splint; additional holes are made in the splint in order to permit forward or backward adjustments. The splint is secured by placing a removable pin in each hole. Connection and disconnection of the splint should be smooth in order to prevent further trauma to the limb.

The splint is fastened to the limb with the leather or Velcro straps (◆ fig. 18.5).

The device is commonly fitted with a raised heel that reduces strain from the stay apparatus. This can be achieved by welding a walking bar to the lower part of the splint or by using a Patten shoe for splint attachment. Alternatively, the horseshoe can be fitted with one or more wedge pads. Depending on the type and severity of the injury, the heels may be raised by 2 to 8 cm. As healing progresses, the heels should be lowered gradually by shortening the raised heels or by removal of wedge pads. As the heels are lowered, the position of the splint relative to the limb may have to be adjusted by shifting the splint forward or backward, changing the angulations of the splint, and adding padding material. The device may be incorporated with a distal limb cast in order to increase the strength of the cast and maintain the limb at the desired position (◆ fig. 18.6).

A variation of the horseshoe-splint combination is a *hinged splint* that permits examination and treatment of the lesion without disconnecting the splint from its attachment; this type provides less stability than the regular device.

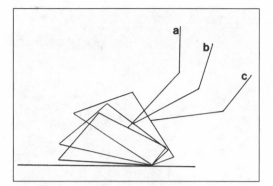

◆ **Fig. 18.7.** Change in position of the digit following laceration injuries, schematic illustration. Laceration to the SDFT (a), SDFT and DDFT (b), and both flexor tendons and SL (c).

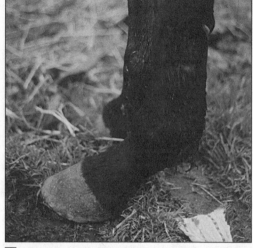

A

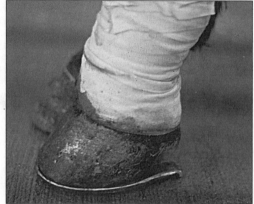

B

◆ **Fig. 18.8.** SDFT laceration in a forelimb. A. The fetlock is dropped slightly and the foot tends to rock backward. B. The same foot following application of extended heel horseshoe that prevents backward rocking of the foot. (Photos by author.)

 ## LACERATIONS OF THE FLEXOR TENDONS AND SUSPENSORY LIGAMENT

LACERATION INJURIES THAT INVOLVE TENDONS and ligaments in the distal limb are relatively common. The injury may result from accidental limb contact, catching a limb in a fence or from kicking a sharp object. Injuries to the palmar/plantar aspect of the distal limb may involve the SDFT, DDFT and SL. The transection of one or more of these structures results in drop of the fetlock joint (Smithcors, 1961c). In cases of severed SDFT, the fetlock drops slightly and the foot remains flat on the ground but may rock backward. In cases of severed SDFT and DDFT there is a pronounced drop of the fetlock and elevation of the toe off the ground, whereas severed flexor tendons and SL result in collapse of the fetlock to the ground and marked elevation of the toe (◆ fig. 18.7).

Emergency treatment of laceration injuries includes control of bleeding and immobilization of the limb. The horse owner should be instructed to control any bleeding with a pressure bandage or other available material such as clothing; a heavy support bandage should be applied to the injured limb. Immediate stabilization of the limb may be achieved with a board splint (Wagner and

Shires, 1986) or with a lower limb splint, if available.

Treatment of laceration injuries includes wound debridement, and in cases where the injury is fresh, suturing of the tendon ends together (Flecker and Wagner, 1986). Cases involving the SDFT alone may be treated by application of an extended heels horseshoe and support bandage. The horseshoe branches should extend 5 to 7 cm from the heels in order to provide adequate palmar/plantar support (◆ fig. 18.8). Heavy horseshoes may

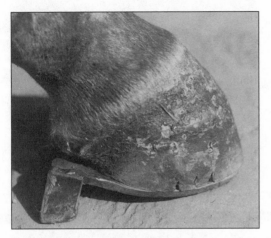

◆ **Fig. 18.9.** Patten shoe applied to a case with chronic lesion at the SDFT. (Photo by author.)

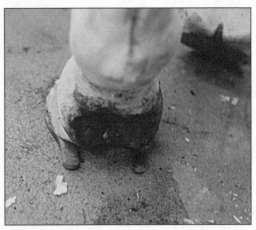

◆ **Fig. 18.10.** Extended heels horseshoe used to protect injury to the heel bulbs. (Photo by author.)

cause further trauma to the limb and should be avoided (McIlwraith 1982). Alternatively, the limb may be fitted with a horseshoe-splint combination or placed in a lower limb cast. Cases involving the SDFT and DDFT are treated by placing the limb in a lower limb cast for three weeks following suturing of the severed ends; the limb should be placed in a slightly flexed position. Following the removal of the cast, the heels should be raised with a Patten shoe or with a horseshoe fitted with several wedge pads. The heels should be raised 5 to 8 cm above the ground (◆ fig. 18.9). The heels are lowered gradually over the next three months in 2 to 3 cm increments per month until they contact the ground. Laceration injuries that involve both the flexor tendons and suspensory ligament are treated similarly (Flecker and Wagner, 1986).

EXTENDED HEELS HORSESHOE

The *extended heels horseshoe* provides palmar/plantar support to the foot by increasing the base distance of the foot (◆ fig. 18.10). The horseshoe is used in cases of stay apparatus injuries, weak suspensory apparatus, chronic laminitis, and following surgical resection of the DDFT. The extended heels horseshoe may be applied following the removal of a lower limb splint, Patten shoe or

fetlock sling shoe. The horseshoe can be fitted with a wedge pad in order to raise the heels and reduce tension from the DDFT. The horseshoe conformation, protection of the heel bulbs in dermatitis cases, bull-nosed hooves and sloping pasterns.

The extended heels horseshoe can be made from a large keg horseshoe or forged from various sizes of bar stock. The amount of extension is dictated by the degree of support that is required, and the extent of risk of the horseshoe being pulled by a hind leg. Depending on the severity of the case and the amount of required support, the branches may extend from 1 cm up to the level of the bulbs of the heels. Alternatively, an extended egg-bar shoe may be used.

PATTEN SHOE

The *Patten shoe* is a device used to relieve strain from the flexor tendons and suspensory ligament by maintaining the digit in a flexed position (Sprinhall, 1964; Smith, 1967). The horseshoe, which was named after the high-heeled footwear worn by women in the 18th century (Springhall, 1964), is also called a rest shoe and a raised–heel shoe. The Patten shoe is applied to the foot following cast or splint removal in cases of flexor tendons and suspensory ligament injuries. Flecker and

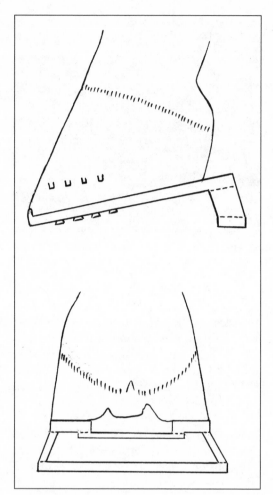

◆ **Fig. 18.11.** Patten shoe, side and plantar views, schematic illustration. See text for details.

Wagner (1986) described the use of a similar device for treatment of lacerated flexor tendons.

The Patten shoe may be forged from 1" x ¼" or ¾" x ¼" bar stock (Springhall, 1964; Manning, 1983; Manning, 1992). The construction of the Patten shoe from bar stock is difficult and requires practice. Under field conditions the device can be constructed relatively fast by fitting an extended heels horseshoe to the hoof, and welding a walking bar to the horseshoe. The degree of heel lift is determined by the stance of the horse. In most cases, it is 4 to 6 cm above the ground. In order to provide stability, the base of the

device should be wider than the horseshoe branches; the base should be flat and in direct contact with the ground (◆ fig. 18.11). Additional stability can be achieved by squaring the toe and adding two side clips that prevent forward movement of the foot (Manning, 1983). As healing progress and the tendon gains strength, the heels are lowered gradually until the device can be replaced with a horseshoe and wedge pad. The Patten shoe may be used for the construction of a horseshoe-splint combination.

The disadvantages of the Patten shoe include excessive weight that is being placed on the palmar/plantar aspect of the foot when the limb is raised; this weight stretches the injured structures and interferes with their healing. In order to prevent excessive tension, the device should be fitted with a wide rubber strap attached to a bar that is welded across the horseshoe branches. The rubber band is incorporated inside the support bandage and maintains the digit in a flexed position when the leg is raised (Manning, 1983). Although no reports on construction of a Patten shoe from aluminum were found, this could solve the weight problem.

🎇 SUSPENSORY APPARATUS FAILURE

Suspensory apparatus failure (SAF) MAY RESULT from traumatic rupture of the suspensory ligament during intense work such as racing. The injury commonly involves the rupture of the ligamentous branches to the sesamoid bones. Rupture of these ligaments, which are part of the fetlock support sling, result in severe pain and collapse of the fetlock to the ground. The prognosis for this type of injury is unfavorable (Wheat and Pascoe, 1980). SAF may also result from weakening of the suspensory ligament in aged animals or from degenerative changes in the ligament. SAF in aged animals is characterized by progressive dropping of the fetlock toward the ground; the fetlock may be grossly enlarged (◆ fig. 8.12). A study on Peruvian Paso horses revealed

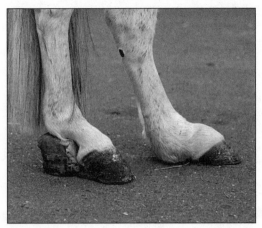

◆ **Fig. 18.12.** Suspensory apparatus failure in the hind limbs of an old horse. The hooves were shod with a fetlock sling shoe made from a combination of a horseshoe and a wooden block. (Photo by author.)

degenerative changes and failure of collagen fibers within the branches of the suspensory ligament in horses with SAF. The disorder, which may develop at any age and in horses that are not working, may have a genetic base (Mero and Pool, 2002).

Farriery of Traumatic Rupture of the Suspensory Ligament

Emergency treatment of *traumatic rupture of the suspensory ligament* includes the application of a splint that holds the fetlock in a flexed position. This may be achieved with a lower limb splint or board splint.

Long-term treatment includes maintenance of the limb in a flexed position with the sole perpendicular to the ground using a board splint, lower limb splint or a horseshoe-splint combination. Supporting limb complications should be prevented by application of a wide-web horseshoe and a wedge pad on the healthy opposite limb (Wheat and Pascoe, 1980). The frog of the opposite limb should be supported with silicone impression material placed between the sole and pad. Alternatively this hoof can be fitted with a solar support boot, or with a wedged hoof boot. The injured limb is supported until fibrosis (scar

tissue) develops and the horse is able to support weight on the limb. This period may take four to six weeks. Removal of the device too early may result in an unstable fetlock joint, and require reapplication of the splint. Leaving the splint on too long may result in excessive fibrosis and/or bone production that prevents the return of the fetlock into normal position (Snyder et al., 1986). Once the horse is able to support weight on the injured limb, the splint is replaced with a Patten shoe. As the fetlock gains strength, the heel of the Patten shoe is gradually lowered (Wheat and Pascoe, 1980). Once the heel approaches the ground, the device is replaced with an extended heels horseshoe and a wedge pad. A fetlock sling shoe should be applied to cases with unstable (dropped) fetlock.

BOARD SPLINT

The *board splint* is a device that is used in the treatment of traumatic rupture of the suspensory ligament, lacerated flexor tendons and tendonitis (◆ fig. 18.13). The splint has been used successfully for postoperative support following surgical repair of severed flexor tendons and suspensory ligaments (Wheat and Pascoe, 1980). The device is simple to construct and is attached to the hoof with iron wire. The splint maintains the fetlock in a flexed position and permits examination and treatment of the injured limb.

The board splint is constructed from a 2.0 cm thick board that is slightly wider than the hoof. The length of the splint should be calculated to be 15 cm below the carpus/tarsus when the digit is flexed. Prior to application of the splint, the hoof is shod with a regular horseshoe. Two holes, 5 to 7 cm apart, are drilled through the horseshoe at the distal toe wall. Equivalent holes are drilled at the end of the board so the board would project 1.5 cm beyond the distal toe wall when applied. The board is padded with a heavy roll of cotton or foam rubber held in place with an elastic adhesive bandage. The limb is wrapped with a support bandage and the splint is wired to the hoof with a heavy iron wire. The splint is positioned along the palmar/plantar aspect of the

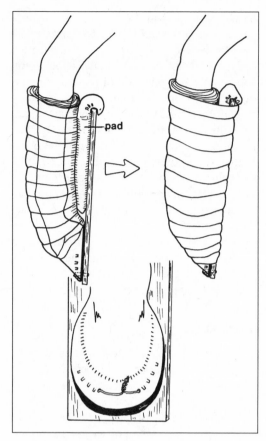

◆ **Fig. 18.13.** Application of board splint,
schematic illustration. See text for details.
(Reprinted by permission from Wheat, J.W. and
Pascoe, J.R. 1980, fig. 5. Figure modified to text.)

limb with the sole at 90° to the ground. The
board is wrapped against the limb with elastic
adhesive bandage (Flecker and Wagner, 1986;
Wheat and Pascoe, 1980; Snyder et al., 1986).
One complication that may result from the
use of a board splint is development of pressure sores (Snyder et al. 1986). This may be
prevented by the use of adequate wrapping
material and daily inspection of the limb.

Farriery of Suspensory Apparatus Failure in Old Horses

Collapse of the suspensory ligament in old
horses is accompanied by scar tissue formation, and permanent "drop" of the fetlock,
which severely restricts the use of the horse.
Farriery of early cases includes the application
of an extended heels horseshoe fitted with a
wedge pad. Alternatively, an aluminum
wedged horseshoe with extended heel or aluminum wedged egg-bar shoe may be applied.
The limbs should be wrapped with support
bandages. Advanced cases may be fitted with
a fetlock sling shoe as the last resort.

FETLOCK SLING SHOE

The *fetlock sling shoe* is a device used to support the fetlock in cases of collapsed suspensory apparatus in old horses (◆ fig. 18.14). The
device, which has several designs, is a combination of a horseshoe and some form of pal-
mar/plantar sling. During weight bearing it

◆ **Fig. 18.14.** Fetlock sling
shoe, side and palmar/plantar
views, schematic illustration.
(Adapted from Wheat and
Pascoe, 1980, fig. 10.)

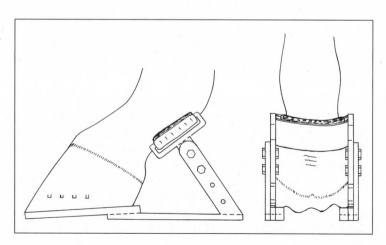

allows the horse to control the amount of
weight placed on the sling. The sling should
be well padded in order to prevent pressure
sores.

🔧 LACERATION OF THE COMMON DIGITAL EXTENSOR TENDON

Laceration injuries TO THE COMMON DIGITAL
extensor tendon are caused by accidents such
as running into a wire fence. Initially, the
injured horse stumbles and knuckles over at
the fetlock. Later, the animal learns to accommodate by flipping the foot forward so it lands
flat (Flecker and Wagner, 1986).

Treatment of extensor tendon laceration
includes wound debridement and medication,
and the application of a heavy support bandage. The limb is fitted with a *dorsal splint* made
from a section of 10 cm (4") diameter PVC
pipe cut lengthwise and fitted over the dorsal
aspect of the lower limb. Two holes are drilled
in the toe wall and equivalent holes are drilled
at the end of the splint. The splint is wired to
the hoof with iron wire and wrapped against
the support bandage with elastic adhesive tape
(Flecker and Wagner, 1986). Following healing, the hoof may be shod with an extended
toe horseshoe that prevents knuckling over at
the fetlock; the toe extension should be angled
upward in order to minimize delay in
breakover and to permit the foot to swing forward during movement (Flecker and Wagner,
1986).

EXTENDED TOE HORSESHOE

The *extended toe horseshoe* is used in cases of
digital extensor tendon lacerations, radial
paralysis, and contracted flexor tendons in
mature horses and foals. The length of the
extension in horseshoes used for mature horses should be 3 to 5 cm, measured from the
center of the toe. Application of the horseshoe
to mature horses with contracted flexor tendons may place excessive tension on the stay
apparatus and cause lameness (fig. 18.15).

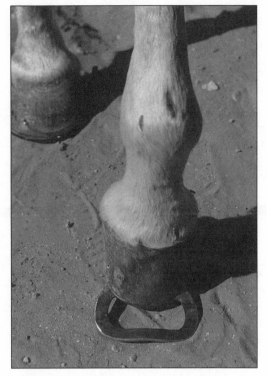

◆ **Fig. 18.15.** Extended toe horseshoe. In this
case, the horseshoe was applied to a mare with
contracted digital flexor tendons, which developed
from prolonged placement of the limb in a cast.
(Photo by author.)

🔧 COLLATERAL LIGAMENT DESMITIS

Collateral ligament desmitis IS AN INFLAMMATION
of the collateral ligaments of the DIP or PIP
joints (McDiarmid, 1998; Dyson et al., 2004;
Turner and Sage, 2002). Damage to the ligament may result from asymmetrical foot
placement that places abnormal tension on
the ligament with consequent tearing of the
ligament at its attachment points to bone
(Dyson et al., 2004).

Predisposing factors for collateral ligament desmitis include mediolateral imbalance, toeing-out or toeing-in, offset pasterns
and uneven ground. Turner et al. (2002) indicated that the condition seems to be more
common in horses involved in Western agili-

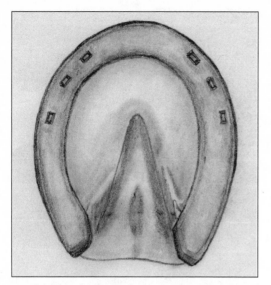

◆ Fig. 18.16. Modified wide-web horseshoe, solar view. The horseshoe is similar to the lateral extension horseshoe but it is fitted along the hoof outline. The wide-web is place on the affected side.

ty competition, and that injuries may be related more to footing than to hoof imbalance.

Little data is available on the farriery of collateral ligament desmitis. Farriery principles include raising the hoof on the affected side; this may include balancing the foot in cases with mediolateral imbalance, or raising the affected side in order to reduce tension from the injured ligament. Muller and Luikart (2006) indicated that raising the affected side by about 1/8" might have a similar effect as reducing the amount of sinking into the ground on that side. They recommended the application of a *modified wide-web horseshoe* that decreases the degree of sinking of the affected side into the ground (◆ fig. 18.16). Turner (2002) recommended the use of half-round horseshoes in cases of collateral ligament desmitis of the DIP joint in order to ease breakover. McDiarmid (1998) described the application of an egg-bar shoe with a lateral extension in one case of damaged collateral ligament. The extension was placed at the affected side and the horse was rested for three months. Alternatively, a horseshoe and

a thick pad, or a glue-on synthetic shoe may be applied in order to increase cushion and protect the limb. A wedge pad place at 90° to the long axis of the foot can be used to raise the affected side of the hoof; however, the degrees available in commercial wedge pads may be too high for that purpose. Alternatively, a shim pad made from plastic or leather can be applied. Glue-on shoes can be used to raise the affected side by tilting the horseshoe to the desired position during curing of the resin. During the recovery period, affected horses should be kept on a level surface.

 ## FARRIERY OF MISCELLANEOUS CONDITIONS ABOVE THE FOOT

APPLICATION OF THERAPEUTIC HORSESHOES TO horses with orthopedic disorders above the foot reduces strain from the limb, encourages healing and allows the horse to walk better during the recovery period. Farriery may include balancing the hooves and application of horseshoes that reduce the hoof lever arm and provide better palmar/plantar support. The following section describes several applications:

radial paralysis. An extended toe horseshoe may be used in cases of *radial paralysis* to assist the horse during hand walking. A short rope is tied to the extension and the rope is pulled forward each time the horse attempts to extend the limb.

inflammation of the distal sesamoidean ligament. Moyer (1982) recommended the use of an egg-bar shoe with a rolled toe in horses with *inflammation of the distal sesamoidean ligament*. The ligament is situated palmar/plantar to the pastern and it connects the sesamoid bones and second phalanx. A predisposing factor for this type of injury (and other stay apparatus injuries) is under-run heels. Prior to application of the horseshoe, the hoof angle should be increased by trimming the toe.

spavin and upward fixation of the patella. Moyer (1990) recommended using a rolled toe horseshoe for *spavin* and *upward fixation of the patella.*

acute dorsal pastern subluxation. *Acute dorsal pastern subluxation* may be treated by application of several wedge pads cut to fit the hoof outline. The pads are placed over the solar area and attached to the hoof with elastic adhesive tape. Raising the heels allows the horse to bear some weight on the limb.

dorsal pastern subluxation. *Dorsal pastern subluxation* of the hind limbs is an orthopedic disorder observed in young horses with legs that are too straight. Lowering the heels resolved the condition in one case (but only for two weeks), and eventually surgery was performed (Shiroma et al., 1989). Lose (1981) recommended using a rolled toe horseshoe following surgical correction. Post-legged horses should be removed from breeding stock.

suspensory ligament desmitis. Bennett (2005) described the application of egg-bar shoes in cases of *suspensory ligament desmitis* (inflammation of the SL), a condition commonly observed in the hind limbs of Western agility competition horses.

stiff-gaited and knee-sprung horses. Asmus (1940) recommended using half-round horseshoes on *stiff-gaited* and *knee-sprung horses.*

rehabilitating horses. Gabel (1982) recommended using flat horseshoes on rehabilitating race horses. Once the horses become nearly sound, a partially worn horseshoes are applied in order to make the transition to racing horseshoes more gradual. The disadvantage of worn horseshoes is that a pair may not have the same weight. Application of new, non-creased, half-round horseshoes can solve this problem; the nail heads should be situated smooth with the ground surface of the horseshoe (Rich, 1907).

More research is required in order to establish protocols for farriery of various orthopedic disorders above the foot. However, proper hoof care of recovering horses is an important part of the treatment, including non-orthopedic cases. During this period the horse may be constrain most of the time in a stable with little exercise. The floor condition may range from dry sawdust to wet urine and manure, which predisposes the feet to contracted heels, thrush and sub-solar abscess. Maintenance of balanced feet will make the horse more comfortable and reduce unnecessary strain from the limbs. Hoof care should include trimming, picking the hooves several times each day and application of pine tar.

APPENDIX A

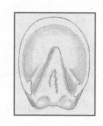

Resources for Farriery Supplies

ACRYLIC RESIN PASTE
Hoof Adhesives
EQUILOX
Pine Island, MN. U.S.A.
www.equilox.com

ACRYLIC RESIN (SOFT, FOR SOLAR SUPPORT)
EQUI-PAK
Vettec Hoof Care Products
Oxnard, CA. U.S.A.
www.vettec.com

ALUMINUM EGG-BAR WEDGED HORSESHOE
G.E. FORGE AND TOOLS INC.
Grover Beach, CA. U.S.A.
bob@geforge.com

BAR SHOES
RGM Bar Shoes
ANVIL BRAND SHOE CO.
Lexington, IL. U.S.A.
www.anvilbrand.com

BELL BOOTS
No-Turn Bell Boot
DAVIS MANUFACTURING
Brandon, WI. U.S.A.
www.davismanufacturing.com

FLAT PADS
Hoofprints
CENTAUR FORGE LLC
Burlington, WI. U.S.A.
www.centaurforge.com

FOOT BOOTS
Easy Boot
EASY CARE INC.
Tucson, AZ. U.S.A.
www.easycareinc.com

FROG SUPPORT PAD
Lily Pad
NANRIC, INC.
Versailles, KY. U.S.A.
www.nanric.com

GLUE-ON FOAL SHOES KIT
Mustad Baby Glue
MUSTAD HOOFCARE SA.
Bulle, Switzerland.
www.mustadhoofcare.com

GLUE-ON SHOES, ALUMINUM CORE
Easy-Glu
MUSTAD HOOFCARE SA.
Bulle, Switzerland.
www.mustadhoofcare.com

GLUE-ON SYNTHETIC SHOES, WIDE-WEB, EGG-BAR
EponaShoe
EPONATECH
Creston, CA. U.S.A.
www.eponashoe.com

HALF-ROUND HORSESHOES
CENTAUR FORGE LLC
Burlington, WI. U.S.A.
www.centaurforge.com

HOOF KNIFE, SHORT BLADE
H. HAUPTNER GMBH & CO. KG
Solingen, Germany
www.hauptner.de

HOOF KNIVES, DETACHABLE BLADES SET
H. HAUPTNER GMBH & CO. KG
Solingen, Germany
www.hauptner.de

HOOF NIPPERS, HALF-ROUND AND RACE
G.E. FORGE AND TOOLS INC.
Grover Beach, CA. U.S.A.
bob@geforge.com

---

* web sites updated June 2007

HOOF PACK, PETROLEUM AND PINE TAR BASE
Forshner's Hoof Packing
Equicare Products
FARNAM COMPANIES, INC.
Phoenix, AZ. U.S.A.
www.farnam.com

HOOF POULTICE
Super-H Poultice
BICKMORE
Brighton, MI. U.S.A.
www.bickmore.com

HOOF TESTERS
G.E. FORGE AND TOOLS INC.
Grover Beach, CA. U.S.A.
bob@geforge.com

HORSESHOE NAILS, RACE #3
CAPEWELL HORSE NAILS, INC.
Bloomfield, CT. U.S.A.
www.capewellhorsenails.com

HORSESHOE NAILS, E-TYPE SLIM
MUSTAD HORSESHOE NAILS
Bloomfield, CT. U.S.A.
www.mustadinc.com

HOT AIR BLOWER
LEISTER PROCESS TECH-
NOLOGIES
Sarnen, Switzerland
www.leister.com

LEATHER PADS, EXTRA HEAVY
CENTAUR FORGE LLC.
Burlington, WI. U.S.A.
www.centaurforge.com

LOWER LIMB SPLINT
Kimzey Splint
KIMZEY WELDING WORKS
Woodland, CA. U.S.A.
www.kimzeymetalproducts.com

MOLD FOR HEART-BAR SHOE
Heartbar mold
VETTEC HOOF CARE PRODUCTS
Oxnard, CA. U.S.A.
www.vettec.com

MOTORIZED BURR
DREMEL TOOL CO.
Racin, WI. U.S.A.
www.dremel.com

NAVICULAR EGG-BAR SHOE
G.E. FORGE AND TOOL INC.
Grover Beach, CA. U.S.A.
bob@geforge.com

NEOPRENE STRIP
Shoe liners
THORO'BREDRACING PLATE CO., INC.
Anaheim, CA. U.S.A.
www.horseshoes.com/thorobred

PADDING FOAM FOR CASTS AND SOLAR SUPPORT
3M CUSTOM SUPPORT FOAM 1467
St. Paul, MN. U.S.A.
www.3m.com

PINE TAR, PURE
BICKMORE
Brighton, MI. U.S.A.
www.bickmore.com

POULTICE BOOT
Davis Barrier Boot
DAVIS MANUFACTURING
Brandon, WI. U.S.A.
www.davismanufacturing.com

RUBBER FLOOR MAT
Durathon
ROBBINS INC.
Cincinnati, OH. U.S.A.
www.robbinsfloor.com

SIDE SUPPORT HORSESHOE
Aluma-Flite
CENTAUR FORGE LLC
Burlington, WI. U.S.A.
www.centaurforge.com

SIDE WEDGE HORSESHOE
Aluma-Flite
CENTAUR FORGE, LLC
Burlington, WI. U.S.A
www.centaurforge.com

SILICONE IMPRESSION MATERIAL
Equisil
THORO'BREDRACING PLATE CO., INC.
Anaheim, CA. U.S.A.
www.horseshoes.com/thorobred

SLING
Munks Sling
Anacortes, WA. U.S.A.
www.livestocksling.com

SOLAR SUPPORT BOOT
Redden Modified Ultimate
NANRIC, INC.
Versailles, KY. U.S.A.
www.nanric.com

TENDON SUPPORT BOOT
Dalmar Tendon Support Boot Ltd
DALMAR IRELAND LTD.,
Glanmire, Ireland
www.simviation.com/dalmar/tre
atment.htm

WEDGE PADS
Colson RCH Wedge Pads
CENTAUR FORGE LLC.
Burlington, WI. U.S.A.
www.centaurforge.com

APPENDIX B

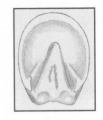

Table of Weights and Measures
(Metric and English Units)

WEIGHTS AND MEASURES
1000 grams = 1 kilogram = 2.2046 pounds
1 pound = 453.59 grams = 0.4536 kilogram
10 millimeters = 1 centimeter = 0.3937 inch
100 centimeters = 1 meter = 39.37 inches or 3.2808 feet
1 inch = 2.54 centimeters

ABBREVIATIONS	
gm	gram
kg	kilogram
mm	millimeter
cm	centimeter
m	meter

APPENDIX C

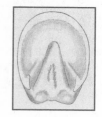

Short Forms

ALD   angular limb deformity
BLM   Bureau of Land Management (U.S.A.)
COM   center of mass
COR   center of rotation
CDET   common digital extensor tendon
DDFM   deep digital flexor muscle
DDFT   deep digital flexor tendon
DL   digital leverage
DIP   distal interphalangeal (joint)
FRC   Farrier Registration Council (U.K.)
GRF   ground reaction force
HLA   hoof lever arm
ICL   inferior check ligament
MCP   metacarpophalangeal (joint, forelimb)
MC   metacarpus (bone, forelimb)
MTP   metatarsophalangeal (joint, hind limb)
MT   metatarsus (bone, hind limb)
NRC   National Research Council (U.S.A.)
N   newton
PDN   palmar/plantar digital nerve
PMMA   polymethyl methacrylate
PIP   proximal interphalangeal (joint)
SDFT   superficial digital flexor tendon
SA   suspensory apparatus
SAF   suspensory apparatus failure
SL   suspensory ligament
SCL   superior check ligament
USDA   United States Department of Agriculture
WLD   white line disease

References

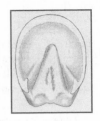

Ackerman N., Garner H.E., Coffman J.R., Clement J.W. 1975. Angiographic appearance of the normal equine foot and alteration in chronic laminitis. *JAVMA* 166(1), 58-62.

Adams O.R. 1974. *Lameness in Horses*. 3rd. ed. Philadelphia: Lea and Febiger.

Aldrich K.M. 1997. Effects determining the ultimate shape of the hoof capsule. *Anvi Mag.* Dec., 24-25.

Allen D., White N.A., Foerner J.F., Gordon B.J. 1986. Surgical management of chronic laminitis in horses: 13 cases (1983-1985). *JAVMA* 189 (12).

Allen D., Korthuis R.J., Clark E.S. 1988. Capillary permeability to endogenous macromolecules in the equine digit. *Am. J. Vet. Res.* 49, 1609.

Anderson A. 1989. Navicular disease. *The Quarter Horse Journal.* April, 36-41.

Anderson G.F. 1992. Evaluation of the hoof and foot relevant to purchase. *Vet. Clin. N. Am. Eq. Pract.* 8 (2), 303-318.

Arabian A.K., Lanovaz J.L., Clayton H.M. 2001. Determination of hoof mass and centre of mass from morphological measurements. *Eq. Vet. J. Suppl.* 33, 46-49.

Ards P. 2006. The farrier in the freezer. *Am. Farriers J.* 32(6), 27-31.

Arnbjerg J. 1972. Orthopedic treatment of foals and cattle with technovit. *Nord. Vet. Med.* 24, 553-558.

Arnbjerg J.1988. Changes in the distal phalanx in foals with deep digital flexor tendon contraction. *Vet. Rad.* 29 (2), 65-69.

Asmus H. 1940. *Horseshoes of interest to veterinarians.* Dep. of Horseshoeing. New York State Veterinary College. Ithaca, New York.

Auer J.A., Martens R.J. 1980. Angular limb deformities in young foals. *Proc AAEP* 26, 81-96.

Auer J.A., Martens R.J., Morris E.L. 1982. Angular limb deformities in foals. Part I. Congenital Factors. *Compend. Cont. Educ. Pract. Vet.* 4 (8), S330-S339.

Auer J.A., Martens R.J., Morris E.L. 1983. Angular limb deformities in foals. Part II. Developmental Factors. *Compend. Cont. Educ. Pract. Vet.* 5 (1), S27-S35.

Avisar Y. 1994. The use of elevated clog for the treatment of unilateral flexural deformity of the distal interphalangeal joint in two foals: case report. *Israel J. of Vet. Med.* 49(4), 169-171.

Avisar Y. 1995. Primary contracted heels: Causes and treatment. *Anvil Mag.* 12, 33-36.

Avisar Y. 1996. Farriery and laminitis. *Anvil Mag.* 10, 34.

Avisar Y. 1997. Corrective trimming and shoeing in contracted tendons in foals. *Anvil Mag.* Sept.

Back J. 1959. *Horses Hitches and Rocky Trails.* Sage Books, Denver. p 45.

Back W., Schamhardt H.C., Hartman W., Barneveld A. 1995. Kinematic differences between the distal portions of the forelimbs and hind limbs of horses at the trot. *Am. J. Vet. Res.* 56, 1522-1528.

Badoux D.M. 1975. General biostatics and biomechanics. In: Getty R., ed. *Sisson and Grossman's The Anatomy of the Domestic Animals.* 5th.ed. Philadelphia, W.B. Saunders, 48-83.

Baird A.N., Seahorn T.L., Morris E.L. 1990. Equine distal phalangeal sequestration. *Vet. Rad.* 31 (4), 210-213.

Balch O., White K. 1985. Degenerative joint disease in the fetlock managed by balanced shoeing: a case report. *Eq. Pract.* 7, 35-40.

Balch O.K., Grant D.B., Ratzlaff M.H., Hyde L.M., Wilson P.D., Cannon J. 1989. Design, application, testing, and use of compressible plastic horseshoes-*Seattle Shoes®. Proc. AAEP* 405-418.

Balch O.K., Metcalf S. 1990. *Farriery for Veterinarians.* Pullman, Wash: S & O Press.

Balch O.K., White K., Butler D. 1991a. Review article: Factors involved in the balancing of equine hooves. *JAVMA* 198 (11), 1980-1989.

Balch O.K., Ratzlaff M.H., Hyde M.L., White K.L. 1991b. Locomotor effects of hoof angle and mediolateral balance of horses exercising on a high-speed treadmill: Preliminary results. *Proc. AAEP* 37, 687-705.

Balch O.K., White K., Butler D. 1993. How lameness is associated with selected aspects of hoof imbalance. *Proc. AAEP* 39, 213-214.

Balch O.K., Clayton H.M., Lanovaz J.L. 1994. Effects of increasing hoof length on limb kinematics of trotting horses. *Proc. AAEP* 40, 73-75.

Balch O.K., Butler K.D.., White K., Metcalf S. 1995a. Hoof balance and lameness: Improper toe length, hoof angle, and mediolateral balance. *Comp. Cont. Educ. Pract. Vet.* 17(10), 1275-1283.

Balch O.K., Butler K. D., White K., Metcalf S. 1995b. Hoof balance and lameness: Foot bruising and limb contact. *Comp. Cont. Educ. Pract. Vet.* 17(12), 1503-1509.

Balch O.K., Clayton H.M., Lanovaz J.L. 1996. Weight and length induced changes in limb kinematics in trotting horses. *Proc. AAEP* 42, 218-219.

Balch O.K., Butler D., Collier M.A. 1997. Balancing the normal foot: hoof preparation, shoe fit and shoe modification in the performance horse. *Eq. Vet. Educ.* 9, 143-154.

Balch O.K., Butler K. D., Collier M.A. 1998a. Part I: Balancing the normal foot: hoof preparation, shoe fit, and shoe modification in the performance horse. *Anvil Mag.* Sept. 20-31.

Balch O.K., Butler K.D., Collier M.A. 1998b. Part II: Balancing the normal foot: hoof preparation, shoe fit, and shoe modification in the performance horse. *Anvil Mag.* Oct., 22-30.

Balch O.K., Helman R.G., Collier M.A. 2001. Underrun heels and toe-grab length as possible risk factors for catastrophic musculoskeletal injuries in Oklahoma racehorses. *Proc. AAEP* 47, 334-338.

Banks W.J. 1986. *Applied Veterinary Histology.* 2nd. Ed. William and Wilkins, Baltimore MD. pp 365-371.

Barrey E. 1990. Investigation of the vertical hoof force distribution in the equine forelimb with an instrumented horseboot. *Eq. Vet. J. Suppl.* 9, 35-38.

Bartel D.L., Schryver H.F., Lowe J.E., Parker R.A. 1978. Locomotion in the horse: A procedure

for computing the internal forces in the digit. *Am. J. Vet. Res.* 39, 1721-1727.

Baxter G.M. 1986. Equine laminitis caused by distal displacement of the distal phalanx: 12 cases (1976-1986). *JAVMA* 189(3).

Baxter G.M. 1992. Equine laminitis. *Eq. Pract.* 14, 13-22.

Baxter G.M., Ingle J.E., Trotter G.W. 1995. Complete navicular bone fractures in horses. *Proc. AAEP* 41. 243-244.

Beeman G.M. 1985. The diagnosis of navicular disease (navicular syndrome). *Proc. AAEP*, 477.

Benedetti F. 1948. The difference in the strength of light and dark hooves in horses. *Annali. Fac. Med. Vet.* (Pisa) 1, 93-106.

Bennett D.G. 2005. Sound in the suspensory. *Performance Horse.* 18(8), 16-17.

Benoit P., Barrey E., Regnalt J.C., Brochet J.L. 1993. Comparison of the damping effect of different shoeing by the measurement of hoof acceleration. *Acta. Anat.* 146, 109-113.

Berns G.E. 1918. Lameness of obscure origin and some of its causes. 55th Annual Meeting, *JAVMA*, 217-222.

Berry R.C., O'Brien R.T., Pool R.R. 1991. Squamous cell carcinoma of the hoof wall in a stallion. *JAVMA* 199(1), 90-92.

Bertram J.E.A., Gosline J.M. 1986. Fracture toughness design in horse hoof keratin. *J. Exp. Biol.* 125, 29-47.

Bertram J.E.A., Gosline J.M., 1987. Functional design of horse hoof keratin: the modulation of mechanical properties through hydration effects. *J. Exp. Biol.* 130, 121-136.

Black J.B. 1992. Palmar digital neurectomy: An alternative surgical approach. *Proc. AAEP* 38, 429-432.

Blackford J.T., Blackford L.A.W., Latimer F.G. 1991. Adjustable tension band stabilization of hoof wall cracks in horses. *Proc. AAEP* 497-512.

Blackford J.T., Latimer F.G., Wan P.Y., Shires G.M.H. 1994. Treating pastern and foot lacerations with a phalangeal cast. *Proc. AAEP* 40, 97.

Blackwell R.B. 1982. Response of acquired flexural deformity of the metacarpophalangeal joint to desmotomy of the inferior check ligament. *Proc. AAEP*, 107-111.

Blombach J. 1994. Rolled toes, rocker toes, square toes. *Am. Farriers J.* Sept./Oct., 40-44.

Booth T.M., Knottenbelt D.C. 1999. Distal limb casts in equine wound management. *Eq. Vet. Edu.* 11(5), 273-280.

Boren S.R., Topliff D.R., Freeman D.W., Bahr R.J., Wagner D.G., Maxwell C.V. 1987. Growth of weanling Quarter horses fed varying energy and protein levels. *Proc. Equine Nutr. Physiol. Symp.* 10, 43-48.

Bosch G., van Schie M.J., Back W. 2004. Retrospective evaluation of surgical versus conservative treatment of keratomas in 41 lame horses (1995-2001). *Tijdschr Diergeneeskd.* 129(21), 700-705.

Bowker R.M., Van Wulfen K.K., Springer S.E., Linder K.E. 1998. Functional anatomy of the cartilages of the distal phalanx and digital cushion in the equine foot and a hemodynamic flow hypothesis of energy dissipation. *Am. J. Vet. Res.* 59(8), 961-968.

Boys Smith S.J., Clegg P.D., Hughes I., Singer E.R. 2006. Complete and partial hoof wall resection for keratoma removal: post operative complications and final outcome in 26 horses (1994-2004). *Eq. Vet. J.* 38(2), 127-133.

Bradley O.C., Grahame T. 1946. *The Topographical Anatomy of the Limbs of the Horse.* W. Green and Son, Ltd. Edinburgh.

Bramlage L.R., Embertson R.M., Libbey C.J. 1991. Resin impregnated foam as a cast liner on the distal equine limb. *Proc. AAEP* 37, 481-485.

Breazile J.E. 1970. Spinal cord and brain stem function. In Swenson M.J. (ed): *Dukes' Physiology of Domestic Animals.* Ithaca, Cornell University press, pp 929-930.

Brown Edwards G. 1973. *Anatomy and Conformation of the Horse.* Dreeman Press Ltd. New York. pp. 163-173.

Bruggink D., Sigafoos R. 1997. Keys to hoof reconstruction. *Am. Farriers J.* Dec.,15-18.

Budras K.D., Schiel C. 1996. A comparison of horn quality of the white line in the domestic horse (*Equus caballus*) and the Przewalski horse (*Equus przewalskii*). *Pferdeheilkunde* 12, 641-645.

Budras K.D., Schiel C., Mulling C. 1998. Horn tubules of the white line: an insufficient barrier against ascending bacterial invasion. *Eq. Vet. Educ.*10(2), 81-85.

Budras K.D., Scheibe K., Patan B., Streich W.J., Kim K. 2001. Laminitis in Przewalski horses kept in a semi-reserve. *J. Vet. Sci.* 2(1), 1-7.

Buffa E.A., Van Den Berg S.S., Verstraete F.J.M., Swart N.G.N. 1992. Effects of dietary biotin supplement on equine hoof horn growth rate and hardness. *Eq. Vet. J.* 24 (6), 472-474.

Bushe T., Turner T.A., Poulos P.W., Harwell N.M. 1987. The effect of hoof angle on coffin, pastern, and fetlock joint angles. *Proc. AAEP* 33, 729-737.

Butler J.L. 1976. The repair of hoof defects using fiberglass and screws. *Proc. AAEP*, 235-237.

Butler K.D. 1977. Practical hoof physiology. *The Arabian Horse.* Aug.

Butler K.D., Hintz H.F. 1977. Effect of level of feed intake and gelatin supplementation on growth and quality of hoofs of ponies. *J. of Am. Sci.* 44(2), 258-261.

Butler K.D. 1983. A flexible heart-bar shoe for founder. *Am. Farriers. J.* 9, 471-473.

Butler K.D. 1985. The prevention of lameness by physiologically-sound horseshoeing. *Proc. AAEP* 31, 465-475.

Butzow R.F. 1961. Anatomy and care of the equine foot. *Illinois Veterinarian* 4(4), 98-103.

Caldwell M. 2001. The horse's foot: Function and symmetry. *Proc. 1st. UK Farriery Convention.* 28-33.

Cannon D. 1979. Common hoof conditions observed in racetrack practice. *Proc. AAEP* 24, 311-314.

Carroll J. 1989. Mushroom and half–mushroom shoes. *Am. Farriers* J. Jan./Feb. 40-43.

Carter K.G. 1990. Supplemental feeding of the normal foal. *Proc. AAEP.* 36, 95-98.

Cauvin E.R.J., Munroe G.A. 1998. Septic osteitis of the distal phalanx: finding and surgical treatment in 18 cases. *Eq. Vet. J.* 30(6), 512-519.

Champagne W. 1998. Glue-on shoeing techniques. *Anvil Mag.,* May, 15-22.

Chapman B., Platt G.W. 1994. Laminitis. *Proc. AAEP* 30, 99-109.

Cheney J.A., Shen C.K., Wheat J.D. 1973. Relationship of racetrack surface to lameness in the Thoroughbred racehorse. *Am. J. Vet. Res.* 34(10), 1285-1289.

Clanton C., Kobluk C., Robinson R.A., Gordon B. 1991. Monitoring surface conditions of a Thoroughbred racetrack. *JAVMA,* 198, 613-620.

Clayton H.M. 1986. Cinematographic analysis of the gait of lame horses. *J. Eq. Vet. Sci.*6, 70-78.

Clayton H.M. 1987. Comparison of the stride of trotting horses trimmed with normal and a broken-back hoof axis. *Proc AAEP* 33, 289-298.

Clayton H.M. 1989. Locomotion, in Jones W.: *Equine Sports Medicine*. Philadelphia, Lea and Febiger, pp 149-187.

Clayton H.M. 1990. The effect of an acute hoof wall angulation on the stride kinematics of trotting horses. *Eq.Vet. J., Suppl.* 9, 86-90.

Clayton H.M., Sigafoos R., Curle R.D. 1990. Effect of three shoe types on the duration of breakover in sound trotting horses. *Eq. Vet. Sci.* 11(2), 129-132.

Coffman J.R., Johnson J.H., Fishburn F.J. 1969. Management of chronic laminitis in the horse. *JAVMA* 155, 45-49.

Coffman J.R., Johnson J.H., Finocchio E.J., Guffy M.M. 1970. Biomechanics of pedal rotation in equine laminitis. *JAVMA* 156(2), 219-221.

Coffman J.R., Garner H.E., Hohn A.W. 1972. Characterization of refractory laminitis, *Proc. AAEP* 18, 351-358.

Coffman J.R. 1973. Bone and muscle defects in foals. *Mod. Vet. Pract.* 54, 67-69.

Colahan P., Lindsey E., Nunier C. 1993. Determination of the center of pressure of the hoofs of the forelimbs of horses standing on a flat level surface. *Acta. Anat.* 146, 175-178.

Colahan P.T. 1994a. University of Florida, College of Vet. Med., Large Animal Clinical Sciences. Personal Communication.

Colahan P. 1994b. Navicular disease vs. navicular syndrome. *Eq. Pract.* 16(3), 20-22.

Colles C.M., Jeffcott L.B. 1977. Laminitis in the horse. *Vet. Rec.* 100, 262-264.

Colles C.M. 1982. Navicular disease and its treatment. *In Pract.* 4, 29-36.

Colles C. M. 1983a. Interpreting radiographs.1. The foot. *Eq. Vet.* J. 15, 297-303.

Colles C. M. 1983b. Concepts of blood flow in the ethiology and treatment of navicular disease. *Proc. AAEP* 29, 265-270.

Colles C. M. 1989a. The relationship of frog pressure to heel expansion. *Equine Vet. J.* 1 (1), 13-16.

Colles C.M. 1989b. A technique for assessing hoof function in the horse. *Equine Vet. J.* 21 (1), 17-22.

Comben N., Clark R.J., Sutherland D.J.B. 1984. Clinical observations on the response of equine hoof defects to dietary supplementation with biotin. *Vet. Rec.*115, 642, 1984.

Cooke H. 2006. Useful application of the G-bar. *Loose Shoe.* 10(2), 13-14.

Corum S.J. 2004. Good/bad effects of antioxidants. *The Horse.* Vol. XXI, No. 7. 99-106.

Craig J.J., Craig M.F., Weltner T.N. 2001. Quantifying conformation of the equine digit from lateromedial radiographs. 21st Annual Meeting of the Assoc. for Equine Sports Medicine.

Craig M.F. Craig J.J. 2003. Personal communication. EponaTech. Creston CA.

Craig. M. 2005. Plastic shoes and foundered hooves. *Am. Farriers J.* 31(6), 93-98.

Cremers H.J.W.M. 1985. The incidence of Chorioptic bovis (Acarina: Psoroptidae) on the feet of horses, sheep, and goats in the Neatherlands. *The Vet. Quart.* 7(4), 283-289.

Crevier-Denoix N., Roosen C., Dardillat C., Pourcelot P., Jerbi H., Sanaa M., Denoix J.-M. 2001. Effects of heel and toe elevation upon the digital joint angles in the standing horse. *Eq. Vet. J. Suppl.* 33, 74-78.

Cripps P.J., Eustace R.A. 1999. Factors involved in the prognosis of equine laminitis in the U.K. *Eq. Vet. J.* 31(5), 433-442.

Cuddeford D. 1994. Artificially dehydrated lucerne for horses. *Vet. Rec.* 135, 426-429.

Cunha T.J. 1991. *Horse Feeding and Nutrition.* Orlando FL, Academic Press, pp 303-317.

Curtis, S.J. 1992. Farriery in the treatment of acquired flexural deformities and discussion on applying shoes to young horses. *Equine Vet. Educ.* 4 (4), 193-197.

Curtis S., Ferguson D.W., Luikart R., Ovnicek G. 1999. Trimming and shoeing the chronically affected horse. In: *Vet. Clin. N. Am.: Eq. Pract.* 15(2), 463-480.

Curtis S.J., Stoneham S. 1999. Effective farriery treatment of hypoflexion tendons (severe digital hyperextension) in a foal. *Eq. Vet. Educ.* 11(5), 256-259.

Cymbaluk N.F., Christinson G.I., Leach D.H. 1990. Longitudinal growth analysis of horses following limited and ad libitum feeding. *Eq. Vet. J.* 22(3) 198-204.

Dart A.J., Pascoe R.R. 1988. A pathogenesis and treatment of osteomyelitis in a stallion after the prolonged topical application of formalin to the distal phalanx. *Australian Vet. J.* 65(6).

Dabareiner R.M., Janicek J.C., Honnas C.H., Crabill M.A. 2004. Heel bulb lacerations in horses: 101 cases. *Proc. AAEP* Vol. 50, 488-491.

Daradka M., Pollitt C.C. 2004. Epidermal cell proliferation in the equine hoof wall. *Eq. Vet. J.*
36(3), 236-241.

Dejardin L.M., Arnoczky S.P., Cloud G.L. 1999. A
method for determination of equine hoof
strain patterns using photoelasticity: an in
vitro study. *Equine Vet. J.* 31, 232-237.

Dejardin L.M., Arnoczky S.P., Cloud G.L., Stick
J.A. 2001. Photoelastic stress analysis of strain
patterns in equine hooves after four-point
trimming. *Am. J. Vet.* Res. 62(4), 467-473.

Denoix J-M. 1999. Functional anatomy of the
equine interphalangeal joint. *Proc. AAEP* 45,
174-177.

Denson N.B. 2004. Synthetic shoes offer advantages. *Am. Farriers J.* 30(3), 63-69.

Dewes H.F., Lowe M.D. 1987. Suspected selenium
poisoning in a horse. *NZ Vet. J.* 35, 53-54.

DeWitt O. 1970. Farrier science for the general
practitioner. *Proc. AAEP* 16, 43-54.

Dickson B., O'Malley J. 1987. Dry-weather hoof
care. *Am. Farriers J.* May/June, 30-34.

Diehl M., Ueltschi G. 1981. Navicular disease; an
occupational disease of the horse? Abstracts.
1st European Conference Medicine and Eques-
trian Sports, Saumur France.

Dinger J.E., Goodwin E.E., Leffel E.C. 1973. Factors affecting hardness of the equine hoof
wall. Scientific Paper No. A2212, Maryland
Experimental Station. College Park, Univ. of
Maryland

Dinger J.E. 1976. Recent findings in hoof physiology. *Am. Farriers J.* Dec. 2 (76), 58.

Donoghue S., Kronfeld D.S. 1980. Vitamin–minerals supplements for horses with emphasis
on vitamin A. *Comp.Cont. Educ.* 2 (8), S121-
S126.

Douglas J.E., Mittal C., Thomason J.J., Jofriet J.C.
1996. The modulus of elasticity of equine
hoof wall: implications for the mechanical
function of the hoof. *J. Expt. Biol.* 199, 1829-
1836.

Dyhre-Poulson P., Smedgegaard H.H., Roed J.,
Korsgaad E. 1994. Equine hoof function investigated by pressure transducers inside the
hoof and accelerometers mounted on the first
phalanx. *Eq. Vet. J.* 26(5), 362-366.

Dyson S. 1988. Variation in the normal radiographic anatomy of equine limbs. *In Practice*.
May, 119-125.

Dyson S.J. 1991. Lameness due to pain associated
with the distal interphalangeal joint: 45 cases.
Eq. Vet. J. 23 (2), 128-135.

Dyson S., Marks D. 2003. Foot pain and the elu-
sive diagnosis. In: *The veterinary Clinics of
North America, Equine Practice, Podiatry*. Ed.
O'Grady S.E., Aug. Vol. 19, No. 2. p 562.

Dyson S.J., Murray R., Schramme M., Branch M.
2004. Collateral desmitis of the distal interphalangeal joint in 18 horses (2001-2002). *Eq.
Vet. J.* 36(2), 160-166.

Eliashar E., McGuigan M.P., Rogers K.A., Wilson
A.M. 2002. A comparison of three horseshoeing styles on the kinetics of breakover in
sound horses. *Eq. Vet. J.* 34(2), 184-190.

Eliashar E., McGuigan M.P., Wilson A.M. 2004.
Relationship of foot conformation and force
applied to the navicular bone of sound horses
at the trot. *Eq. Vet. J.* 36(5), 431-435.

Ellis D.R. 1998. Condition of the hoof wall in
young horses and corrective farriery with
regard to limb deformities. *Eq. Vet. Educ.*
Manual No. 4, 42-47.

Emery L., Miller J., Van Hoosen N. 1977. *Horseshoeing Theory and Hoof Care*, 1st ed. Lea and
Febiger, Philadelphia.

Eustace R.E., Caldwell M.N. 1989a. The construction of the heart bar shoe and technique of
dorsal wall resection. *Eq. Vet. J.* 21(5), 367-369.

Eustace R.E., Caldwell M.N. 1989b. Treatment of
solar prolapse using the heart bar shoe and
dorsal hoof wall resection technique. *Equine
Vet. J.* 21(5) 370-372.

Eustace R.A. 1992. Adjustable glue-on heart bar
shoe. *Hoofcare and Lameness Mag.* 57/914,
13-14.

Eustace R.A. 2001a. Aetiopathogenesis of laminitis. *Proc. 1st. UK Farriery Convention*. 51-52.

Eustace R.A. 2001b. Diagnosis and classification
of equine laminitis in relation to prognosis.
Proc. 1st. UK Farriery Convention. 49-50.

Evans H.L., Jenny J., Raker W.C. 1966. The repair
of hoof cracks with acrylic. *JAVMA* 148(4).

Fackelman G.E. 1979. Flexoral deformity of the
metacarpophalangeal joint in growing horses.
Comp. Cont. Educ. Pract. Vet. 1(9), 51-58.

Fackelman G.E. 1980. Equine flexural deformities
of developmental origine. *Proc. AAEP* 26, 97-
105.

Fackelman G.E., Auer J.A., Orsini J., Salis B.
1983a. Surgical treatment of severe flexural

deformity of the distal interphalangeal joint in young horses. *JAVMA* 182(9), 949-952.

Fackelman G.E. 1983b. Tendon surgery. In: *Vet. Clin. North Am.*:Large Animal Pract. 381-390.

Ferguson J. 1994. University of Florida, College of Vet. Med. Large Animal Clinical Sciences. Personal communication.

Fessler J.F. 1971a. Surgical management of equine foot injuries. *Modern Vet. Pract.* February. 41-46.

Fessler J.F. 1971b. Surgical management of equine foot problems. *Modern Vet. pract.* March. 45-49.

Fessler, J.F. 1977. Tendon disorders of the young horse. *Arch. Am. Coll. Vet. Surg.* 6, 19-23.

Fessler J.F. 1989. Hoof injuries. In: *Wound Management. Vet. Clinic. of N. Am.: Eq. Pract.* 5 (3), 643-664.

Finnegan D., Rumph J. 1991. Hoof management: Balancing act. *Large Anim. Vet.* Sept./Oct.

Firth E.C., Schamhardt H.C., Hartman W. 1988. Measurements of bone strain in foals with altered foot balance. *Am. J. Vet. Res.* 49(2), 261-265.

Flecker H.R., Wagner C.P. 1986. Therapy and corrective shoeing for equine tendon disorders. *Comp. Cont. Educ.* 8(12), 970-976.

Floyd A.E. 2003. Malignant melanoma in the foot of a bay horse. *Eq. Vet. Edu.* 5(6), 379-381.

Forssell G. 1943. The diagnosis of lameness. Lectures at the Royal Veterinary College, Stockholm, Sweden.

Frandson R.D., Lebel J.L., Slade L.M., Barbalace R.C. 1976. Effect of slope of equine hoof on concussion and phalangeal angulation. *Am. Farriers* J. 4, 72-73.

Frank E.R. 1953. *Veterinary Surgery.* Minneapolis, Burgess Publishing Compnay.

Fraser R.D.B., MacRae T.P., Rogers G.E. 1972. *Keratins.* Springfield Ill. Charles C. Thomas Publ. pp. 139-143.

Fredricson I., Dalin G., Drevemo S., Hjerten G. 1975b. A biotechnical approach to the geometric design of racetracks. *Eq. Vet.* J. 7, 91-96.

Gabel A.A. 1982. Prevention, diagnosis and treatment of inflammation of the distal hock. *Proc. AAEP* 28, 287-298.

Gabel A.A., Bukowieki C.F. 1983. Fractures of the Phalanges. *Vet Clin. N. Am. Large Anim.* Pract. 5, 233-60.

Galey F.D., Whiteley H.E., Goetz T.E., Kuenstler A.R., Davis C.A., Beasley V.R. 1991. Black walnut (Juglans nigra) toxicosis: A model for equine laminitis. *J. Comp. Pathol.* 104, 313-326.

Garner H.E. 1975. Equine laminitis of alimentary origin: an experimental model. *Am. J. Vet. Res.* 36, 441-444.

Garner H.E., Sprouse R.F., Moore J.N., Coffman J.R. 1981. A mechanistic approach to prevention and treatment of acute equine laminitis. *Proc. AAEP* 40, 489.

Gauthier T. 2001. Putting hoof adhesives to the test. *Anvil Mag.* June.

Geary J.E. Jr 1975. The dynamics of the equine foreleg. MMAE thesis, Univ. of Delaware.

Gee S. 2006. USDA to Walking Horses industry: "Step up or we will". *Horse Illustrated*, 30(6), 42-49.

Gelatt K.J., Neuwirth L., Hawkins D.L., Woodard J.C. 1996. Haemangioma of the distal phalanx in a colt. *Vet. Radiol. Ultrasound* 37, 275-280.

Gerring E.L. 1980. Unusual case of pedal bone fracture in the horse. *Equine Vet.* J. 12, 150-151.

Geyer H., Schultz J. 1994. The long term influence of biotin supplementation on hoof horn quality in horses. *Schweiz. Arch. Tierheilk.* 136 (4), 137-149.

Geyer H. 1999. Structural alterations of the white line. *Europ. Farriers J.* April, 77, 8-21.

Geyer H. 2005. Personal communication. Veterinär-Anatomisches Institut, Univ. Zürich

Gibson K.T., McIlwraith C.W., Park R.D. 1990. A radiographic study of the distal interphalangeal joint and navicular bursa of the horse. *Vet. Rad.* 31(1).

Glade M.J., Salzman R.A. 1985. Effects of toe angle on hoof growth and contraction in the horse. *J. Eq. Vet. Sci.* 5 (1), 45-50.

Gnegy B.D. 2003. Consider the whole working foot. *Am. Farriers J.* Dec. 29, 93-100.

Goetz T.E., Comstock C.M. 1985. The use of adjustable heart-bar shoes in the treatment of laminitis in horses. *Proc. AAEP* 31, 605-616.

Goetz T.E. 1987. Anatomic, hoof, and shoeing considerations for the treatment of laminitis in horses. *JAVMA* 190(10), 1323-1332.

Goubaux A., Barrier G. 1892. *The Exterior of the Horse.* Translated and edited by Harger S.J.J. Philadelphia and London. J.B. Lippincott Co.

Gower J. 2000. *Horse Color Explained, A Breeder's Perspective*. Trafalgar Square publishing, North Pomfret, Vermont. pp. 90, 102.

Graham C. W. 1965a. Care of the horse's foot (from a veterinarian point of view). *Vet. Med/SAC* 60(3), 255-261.

Graham C.W. 1965b. Postoperative results of plastic hoof repair. *Proc. AAEP* 41-55.

Gregory C. 2004a. The Z-bar factor. *Am. Farriers J.* May/June, (30)4, 54-58.

Gregory C. 2004b. Building the Z-bar. *Am. Farriers J.* July/Aug., (30)5, 64-69.

Grosenbaugh D.A., Hood D.M. 1993. Practical equine hoof wall biochemistry. *Eq. Pract.* 15(8), 8-14.Gross K.D., Stover S.M., Hill A. E., Gardner I.A. 2004. Evaluation of forelimb horseshoe characteristics of Thoroughbreds racing on dirt surfaces. *Am. J. Vet. Res.* 65(7), 1021-1030.

Grubb L., Kane A.J. 1997. Study reveals link between toe grabs and injuries at the racetrack. *Anvil Magazine*, (4), 34-35.

Gubert K.P. 1989. The flail heel syndrome. *Am. Farriers J.* July/Aug. 16-21.

Guyton A.C. 1986. The stretch reflex. In: *Textbook of Medical Physiology*, 7th. ed. W.B. Saunders. pp 609-613.

Hackett R.P.1982. Delayed Wound Closure: A review and report of the use of the technique on three equine limb wounds. *Vet. Surg.* 12, 48-53.

Hamir A.N., Kunz C., Evans L.H. 1992. Equine keratoma. *J. Vet. Diagn. Invest.* 4, 99-100.

Hammill D. 2005. Scratches and leg mange in horses. *Small Farmer's J.* 116, 23-25.

Harman J., Ward M. 2001. The role of nutritional therapy in the treatment of equine Cushing's syndrome and laminitis. *Alt. Med. Rev.* Sept. Vol. 6, Suppl. S4 -S16.

Helms J., Pleasant R.S., Modransky P.D. 1994. Management of a keratoma in a horse. *Eq. Pract.* 16(7), 35-38.

Hennig G.E., Kraus B.H., Fister R., King V.L., Steckel R.R., Kirker-Head C.A. 2001. Comparison of two methods for presurgical disinfection of the equine hoof. *Vet. Surg.* 30, 366-373.

Henninger R.W., Owen D.L. 1986. Management of hoof-wall disease in horses. Part 1: diagnosis and surgical treatment. *Mod. Vet. Pract.* 141-146.

Hermans W.A. 1987. *Hoefverzorging en Hoefbeslag.* Groene Reeks. Uitgeverij Terra Zutphen.

Hickman J. 1964. Injuries and disease of the hoof and claw. *Veterinary Orthopedics.* Philadelphia. J.B. Lippincott Co.

Higami A. 1999. Occurrence of white line disease in performance horses fed low-zinc and low-copper diets. *J. Equine Sci.* 10(1), 1-5.

Hildebrand M. 1959. Motions of the running cheetah and horse. *J. of Mammalogy* 40(4), 481-495.

Hildebrand M. 1960. How animals run. *Scientific American* 202 (5), 148-157.

Hildebrand M. 1982. In: *Analysis of Verterbrate Structure.* Mechanics of support and movement. 2nd. ed. John Wiley and Sons, Inc. pp. 425-427.

Hildebrand M. 1987. The mechanics of the horse legs. *Am. Sci.* 75, 594-601.

Hill C., Klimesh R. 1989. Shoeing requirements of the long-distance horse. *Am. Farriers J.* Sept/Oct., 28-41.

Hinterhofer C., Stanek C., Haider H. 2001. Finite element analysis (FEA) as a model to predict effects of farriery on the equine hoof. *Eq. Vet. J. Suppl.* 33, 58-62.

Hintz H.F. 1978. Growth Rate of Horses. *Proc. AAEP.* 455-459.

Hintz H.F. 1983. *Horse Nutrition. A Practical Guide.* New York, pp 178-193.

Honnas C.M., O'Brien T.R., Linford R.L. 1988a. Distal phalanx fractures in horses. A survey of 274 horses wth radiographic assesment of healing in 36 horses. *Vet. Rad.* 29(3), 98-107.

Honnas C.M., O'Brien T.R., Linford R.L. 1988b. Solar margin fractures of the equine distal phalanx. *Proc. AAEP* 33, 399-411.

Honnas C.M., Ragle A.C., Meagher M.D. 1988c. Necrosis of the collateral cartilage of the distal phalanx in horses: 16 cases (1970-1985). *JAVMA* 193(10).

Honnas C.M., Meagher D.M., Linford R.L. 1988d. Surgical management of difficult foot problems in the horse: current concepts. *Proc. AAEP* 34, 249-262.

Honnas C.M., Liskey C.C., Meagher M.D., Brown D., Luck E.E. 1990. Malignant melanoma in the foot of a horse. *JAVMA* 197(6), 756-758.

Honnas C.M., Welch D.R., Ford S.T., Watkins P.J. 1992. Septic arthritis of the distal interphalangeal joint in 12 horses. *Vet. Surg.* 21(4), 261-268.

Honnas C.M. 1998. Keratomas of the equine digit. *Eq. Vet. Educ.* Manual No.4, 68-72.

Honnas C.M., Moyer W. 2000. How to approach hoof wall surgery in the horse. Proc. AAEP 46, 153-155.

Hood D.M., Grosenbaugh D.A., Slater M.R. 1994a. Vascular perfusion in horses with chronic laminitis. *Eq. Vet. J.* 26 (3), 191-196.

Hood D.M., Beckman A.S., Walker M.A., Morgan S.J. 1994b. Genetic predisposition to chronic laminitis in horses. *Proc. AAEP* 40.

Hood D.M., Beckham A.S., Chaffin M.K., Hunter J.F., Matthew N.S., Moyer W., Slater M.R. 1995. Comparison of phenylbutazone, Lily pads, and trimming on expressed pain in horses with chronic laminitis. *Proc. AAEP* 41, 248-250.

Hunt R.J. 1993. A retrospective evaluation of laminitis in horses. *Eq. Vet. J.* 25, 61-65.

Hunting W. 1898. *The Art of Horseshoeing – A Manual for Farriers*. William R. Jenkins, New York.

Jackson S.G. 1996. Nutrition and the equine foot: Some things to think about. *Anvil Mag.* June.

Jackson J. 1997. *The Natural Horse.* 2nd.ed. Harrison A.R. Star Riding Publishing.

Janicek J.C., Dabareiner R.M., Honnas C.M., Crabill M.A. 2005. Heel bulb lacerations in horses: 101 cases (1988-1994). *J. Am. Vet. Assoc.* 226(3), 418-423.

Jann H.W., Williams J.A., Whitfield C.C., Henry G. Alley S. 1997. Surgical treatment of chronic refractory laminitis: Deep digital flexor tenotomy. *Eq. Pract.* 19(9), 26-32.

Jenny J., Evans L.H., Raker C.W. 1965. Hoof repair with plastics. *JAVMA*, 147(12), 1340-1345.

Johnson E.L., Asquith R.L. 1993. Anatomy and topography of the equine foot. Univ. of Florida. Extension bulletin AS-28.

Johnson J.H. 1970. Puncture wounds of the foot. *Vet. Med/ Small Anim. Clin.* 65, 147-152.

Johnson J.H. 1972. Septic Conditions of the equine foot. *JAVMA* 161(11), 1276-1279.

Johnson J.H. 1973. Contracted tendons. *Mod. Vet. Pract.* May, 67-69.

Johnson J.H. 1982. The foot. In: *Equine Medicine and Surgery*, Ed. Mansmann R.A. and McAllister E.S. American Veterinary publication, Santa Barbara, CA.

Jones E.L., Collier A.M. 1983. Therapeutic horseshoeing: Corrective shoeing in specific conditions. *Mod. Vet. Pract.* July, 567-574.

Jongbloets A.M., Sloet van Oldruitenborgh-Oosterbaan M.M., Meeus P.J., Back W. 2005. Equine exudative canker: An (auto-) immune disease? *Tijdschr Diergeneeskd.* 130(4), 106-109.

Josseck H. 1991. Hufhornveränderungen bei Lipizzanerpferden und ein Beandlungsversuch mit Biotin. Untersuchungen des makroskopischen Hufstatus und des Hornwachstums sowie zum Verlauf des Plasmsbiotinspiegels und der genetischen Grundlagen der Hufhornschäden. *Diss. Med. Vet.* Zürich.

Josseck H., Zenker W., Geyer H. 1995. Hoof horn abnormalities in Lipizzaner horses and the effect of dietary biotin on macroscopic aspects of hoof horn quality. *Eq. Vet. J.* 27(3), 175-182.

Juell A. 1998. Glueing on aluminum horseshoes. *Anvil Mag.* Nov., 24-30.

Kai M., Takahashi T., Aoki O., Oki H. 1999. Influence of rough track surfaces on components of vertical forces in cantering Thoroughbred horses. *Eq. Vet. J. Suppl.* 30, 241-217.

Kainer R.A. 1989. Clinical anatomy of the equine foot. In: *Vet. Clin. N. Am. Eq. Pract.* 5, 1-27.

Kane A.J., Stover S.M., Gardner I.A., Case J.T., Johnson B.J., Read D.H., Ardans A.A. 1996a. Horseshoe characteristics as possible risk factors for fatal musculoskeletal injury of Thoroughbred racehorses. *Am. Vet. Res.* 57(8), 1147-1152.

Kane A.J. 1996b. Toe grabs and rim shoes as possible risk factors for catastrophic injury of Thoroughbred racehorses. *Proc. AAEP* 42, 286-288.

Kane A.J., Stover S.M., Gardner I.A. Bock K.B., Case J.T., Johnson B.J., Anderson M.L., Barr B.C., Daft B.M., Kinde H., Larochelle D., Moore J., Mysore J., Stoltz J., Woods L., Read D.H., Ardans A.A. 1998. Hoof size, shape, and balance as possible risk factors for catastrophic musculoskeletal injury of Thoroughbred racehorses. *Am. J. Vet. Res.* 59 (12), 1545-1552.

Kane A.J., Stover S.M., Bock K.B., Gardner I.A. 1999. New technique for quantitative measurement of hoof balance. *Am. Farriers J.* Sept./Oct. 65-71.

Kaneps A.J., O'brien T.R., Redden R.F., Stover S.M., Pool R.R. 1993. Characterisation of osseous bodies of the distal phlanx of foals. *Eq. Vet. J.* 25(4), 285-292.

Kaneps A.J., O'Brien T.R., Willits N.H., Dykes J.E., Stover S.M. 1998. Effect of hoof trimming on the occurrence of distal phalangeal palmar process fractures in foals. *Eq. Vet. J. Suppl.* 26, 36-45.

Kasapi M.A., Gosline J.M. 1997. Design complexity and fracture control in the equine hoof wall. *J. Expt. Biol.* 200, 1639-1659.

Kasapi M.A., Gosline J.M. 1998. Exploring the possible function of equine hoof wall tubules. *Eq. Vet. J.* suppl. 26, 10-14.

Keegan G.K., Baker J.G., Boero J.M., Pijanowski J.G., Phillips W. J. 1992. Evaluation of support bandaging during measurement of proximal seasamoidean ligament strain in horses by use of a mercury gauge. *Am. J. Vet. Res.* 53 (7), 1203-1208.

Keller M., Krehon S., Stanek C., Rosengarten R. 2000. Keratinopathogenic mould fungi and dermatophytes in healthy and diseased hooves of horses. *Vet. Rec.* Nov. 147 (22), 619-622.

Kelly N.J., Watrous B.J., Wagner P.C. 1987. Comparison of splinting and casting on the degree of laxity induced in the thoracic limb in young horses. *Eq. Pract.* 10, 10-16.

Kempson S.A. 1987. Scanning electron microscope observation of hoof horn from horse with brittle feet. *Vet. Rec.* 120, 568-570.

Kempson S.A. 1994. Promoting good quality hoof horn. In: *No Foot – No Horse* II. Ed. Clarke A. Ontario, Univ. of Guelph. pp 8-14.

Kempson S.A. 1996. Why dietary excesses are bad for horses. *Am. Farriers* J. 22, 29-34.

Kilby E., Leach D. 1982. Ingenious engineering. *Equus.* June 1982. 34-43.

Kempson S.A., Campbell E.H. 1998. A permeability barrier in the dorsal wall of the equine hoof capsule. *Eq. Vet. J. Suppl.* 26, 15-21.

Kempson S.A. 2004. Use of a topical disinfectant as part of a hoof care program for horses with diseases of the hoof capsule. *Vet. Rec.* 154, 647-652.

King M. 2002. Hoof dressings: What studies show. *The Horse*, Oct. 81-84.

Klimesh R. 1997. Squared toes to the rescue: How to make and use a squaring block. *Anvil Mag.* May, 18-24.

Knight A.D., Weisbrode E.S., Schmall M.L., Reed M.S., Gabel A.A., Bramlage R.L., Tyznik I.W. 1990. The effect of copper supplementation on the prevalence of cartilage lesions in foals. *Eq. Vet. J.* 22(6), 426-432.

Knottenbelt D. 2006. Pemphigus: The body under attack. *Hoofcare and Lameness Magazine* 77, 17-20.

Kobluk C.N., Robinson R.A., Gordon B.J., Clanton C.J., Trent A.M., Ames T.R. 1990. The effect of conformation and shoeing: A cohort study of 95 Thoroughbred Racehorses. *Proc. AAEP* 36, 259-274.

Koepisch W.F. 1998a. Using the aluminum wedge shoe. *Anvil Mag.* Feb. 23-31.

Koepisch W.F. 1998b. The Roller Motion Shoe. *Anvil Mag.* Dec. 37-39.

Konig B., Budras K.D. 2003. Structure and clinical implications of the coronet horn stratification with special consideration of horn maturation, ageing and decay in the equine hoof. *Dtsch Tierarztl Wochenschr.* 110(11), 438-444.

Krpan M.K., Crawley G.R. 1986. Management of hoof-wall disease in horses. Part 2: Repair of hoof wall defects. *Mod. Vet. Pract.* 2, 147-151.

Kruzel M.K, Mackay-Smith M. 1982. Best feet forward. *Equus* 56, 68-73.

Küng M. 1991. Die Zugfestigkeit des Hufhorns von Pferden. *Diss. Med. Vet. Univ.* Zürich.

Kunze D.J., Monticello T.M., Jakob T.P. 1986. Malignant melanoma of the coronary band in a horse. *JAVMA* 188, 297-298.

Kuwano A., Oikawa M., Takatori K. 1996. Pathomorphological findings in a case of onychomycosis of a racehorse. *J. Vet. Med. Sci.* 58(11), 1117-1120.

Kuwano A., Yoshihara T., Takatori K., Kosuge J. 1998. Onychomycosis in white line disease in horses: pathology, mycology and clinical features. *Eq. Vet. J. Suppl.* 26, 27-35.

Kuwano A., Tanaka K., Kawabata M., Ooi Y., Takahashi T., Yoshihara T., Reilly D. 1999. A survey of white line disease in Japanese racehorses. *Eq. Vet. J.* 31(6), 515-518.

Kuwano A., Katayama Y., Kasashima Y., Okada K., Rei J.D. 2002. A gross and histopathological study of an ectopic white line development in equine laminitis. *J. Vet. Med. Sci.* 64(10), 893-900.

Lambert F. 1966. The role of moisture in the physiology of the hoof of the harness horse. *Vet. Med./Sm. An. Clin.*, 61(4), 342-347.

Lambert F. 1968. An experiment demonstrating rapid contraction of a Standardbred horse hooves from moisture loss during flooring. *Vet. Med./ Sm. Anim. Clin.* 63, 878-881.

Lambert F. 1971. Some observable physical principles of shock diffusion in the horse hoof. *Vet Med./Sm. Anim. Clin.*, 71, (6) 601-604.

Landeau J.L., Barret D.J., Batterman S.C. 1983. Mechanical properties of equine hooves. *Am. J.Vet. Res.*44(1).

Lanovaz J.L., Clayton H.M., Watson L.G. 1998. In vitro attenuation of impact shock in equine digits. *Eq. Vet. J.* Suppl. 26, 96-102.

Lawrence J.M., Huddleston N. 1951. *American Livestock Biographies*. News Publishing Company, Sacramento, CA.

Layton W.E. 1965. Care of the horse's foot (from a farrier's point of view). *Vet. Med./Sm. Anim. Clin.*, 60 (3), 248-254.

Leach D.H. 1980. The structure and function of the equine hoof wall. PhD Thesis, University of Saskatchewan, Saskatoon.

Leach D.H. 1983. Biomechanical considerations in raising and lowering the heel. *Proc. AAEP.* 28, 333-342.

Leach D.H., Oliphant L.W. 1983. Ultrastructure of the equine hoof wall secondary epidermal lamellae. *Am. J.Vet. Res.* 44(8), 1561-1570.

Leach D.H., Zoerb G.C. 1983. Mechanical properties of equine hoof wall tissue. *Am. J.Vet. Res.* 44(11), 2190-2194.

Leach D. 1986a. Navicular disease. *FYI Newsletter*, Fran Jurga, Publisher.

Leach D.H. 1986b. Locomotion-understanding the concepts and terminology. *Proc. Int. Conf. Equine Sports Med.* pp 3-8.

Lewis L.D. 1982. *Feeding and Care of the Horse*. Lea and Febiger. Philadelphia.

Ley W.B., Scott Pleasant R., Dunnington E.A. 1998. Effects of season and diet on tensile strength and mineral content of the equine hoof wall. *Eq. Vet. J.* Suppl. 26, 46-50.

Linford L.R. 1990. Laminitis (founder). In: *Large Animal Internal Medicine*. Ed. Smith P.B. Mosby. pp 1158-1168.

Lloyd C.K., Peterson P.R., Wheat D.J., Ryan E.A., Clark H.J. 1988. Keratomas in horses: Seven cases (1975-1986). *JAVMA* 193(8).

Lochner F.K., Milne D.W. Mills E.J. Groom J.J. 1980. In vivo and in vitro measurements of tendon strain in the horse. *Am. J.Vet. Res.* 41(12), 1929-1937.

Lockard A.J., Reinertson E.L. 1986. Stimulation of equine hoof growth using a counter-irritant. *Iowa State Univ. Vet.* 48(2), 99-101.

Loomis E.C., Hughes J.P., Bramhall E.L. 1975. *The Common Parasites of Horses*. Division of Agricultural Sciences, University of California, publication No. 4006.

Longland A.C., Cairns A.J. 2000. Fructans and their implications in the aetiology of laminitis. Proc. 3rd. Intern. Conf. on Feeding Horses, 52-55.

Lose M.P. 1981. Correction of hindleg pastern subluxation. *Mod. Vet. Pract.* 62(2), 156.

Lose M.P., Hopkins E.F., Franchette D. 1981. Equine contraction. *Vet. Med./ Sm. Anim. Clin.* 76(7), 1023-1031.

Loving N.S. 1997. *Conformation and Performance. A Guide to the Performance Consequences of Common Conformation Points*. Breakthrough Publications, Ossining NY. pp 131-148.

Ludford J. 2004. Increase your odds of success by knowing the basics of glue-ons. *Am. Farriers J.* 30(5), 47-50.

Luikart R. 1993. *Standards for Judging Farriery*. Lexington, Kentucky, American Farrier's Association Publishing, pp 10-13.

Lungwitz A. 1891. The changes in the form of the horse's hoof under the action of the body-weight. *J. Comp. Path. Therap.* 4 (3), 191-211.

Lungwitz A. 1966. *Defects of the hoof. In: A Textbook of Horseshoeing*, 11th ed. Trans. J.W. Adams. Oregon State University Press, Corvallis, OR. pp 185-190.

Lyon W.E. 1934. *First Aid Hints for the Horse Owner*. Charles Scribner's Sons, New York. pp 43-44.

MacFadden B.J. 2005. Fossile horses-Evidence for evolution. *Science*. March 18, Vol. 307. 1728-1730.

MacGregor T. 1998. Solar puncture: 'Big' hole vs. 'Little' hole. *Anvil Mag*. March, 20-25.

Mackay-Smith P.M. 1993. Hoof management: what horses tells us. *Proc. AAEP* 39, 231.

Madsen L.L. 1942. In: *Keeping Livestock Healthy*. Editor: Hambidge G. Nutritional diseases of farm animals, vitamin A. pp. 339-343. USDA.

Magner D. 1980. *The Classic Encyclopedia of the Horse.* Bonanza Books, New York.

Manning C.D. 1983. Making and using the Patten shoe. *Am. Farriers J.* Jan./Feb., 24-30.

Manning C.D. 1992. The Patten Shoe revisited. *Am. Farriers J.* Dec., 38-41.

Mansmann R.A., King C., Stewart E. 2000. How to develop a preventive foot care program – A model. Proc. *AAEP* 46, 156-161.

Marianne Y. 1986. Clinicians guide to equine laminitis. *Eq. Vet. J.* 18(2), 156-158.

Markel D.M., Richardson G.L., Peterson P.R., Meagher D.M. 1987. Surgical reconstruction of chronic coronary band avulsions in three horses. *JAVMA* 190(6),687-688.

Marks D., Mackay-Smith M.P., Cushing L.S., Leslie J.A. 1971. Use of an elastomer to reduce concussion to horse's feet. *JAVMA* 158(8), 1361-1365.

Marks D. 2000. Conformation and soundness. Proc. *AAEP* 46, 39-45.

Martinelli M.J., Ferrie J.T. 1998. Farrier primer for the student and practicing veterinarian. *Eq. Vet. Ed. Manual* No. 4. 16-24.

McClinchey H.L., Thomason J.J., Runciman R.J. . 2004. Grip and slippage of the horse's hoof on solid substrates measured ex vivo. *Biosyst. Eng.* 89 (4), 485-494.

McCunn J. 1951. Lameness in the horse, with special reference to surgical shoeing. *The Vet. Rec.* 40(63), 629-634.

McDiarmid A.M. 1998. Distal interphalangeal joint lameness in a horse associated with damage to the insertion of the lateral collateral ligament. *Eq. Vet. Edu.* 10(3), 114-118.

McGladdery, A.J. 1992. Three cases of acquired flexural deformity of the distal interphalangeal joint in growing foals on a stud farm. *Equine Vet. Educ.* 4(40), 173-176.

McIlwraith, C.W., Fessler, J.F. 1978. Evaluation of inferior check ligament desmotomy for treatment of acquired flexor tendon contracture in the horse. *JAVMA* 172(3).

McIlwraith C.W., James L.F. 1982. Limb deformities in foals associated with ingestion of locoweed by mares. *JAVMA* 181(3), 255-258.

Meershoek L.S., Lanovaz J.L., Schamhardt H.C. 2002. Calculated forelimb flexor tendon forces in horses with experimentally induced superficial digital flexor tendonitis and the effects of application of heel wedges. *Am. J. Vet. Res.* 63(3), 432-437.

Menzies-Gow N.J., Bond R., Patterson-Kane J.C., McGowan C.M. 2002. Coronary band dystrophy in 2 horses. *Vet. Rec.* 150, 665-668.

Merillat A.L. 1911. *Veterinary Surgical Operations.* Alexander Eger, Chicago.

Merkens H.W., Schamhardt H.C., Van Osch G.J.V.M., Van Den Bogert A.J. 1993. Ground reaction force patterns of Dutch Warmblood horses at normal trot. *Eq. Vet. J.* 25(2), 134-137.

Mero J.L., Pool R.R. 2002. Twenty cases of degenerative suspensory ligament desmitis in Peruvian Paso horses. Proc. *AAEP* 48, 329-334.

Messer N.T. 1981. Tibiotarsal effusion associated with chronic zinc intoxication in three horses. *JAVMA* 178, 294-297.

Metcalf S., Wagner P.C., Balch-Burnett O. 1982. Corrective trimming and shoeing in the treatment of tendon disorders of young horses. *Eq. Pract.* 4(9), 6-15.

Meyers V.S. 1976. Ruptured common digital extensor tendons associated with contracted flexor tendons in foals. Proc. *AAEP* 22, 67-73.

Miles W.J. 1846. *On the Horse's Foot.* Longman, Brown, Green and Longman.

Miller M.R. 1994. An effective shoe for navicular disease. *Eq. Vet. Sci.* 14(6).

Miller W.C., Robertson E.D.S. 1943. *Practical Animal Husbandry.* 3rd. ed. Oliver and Boyd Ltd. London. pp. 279-323.

Millman J. 1998. Bar shoes–when and how to use them. *Am. Farriers J.* March/Apr. Insert.

Milne F.J. 1967. Clinical examination and diagnosis of the diseased equine foot. *JAVMA* 151, 1599-1608.

Miyaki H., Ohnishi T., Yamamoto T. et. al. 1974. Measurements of the water content of the hoof wall, sole and frog in horses. *Exp. Reports Equine Health Res. Lab.* 11:15-20.

Monhart B. 2002. Die Einwirkung von Umgebungsfaktoren auf das Hufhorn des Pferdes. *Inaugural-Dissertation*, Med. Vet. Univ. Zürich.

Moore N. J., Allen A. D. 1995. *A Guide to Equine Acute Laminitis.* Veterinary Learning systems, Trenton NJ.

Moore R.C. 1916. Equine laminitis or pododermatitis. *Am. J. Vet. Med.*, 11, 281-292.

Moyer W., Anderson J.P. 1975a. Lameness caused by improper shoeing. *JAVMA* 166, 47-53.

Moyer W., Anderson J.P. 1975b. Sheared heels: Diagnosis and treatment. *JAVMA* 166(1), 53-55.

Moyer W. 1979. Diseases of the equine heel. *Proc. AAEP* 25, 21-29.

Moyer W. 1980. The basics of corrective shoeing. *Compend. Cont. Educ. Pract. Vet.* 11(10), S193-S199.

Moyer W. 1981. Therapeutic principles of diseases of the foot. *Proc. AAEP* 27, 453-466.

Moyer W. 1982. Distal sesamoidean desmitis. *Proc. AAEP* 28, 245-251.

Moyer W. 1983. Repairing hoof cracks in horses: A review and report of a new technique. *Comp. Cont. Educ. Pract. Vet.* 5(9), S495-S500.

Moyer W. 1988a. Chronic sub-solar bruising. *Proc. AAEP* 34, 333-335.

Moyer W. 1988b. Management of proximal incomplete quarter cracks in Standardbred racehorses. *Proc. AAEP*, 329-332.

Moyer W., Sigafoos R. 1988. Treatment of distal phalanx fractures in racehorses using a continuous rim-type shoe. *Proc. AAEP* 34, 325-328.

Moyer W. 1989a. Corrective shoeing. *Vet. Clin. North Am.: Large Anim. Pract.* 2,3.

Moyer W., Redden R.R. 1989b. Chronic and severe laminitis : a critique of therapy with heart-bar shoes and hoof wall resection. *Equine Vet. J.* 21(5) 317-318.

Moyer W. 1990. Pathogenesis of foot problems. In: *Equine Lameness and Foot Conditions.* University of Sydney, Sydney Australia. pp 261-262.

Moyer W., Sigafoos D.R. 1991. Preliminary experience and uses of composite hoof wall repair. *Proc. AAEP* 681-686.

Moyer W., Sigafoos D.R. 1993. *A Guide to Equine Hoof Wall Repair.* Veterinary Learning Systems, Trenton N.J.

Moyer W., O'Brien T.R., Walker M. 1999. Nonseptic pedal osteitis: A cause of lameness and a diagnosis? *Proc. AAEP* 45, 178-179.

Muller N., Luikart R. 2006. Teaming up against coffin joint ligament injuries. *Am. Farriers J.* 32(2), 83-86.

Munzinger K. 2005. Die Hufhornqualität von Lipizzanerpferden und Einflüsse von Futterzusätzen und Umgebungsfaktoren. Inaugural-Dissertation, Med. Vet. Univ. Zürich.

Muybridge E. 1957. *Animals in Motion.* Dover Publ. New York.

Nagamine C.M., Castro F., Buchanan B., Schumacher J., Craig L.E., 2005. Proliferative pododermatitis (canker) with intralesional spirochetes in three horses. *Vet. Diagn. Invest.* 17(3), 269-271.

National Research Council 1989. *Nutrient requirements of horses,* 5th. Ed. Washington, DC, National Academy of Science.

Naylor J.M., Ralston S.L. 1991. *Large Animal Clinical Nutrition.* Mosby Year Book. St. Louis, Missori. pp 83-84.

Newlyn H.A., Collins S.N., Cope B.C., Hopegood L., Latham R.J., Reilly J.D. 1998. Finite element analysis of static loading in donkey hoof wall. *Eq. Vet. J. Suppl.* 26, 103-110.

Nickel R. 1938. Über den Bau der Hufröhrchen und seine Bedeutung fur den Mechanismus des Pferdehufes. *DTW* 46, 449-552.

Nickel R., Schummer A., Seiferle E. 1986. *The Anatomy of the Domestic Animals.* Vol. 1: The Locomotor System of the Domestic Mammals. Springer –Verlag, New York.

Nyland H. 2006. The grass-laminitis connection. *Western Horseman.* Apr. 71(4), 80-92.

O'Brien J.C. 1968. Bits, boots and bridles. In: *Care and Training of the Trotter and Pacer.* Written by Harrison J.C. 1st ed. Columbus OH. The United States Trotting Association. pp 418-517.

O'Connor J.J. 1960. In: *Dollar's Veterinary Surgery.* 4th. ed. Bailliere, Tindalland Cox, London.

O'Grady S.E. 1993a. A practical approach to treating laminitis. *Vet. Med.* Sept., 867-875.

O'Grady S.E. 1993b. White line disease. *Am. Farriers J.* July/Aug. 22-26.

O'Grady S.E. 1995a. Fresh look at foal care. *Am. Farriers J.* May/June, 75-80.

O'Grady S.E. 1995b. Long-toe low-heel syndrome-A growing problem. *Am. Farriers J.* Jan/Feb. 31-34.

O'Grady S.E. 1996. Chronic foot soaking. *Am. Farriers J.* Sept./Oct., 51-56.

O'Grady S.E., Watson E.W. 1999. How to glue on therapeutic shoes. *Proc. AAEP* 45, 115-119.

O'Grady S.E. 2000. White line disease update. *Am. Farriers J.* July/Aug. 29-36

O'Grady S.E., Horne P.A. 2001. Lameness caused by a solar keratoma: a challenging differential diagnosis. *Eq. Vet. Educ.* 13(2), 87-89.

O'Grady S.E. 2001. How to repair a quarter crack. Proc. *AAEP* 47, 287-290.

O'Grady S.E. 2004. Glue-on shoes. *Am. Farriers J.* 30 (2), 73-80.

O'Grady S.E., Madison J.B. 2004. How to treat equine canker. *Proc. AAEP* Vol. 50, 202-205.

O'Grady S.E. 2004. Glue-on shoes. Best for realigning P3 in horses with chronic laminitis. *Am. Farriers J.* 3(2), 73-80.

Oikawa M., Kasashima Y. 2002. The Japanese experience with tendonitis in racehorses. *J. Eq. Sci.* 13(2), 41-56.

Oke R.A. 2003. Unilateral white line disease and laminitis in a quarter horse mare. *Can. Vet. J.* 44(2) 145-146.

Østblom L. C., Lund C., Melsen F. 1982. Histological study of navicular bone disease. *Eq. Vet. J.* 14, 199-202.

Østblom L. C., Lund C., Melsen F. 1984. Navicular bone disease: Results of treatment using egg-bar shoeing technique. *Equine Vet. J.* 16(3), 203-206.

Østblom L.C. 1984. Egg-bar shoeing technique for treatment of navicular disease. *Eq. Vet. J.* 16(3), 206.

O'Toole D., Raisbeck M.F. 1995. Pathology of experimentally-induced chronic selenosis (" alkali disease) in yearling cattle. *J. Vet. Diag. Invest.* 7, 364-373.

Ovnicek G. 1996. Wild horse hoof pattern offers help for domestic hoof problems. *Am. Farriers J.* March/April, 15-18.

Owen J.M. 1975. Abnormal flexion of the corono-pedal joint or "contracted tendons" in unweaned foals. *Eq. Vet. J.* 7, 40-45.

Page B., Anderson F.G. 1992. Diagonal imbalance of the equine foot: A cause of lameness. *Proc. AAEP* 38, 413-417.

Painter J.H. 1996. Use of polyvinylchloride pipe to create hoof extensions for foals. *Proc. AAEP.* 42, 216.

Painter J., Schumacher J. 1997. Try PVC pipe for quick, inexpensive hoof extension. *Am. Farriers J.* March/April, 24-26.

Pardoe C.H., Wilson A.M. 1999. In vitro mechanical properties of different equine hoof wall crack fixation techniques. *Eq. Vet. J.* 31(6), 506-509.

Pardoe C.H., McGuigan M.P., Rogers K.M., Rowe L.L., Wilson A.M. 2001. The effect of shoe material on the kinetics and kinematics of foot slip at impact on concrete. *Eq. Vet. J. Suppl.* 33, 70-73.

Parks A.H. 1999. Equine foot wounds: General principles of healing and treatment. *Proc. AAEP* 45, 180-187.

Peacock E.E., VanWinkle W. 1976. *Wound Repair,* 2nd. ed. W.B. Saunders Co. Philadelphia. pp 204-270.

Pearson L., Huidekoper R.S., Michener CH.B., Harbaugh W.H., Law J., Trumbower M.R., Liautard A., Holocombe A.A., Adams J.W., Mohler J.R. 1942. *Special Report on the Diseases of the Horse.* USDA Bureau of Animal Industry, U.S.A.

Peloso J.G., Cohen N.D., Walker M.A. 1996. Case-control study of risk factors for the development of laminitis in the contralateral limb in Equidae with unilateral lameness. *J. Am. Vet. Med. Assoc.* 290, 1746-1749.

Percivall W. 1855. *Hippopathology, A Systematic Treatise on the Disorders and Lameness of the Horse.* Vol. I. Longman, Brown, Green and Longmans, London. pp 236-238.

Percivall W. 1865. *Hippopathology, Lameness in the Horse.* Part I, Vol. IV. Longman, Green, Longman, Roberts and Green, London. pp 263-271.

Peremans K., Verschooten F., De Moor A., Desmet P. 1991. Laminitis in the pony: conservative treatment vs. dorsal hoof wall resection. *Equine Vet. J.* 23 (4), 243-246.

Pickersgill C.H. 2000. Recurrent white line abscessation associated with a keratoma in a riding pony. *Eq. Vet. Educ.* 12(6), 286-291.

Podoll M. 2005. Heart bar mold saves time, money, mess. *Am. Farriers J.* April, 31(3), 29-31.

Podol M. 2006. Super soaker. *Am. Farriers J.* 32(4), 45-49.

Pollitt C.C. 1986. Laminitis and hoof conditions in the horse, Univ. of Qld. Post Grad. *Comm. in Vet. Sc.*

Pollitt C.C. 1995. *Color Atlas of the Horse's Foot.* Mosby-Wolfe Publishing.

Pollitt C.C. 1999. Equine laminitis: A revised pathophysiology. *Proc. AAEP* 45, 188-192.

Pollitt C.C., Daradka M. 2004. Hoof wall wound repair. *Eq. Vet. J.* 36(3), 210-215.

Pool R.R., Meagher D.M., Stover S.M. 1989. Pathophysiology of navicular syndrom. In: *Vet. Clin. N. Am.: Eq. Pract.* 5, 109-129.

Prescott C.W. 1970. Canker in the hoof of a horse. *Aust. Vet. J.* 46, 449-451.

Pugh D.G., Williams M.A. 1992. Feeding foals from birth to weaning. *Comp. Cont. Educ. Pract. Vet.* 14 (4), 526-533.

Pugh D.G., Schumacher J. 1993. Feeding and nutrition of brood mares. *Comp. Cont. Educ. Pract. Vet.* 15 (1), 106-115.

Quddus M.A., Kingbury H.B., Rooney J.R. 1978. A force and motion study of the foreleg of a Standardbred trotter. *J. Eq. Med. Surg.* 2, 233-242.

Raisbeck F.M. 2000. Selenosis. In: *Vet. Clin. N. Am.: Eq. Pract.* Ed. Osweiler D.G., Galey D.F. W.B.Saunders Co. pp. 465-480.

Ratzlaff M.H., Shindell R.M., DeBowes R.M. 1985. Changes in digital venous pressures of horses moving at the walk and trot. *Am. J. Vet. Res.* 46 (7), 1545-1549.

Ratzlaff M.H., Grant B.D. 1986. The use of electrogoniometry and cinematography in the diagnosis and evaluation of forelimb lameness. *Proc. AAEP* 31, 183-199.

Ratzlaff M.H. 1988. Current methods for the analysis of locomotion and their potential clinical application. *Proc. AAEP* 34, 99-127.

Ratzlaff M.H., Hyde M.L., Grant B. et al. 1990. Measurement of vertical forces and temporal components of the strides of galloping horses using instrumented shoes. *J. Eq. Vet. Sci.* 10 (1), 23-35.

Redden R.F. 1986. Minimizing complications of laminitis in horses. *Mod. Vet. Pract.* May, 446-450.

Redden R.F. 1987. Hoof wall resection as a treatment in laminitis. *Proc. AAEP* 32, 647-656.

Redden R.F. 1988. Complicated laminitis. *Proc. AAEP* 34, 311-319.

Redden R.F. 1990. White line disease. *Eq. Pract.* 12(6), 14-15,18.

Redden R.F. 1992. 18° Elevation of the heels as an aid in treating acute and chronic laminitis. *Proc. AAEP* 38, 375-379.

Redden R.F. 1998. Shoeing the laminitic horse. In: *Understanding Laminitis*. Ed. R. Redden. The blood-Horse Inc. pp 60-79.

Redden R.F. 2003a. Preventing laminitis in the contralateral limb of horses with non-weight-bearing lameness. *Proc. AAEP* 49, 320-327.

Redden R.F. 2003b. Hoof capsule distortion: understanding the mechanism as a basis for rational management. In: *The Veterinary Clinics of North America, Equine Practice, Podiatry.* Ed. O'Grady S.E., Aug. Vol. 19, No. 2. p 453-455.

Reeves M.J., Yovich J.V., Turner S. 1989. Miscellaneous conditions of the equine foot. In: The Equine Foot Ed. Yovich J.V. *The Vet Clin. N. Am. Eq. Pract.* 5(1), 239-241.

Reilly J.D., Cottrell D.F., Martin R.J., Cuddeford D. 1996. Tubule density in equine hoof horn. *Biomimetics.* 4, 23-35.

Reilly J.D., Collins S.N., Cope B.C., Hopegood L., Latham R.J. 1998a. Tubule density of the stratum medium of horse hoof. *Eq. Vet. J. Suppl.* 26, 4-9.

Reilly J.D., Cottrell D.F., Martin R.J., Cuddeford D.J. 1998b. Effect of supplementary dietary biotin on hoof growth and hoof growth rate in ponies: a controlled trial. *Eq. Vet. J. Suppl.* 26, 51-57.

Renchin R., Sigafoos R. Redden R. 1995. Dremel tool makes hoof work easy. *Am. Farriers J.* Sept./Oct.

Richardson G.L., O'Brien T.R. 1985. Puncture wounds into the navicular bursa of the horse: Role of radiographic evaluation. *Vet. Rad.* 26(6), 203-207.

Richardson G.L., Pascoe J.R., Meagher D.M. 1986a. Puncture wounds of the foot in horses: Diagnosis and treatment. *Comp. Cont. Educ. Pract. Vet.* 8, S379-S388.

Richardson G.L., O'Brien T.R., Pascoe J.R. 1986b. Puncture wounds of the navicular bursae in 38 horses: A retrospective study. *Vet. Surg.* 15(2), 156-160.

Richardson G.L. 1999. Surgical management of penetrating wounds to the equine foot. *Proc. AAEP* 45, 198-199.

Rick G.E. 1907. *Rick's New Artistic Horseshoeing*, 1st ed. The Commercial Printing Co. Akron, Ohio.

Ridley J. 2004. Battling a white line case caused by bad shoeing. *Am. Farriers J.* 30(8), 77-79.

Riemersma D.J., Van Den Bogert A.J., Jansen M.O., Schamhardt H.C. 1996. Influence of shoeing on ground reaction forces and tendon strains in the forelimb of ponies. *Eq. Vet. J.* 28(2), 126-132.

Rijkenhuizen A.B.M. 2006. Navicular disease: A review of what's new. *Eq. Vet. J.* 38(1), 82-88.

Ritmeester A.M., Ferguson D. 1996. Coronary grooving promotes dorsal hoof wall growth in horses with chronic laminitis. *Proc. AAEP* 42, 212.

Ritmeester A.M., Denicola D.B., Blevins W.E., Christian J.A. 1997. Primary intraosseous mast cell tumour of the third phalanx in a Quarter Horse. *Eq. Vet. J.* 29(2), 151-152.

Ritmeester A.M., Blevins W.E., Ferguson D.W., Adams S.B. 1998. Digital perfusion, evaluated scintigraphically, and hoof wall growth in horses with chronic laminitis treated with egg bar-heart bar shoeing and coronary grooving. *Eq. Vet. J. Suppl.* 26, 111-118.

Roberts E.D., Ochoa R., Haynes P.F. 1980. Correlation of dermal-epidermal laminar lesions of equine hoof with various disease conditions. *Vet. Pathol.* 17, 656-666.

Robertson I.P., Hood D.M. 1996. Ability of commercial hoof wall products to maintain hydration of the equine hoof wall. *Proc. AAEP* 42, 208-211.

Robinson N.E., Dabney J.M., Weinder W.J. 1975. Vascular responses in the equine digit. *Am. J. Vet. Res.* 36:1249.

Roepstorff L., Johnston C., Drevemo S. 2001. In vivo and in vitro heel expansion in relation to shoeing and frog pressure. *Eq. Vet. J. Suppl.* 33, 54-57.

Roland E., Susan S.M., Hull M.L., Dorsch K. 2003. Geometric symmetry of the solar surface of hooves of Thoroughbred racehorses. *Am. J. Vet. Res.* 64(8), 1030-1039.

Rooney J.R. 1974a. *The Lame Horse, Causes, Symptomes and Treatment.* 1st ed., A.S. Barnes. New Jersey.

Rooney J.R. 1974b. The cutting-in mechanism of the equine hoof. *Mod.Vet. Pract.* 55(3), 217-220.

Rooney J.R. 1977a. *Autopsy of the Horse.* Krieger, Huntington, New York.

Rooney J.R. 1977b. Interaction of hoof with ground. *Mod. Vet. Pract.* 58, 624-625.

Rooney, J.R. 1977c. Forelimb contracture in the young horse. *J. Eq. Med. Surg.* 1, 350-351.

Rooney J.R. 1978. Road founder. *Mod. Vet. Pract.* 59(5), 391-392.

Rooney J.R., Quddus M.A., Kingsbury H.B. 1978. A laboratory investigation of the function of the stay apparatus of the equine foreleg. *J. Eq. Med. Surg.* 2, 173-180.

Rooney J.R. 1981a. *The Mechanics of the Horse.* Krieger, Huntington New York.

Rooney J.R. 1981b. Ringbone vs. pyramidal disease. *Eq.Vet. Sci.* Jan./Feb., 23-24.

Rooney J.R. 1984. The angulation of the forefoot and pastern of the horse. *J. Equine Vet. Sci.* 4, 138-143.

Rooney R. 1999a. Surface, friction, and the shape of the equine hoof. Online *J. Vet. Res.* 4, 73-93.

Rooney J. 1999b. Rings of the hoof wall of Equids. *Anvil Mag.* Dec. 24-27.

Runciman R.J., Thomason J.J., Springett G., Bullock S. Sears W. 2004. Horseshoe fixation versus hoof colour, a comparative study. *Biosyst. Eng.* 89(3), 377-382.

Ruohoniemi M., Mäkelä O., Eskonen T. 2004. Clinical significance of ossification of the cartilage of the front feet based on nuclear bone scintigraphy, radiography and lameness examination in 21 Finnhorses. *Eq. Vet. J.* 36(2), 143-148.

Russel W. 1882. *Russell on Scientific Horseshoeing for the Different Diseases of the Foot.* Cincinnati, Robert Clarke & CO.

Sack W.O., Habel R.E. 1977. *Rooney's Guide to the Dissection of the Horse.* Veterinary Textbooks, Ithaca, N.Y.

Sahay P.N., Dals L.L., Singh D.P. 1984. Acrylic agent in the management of sand crack in horse. *Indian Vet. J.* 61, Nov. 995.

Sarasin A. 1994. An in vitro model for organotypic epidermal differentiation: effects of biotin. *Dissertation*, Vet. Med. Fac. Univ. of Zurich, Switzerland.

Scheffer C.J.W., Back.W. 2001. Effects of 'navicular shoeing' on equine distal forelimb kinematics on different track surface. *The Vet. Quarterly* 23(4), 191-195.

Schmitt A. 1998. Verlaufsuntersuchungen zum Hufstatus von Lippizzanerpferden mit und ohne Biotinbehandlung. *Diss.* Med. Vet. Univ. Zürich.

Schmotzer W., Wagner P.C., Bewley L 1988. The mushroom shoe: Corrective trimming and shoeing in the treatment of DDF tendon disorders of young horses. *Am. Farriers J.* March/April, 29-31.

Schoonover M.J., Jann H.W., Blaik M.A. 2005. Quantitative comparison of three commonly used treatments for navicular syndrome in horses. *Am. J. Vet. Res.* 66(7), 1247-1251.

Schryver H.F., Bartel D.L., Langrana N., Lowe J.E. 1978. Locomotion in the horse: Kinematicts and external and internal forces in the normal equine digit in the walk and trot. *Am. J. Vet. Res.* 39(11).

Schumacher J., Schumacher J., Schramme M.C., DeGraves F.J., Smith R., Coker M. 2004. Diagnostic analgesia of the equine forefoot. *Eq. Vet. Educ.* June, 199-206.

Scott E.A., McDole M., Shires M.H. 1979a. A review of third phalanx fractures in the horse: Sixty-five cases. *JAVMA* 174(12), 1337-1343.

Scott E.A., McDole M., Shires M.H., Lamar A.M. 1979b. Fractures of the third phalanx (P3) in the horse at Michigan State University, 1964-1979. 25th *Proc. AAEP*, 439-450.

Sellnow L. 2002. Healing hoof cracks. *The Horse.* Vol. XIX, No.12, 59-64.

Sellnow L. 2004. Safe and sound. *The Horse.* Vol. XXI, No.7, 91-98.

Sherman R.A., Morrison S. Ng D. 2006. Maggot debridement therapy for serious horse wounds – A survey of practitioners. *The Vet. J.* Jul. 8.

Shiroma J.T., Engel H.N., Wagner P.C., Watrous B.J. 1989. Dorsal subluxation of the proximal intephalangeal joint in the pelvic limb of three horses. *JAVMA* 195(6), 777-780.

Shively M.J. 1982a. Equine-English dictionary: Part I- Standing conformation. *Eq. Pract.* 4(5), 10-27.

Shively M.J. 1982b. Equine-English dictionary: Part II- Locomotion (ways of going). *Eq. Pract.* 4(8), 11-20.

Shively M.J. 1983. Functional and clinical significance of the check ligaments. *Eq. Pract.* 5(2), 37-42.

Sigafoos R. 1986. The continuous rim-type shoe. *Am. Farriers J.* July/Aug., 21-34.

Sigafoos R. 1989. Determining the angle of the wedge shoe. *Am. Farriers J.* Dec., 46-47.

Sigafoos D.R. 1991. Composite reconstruction of equine underrun heels. *Proc. AAEP* 673-680.

Sigafoos R. 1995. Polymeric composite repair for acute and chronic refractory hoof injuries in horses. *Proc. AAEP* 41, 253-257.

Silver A. 1973. Some factors affecting wound healing. *Eq. Vet. J.* 5, 47.

Simpson G.G. 1951. *Horses-The Story of the Horse Family in the Modern World and through Sixty Million Years of History.* Oxford University Press. New York.

Simpson J.F. 1968. The theory of shoeing and balancing. In: *Care and Training of the Trotter and Pacer.* Written by Harrison J.C. 1st ed. Columbus OH. The United States Trotting Association. pp 292-373.

Singh S.S., Ward W.R., Murray R.D. 1993. Technique of hoof biopsy in cattle. *Vet. Rec.* 133, 190-191.

Sisson S., Grossman J.D. 1953. *The Anatomy of the Domestic Animals.* 4th ed. W.B. Saunders Company, Philadelphia, PA.

Smith A.P. 1967. Corrective shoeing for bowed tendon. *Mod. Vet. Pract.* 48(2), 53.

Smith R.K.W., McGuigan M.P., Hyde J.T., Daly A.S.G., Pardoe C.H., Lock.A.N., Wilson A.M. 2002. In vitro evaluation of nonrigid support system for the equine metacarpophalangeal joint. *Eq. Vet. J.* 34(7), 726-731.

Smithcors J.F. 1961a. The Equine leg. *Mod. Vet. Pract.* 42, 24.

Smithcors J.F. 1961b. The Equine leg. *Mod. Vet. Pract.* 42, 31.

Smithcors J.F. 1961c. The Equine leg. *Mod. Vet. Pract.* 42, 33.

Smythe R.H, Goody P.C. 1972. *The Horse Structure and Movement.* Second ed. J.A. Allen & Co Ltd. London, pp.180-184.

Snow V.E. 1984. Foot problems in horses. *Mod.Vet. Pract.* Sept., 735-737.

Snow V.E., Birdsall P. D. 1990. Specific parameters used to evaluate hoof balance and support. *Proc. AAEP* 36, 299-311.

Snyder J.R., Wheat J.D., Bleifer D. 1986. Conservative management of metacarpophalangeal instability. *32nd Proc. AAEP*, 357-364.

Sønnichsen H.V. 1982. Subcarpal check ligament desmotomy for the treatment of contracted deep flexor tendon in foals. *Eq.Vet. J.* 14(3), 256-257.

Sparks J.M. 1970. Prevention of lameness in horses. *Proc. AAEP* 16, 67-82.

Springhall J.A. 1964. Special shoes and their uses. In: *Elements of Horseshoeing.* Univ. of Queensland Press. 39-43.

Stanley S. 2004. Shoeing for the 21st century. *Am. Farriers J.* July/Aug. (30) 5. 102-106.

Stashak T.S. 1987. *Adams' Lameness in Horses,* 4th ed. Lea and Febiger, Philadelphia.

Stashak T.S. 1989. Management of lacerations and avulsion injuries of the foot and pastern region and hoof wall cracks. *Vet. Clin. N. Am.: Eq. Pract.* 5, 195-220.

Stashak T. S. 1991. *Equine Wound Management.* Lea and Febiger, Philadelphia. Pp24-27.

Steckel R.R., Fessler J.F. 1983. Surgical management of severe hoof wounds in the horse: A retrospective study of 30 cases. *Comp. Cont. Educ. Pract. Vet.* 5(8), S435-S443.

Steckel R.R. 1987. Puncture wounds, abscesses, thrush, and canker. In: *Robinson N.E.: Current Therapy in Equine Medicine.* Philadelphia, WB Saunders. p 266.

Steckel R.R., Fessler F.J., Huston C.L. 1989. Deep puncture wounds of the equine hoof: A review of 50 cases. *Proc. AAEP* 167-176.

Steindler A. 1955. *Kinesiology of the Human Body.* Springfield Ill.: C.C. Thomas.

Stephens S. 2003. Hoof cracks. *Equus.* No. 308, June. 67-76.

Stewart-Spears G. 2004. Managing thin, shelly feet. *The Horse.* March, Vol. 21, No.3. 119-126.

Stick J.A., Jann H.W., Scott E.A., Robinson N.E. 1982. Pedal bone rotation as a prognostic sign in laminitis of horses. *JAVMA* 180(3), 251-252 .

Stick J.A., Nickels F.A., Williams A.M. 1992. Long term effect of desmotomy of the accessory ligament of the deep digital flexor muscle in Standardbreds: 23 cases (1979-1989). *JAVMA* 200(8), 1131-1132.

Stokes M., Hendrickson A., Wittern C. 1998. Use of an elevated boot to reduce contralateral support limb complications secondary to cast application in the horse. *Eq. Pract.* 20(6), 14 - 16.

Storer T.I., Stebbins R.C., Usinger R.L., Nybakken J.W. 1974. *General Zoology* 6th ed. McGraw-Hill Book Company. New York.

Strickland C. 2001. Nail-free equine footwear. *The Horse.* Dec. 75-79.

Stump J.E. 1967. Anatomy of the normal equine foot, including microscopic features of the laminar region. *JAVMA* 151 (12), 1588-1598.

Suchorski-Tremblay A.M., Kok R., Thomason J.J. 2001. Modelling horse hoof cracking with artificial neural networks. Canadian Biosystem Engineering. 43, 7.17-7.22.

Sutton B., Butler D. 1980. Selenium toxicity in horses. *Am. Farriers J.* June, 44-46.

Sweeny C.R., Habecker P.L., Russell G.E. 2000. Effect of sodium bisulfate on skin and hooves of horses. *Am. J. Vet. Res.* 61(11), 1418-1421.

Tanaka K. 1998. Tendonitis and the hoof. *Am. Farriers.* J. May/June. 74-76.

Tanaka K., Onishi T., Hirano S. 2002. A case study of laminitis in racehorses: Recovery from prolapse of the solar corium. *J. Eq. Sci.* 13(1), 1-7.

Taylor T.S., Vaughan J.T. 1980. Effects of denervation of the digit of the horse. *JAVMA* 177 (10), 1033-1039.

Taylor D.D., Hood D.M., Wagner I.P., 2002. Short-term effect of therapeutic shoeing on severity of lameness in horses with chronic laminitis. *Am. J. Vet. Res.* 63(12), 1629-1633.

Taylor D.D., Hood D.M., Potter G.D., Hogan H.A., Honnas C.M. 2005. Evaluation of displacement of the digital cushion in response to vertical loading in equine forelimb. *Am. J. of Vet. Res.* 66(4), 623-629.

Tearney P. 2005. Arming yourself for the battle with laminitis. *Am. Farriers J.* 31(8), 74-77.

Tearney P. 2006. From foal barns to the red mile. *Am. Farriers J.* 32(1), 31-40.

"The Farriers Guide". 1986. *Farrier Craft and Business Guide*, The Farrier Registration Council. England. www.farrier-reg.gov.uk.

The Horseshoer 1966. Normal, special and corrective shoeing. U.S. War Department. California Polytechnic State University, San Luis Obispo, CA.

Thomas H.S. 1998. Sole armor. *Anvil Mag.* Aug., 32-34.

Thomas H.S. 2001. Remedy for "scratches." *Anvil Mag.* Jan.

Thomason J.J., Biewener A.A., Bertram J.E.A. 1992. Surface strain on the equine hoof wall in vivo: Implications for the material design and functional morphology of the wall, *J. Exp. Biol.* 166, 145-165.

Thomason J.J. 1998. Variation in surface strain on the equine hoof wall at the midstep with shoeing, gait, substrate, direction of travel, and hoof shape. *Eq. Vet. J. Suppl.* 26, 86-95.

Thompson K.N. et al 1992. The influence of toe angle on strain characteristics of the deep digital flexor tendon, superficial flexor tendon, suspensory ligament, and hoof wall. *Eq. Athlete* 5(6), 1,6-8.

Thompson K.N., Cheung T.K., Silverman M. 1993. The effect of toe angle on tendon, ligament and hoof wall strains in vitro. *J. Eq. Vet. Sci.* 13 (11), 651-654.

Thompson K.N., Herring L.S. 1994. Metacarpophalangeal and phalangeal joint kinematics in horses shod with hoof calks. *J. Eq. Vet. Sci.,* 14(6).

Thompson K.N. 1998. Heel wedges: Their effect on tendon and ligament strains. *Anvil Mag.* Feb. 32,33.

Tjalsma E.J., Van Mauric J.M. 1995. The abnormal white line and hollow wall in the horse, a comparative mycological study. *Tijdschrift voor Diergeneeskunde* 120, 526-529.

True R.G., Lowe J.E., Heissen J., Bradley W. 1978. Black walnut shavings as a cause of acute laminitis. *Proc. AAEP* 24, 511-515.

Turner T.A. 1986a. Shoeing principles for the management of navicular disease. *JAVMA* 189, 298-301.

Turner T.A. 1986b. Navicular disease management: Shoeing principles. *Proc. AAEP* 32, 625-633.

Turner T.A. 1988. Hoof abnormalities and their relation to lameness. *Proc. AAEP* 34, 293-297.

Turner T.A. 1992. The use of hoof measurements for the objective assessment of hoof balance. *Proc. AAEP* 38, 389-395.

Turner A., Malone E. 1997. How to treat navicular bone fractures. *Proc. AAEP* 43, 370-371.

Turner T.A. 1998. White line disease. *Eq. Vet. Educ.* Manual No.4, 73-76.

Turner T.A., Sage A.M. 2002. Desmitis of the distal interphalangeal collateral ligaments: 22 cases. *Proc. AAEP* 48, 343-346.

Turoff D. 1998. The use of hoof testers. *Anvil Mag.* April, 40-43.

Valdez H. 1980. A hydrogel preparation for cleansing and protecting equine wounds. *Eq. Pract.* 2(33).

van den Belt, A.J., Dik K.J., van den Broek J. 2003. The use of radiography as a tool for the efficacy of selective breeding of a poor radiographic navicular bone condition (grades 3 and 4). *Proc. of the 13th Int. Vet. Radiol. Soc.,* Midrand, South Africa.

van Eps A. W., Pollitt C.C. 2004. Equine laminitis: Cryotherapy reduces the severity of the acute lesion. *Eq. Vet. J.* 36(3), 255-260.

van Heel M.C.V., van Weeren P.R., Back W. 2006. Shoeing sound Warmblood horses with rolled toe optimises hoof-unrollment and lowers peak loading during breakover. *Eq. Vet. J.* 38(3), 258-262.

Vanschepdael P. 2006. The Mechanical properties of various ground types and their shoeing implications. *The Farriers J.* No. 119.

Vaughan J.T., Allen R. 1987. Restraint of horses: Part 2 – Foot restraint. *Mod.Vet. Pract.* July/Aug., 440-444.

Verschooten F. 1994. An unusual case of overgrowth of the hooves in a pony. *J. Eq. Vet. Res.* 14(6), 324-328.

Verschooten F., van Waerebeek B. 1994. The ossification of the cartilages of the distal phalanx in the horse. *Vet. Radiol. Ultrasound,* 35.

Viitanen M.J., Wilson A.M., McGuigan H.P., Rogers K.D., May S.A. 2003. Effect of foot balance on the intra-articular pressure in the distal interphalangeal joint in vitro. *Eq. Vet. J.* 35(2), 184-189.

Wagner P.C., Reed S.M. and Hegreberg G.A. 1982. Contracted tendons (flexural deformities) in the young horse. Compend. *Cont. Educ. Pract. Vet.* 4, S101-S110.

Wagner P.C., Grant B.D., Knapes A.J. and Watrous, B.J. 1985a. Long term results of desmotomy of the accessory ligament of the deep digital flexor tendon (distal check ligament) in horses. *JAVMA* 187(12).

Wagner P.C., Shires M.H., Watrous B.J., Kaneps A.J., Schmotzer W.B. and Riebold T.W. 1985b. Management of acquired flexural deformity of the metacarpophalangeal joint in Equidae. *JAVMA* 187(9).

Wagner P.C., Balch-Burnett O. 1986. Surgical management of keratomas in the foot of the horse. *Eq. Pract.* 8(5).

Wagner P.C., Shires G.M.H. 1986. Laceration of flexor tendons in the horse: Treatment to maximize athletic function. *Equine Pract.* 8(7), 10-14.

Wagner P.C., Waltrous J.B. 1990a. Equine pediatric orthopedics: Clinical, radiographic, and therapeutic aspects; Part 1- Osteochondrosis. *Eq. Pract.* 12(4), 32-37.

Wagner P.C., Waltrous J.B. 1990b. Equine pediatric orthopedics: Part 2-Flexural limb deformities (tendon contracture). *Eq. Pract.* 12(5), 27-33.

Wagner P.C. and Watrous J.B. 1990c. Equine pediatric orthopedics: Part 3-Tendon laxity and rupture. *Eq. Prac.* 12(6).

Wagner P.C. von Matthiessen 1994. Case selection and management of flexural limb deformities in horses: Congenital fleural limb deformities, part 2. *Eq. Pract.* (16)1, 7-11.

Wagner I.P., Hood D.M., Hogan H.A. 2001. Comparison of bending modulus and yield strength between outer stratum medium and stratum medium zona alba in equine hooves. *Am. J. Vet. Res.* 62(5), 745-751.

Wagner I.P., Hood D.M. 2002. Effect of prolonged water immersion on equine hoof epidermis in vitro. *Am. J. Vet. Res.* 63(8), 1140-1144.

Weisenberg H. 1990. Personal communication. Equine Veterinary Services, Hod Hasharon, Israel.

Weiser M., Stöckle W., Walch H., Brenner G. 1965. Über die Verteilung von Natrium, Kalium, Kalzium, phosphor, magnesium, kupfer und zink im hufhorn von pferd. *Arch. Exp. Veterinarmed.* 19, 927-931.

Weiss R.A., Eichenr R., Sun T. 1984. T. Monoclonal antibody analysis of keratin expression in epidermal diseases: A 48 and 56 kdalton keratin as molecular markers for hyperproliferative keratinocytes. *J. Cell Biol.* 98, 1397-1406.

West C. 2004. Gaining a foothold. *The Horse* Vol. XXI, No. 8. 30-46.

Wiseman R.F. 1968. *The Complete Horseshoeing Guide.* Univ. of Oklahoma Press. pp 204-208.

Wheat J.W., Pascoe J.R. 1980. A technique for management of traumatic rupture of the equine suspensory apparatus. *JAVMA* 176(3), 205-210.

White N.A., Baggett N. 1983. A method of corrective shoeing for laminitis in horses. *Vet. Med./Sm. Anim. Clin.* 775-778.

White S.L., Rowland G.N., Whitlock R.H. 1984. Radiographic, macroscopic and microscopic changes in growth plates of calves raised on hard flooring. *Am.J. Vet. Res.* 45, 633-639.

Whitehead C.C. 1981. The assessement of biotin status in man and animals. *Proc.Nutr. Soc.* 40, 165.

Wildenstein M.J. 2004. Treating hoof cracks and other hoof maladies. *Am. Farriers J.* Sept./Oct. 81-85.

Willemen M.A. 1994. The effect of toe weight on linear and temporal stride characteristics of Standardbreds trotters. *The Vet. Quarterly Suppl.* May, 16 (2).

Willemen M.A., Savelberg H.H.C.M., Barneveld A. 1997. The improvement of the gait quality of sound trotting Warmblood horses by normal shoeing and its effect on the load on the lower forelimb. *Livestock Production Science.* 52, 145-153.

Willemen M.A., Savelberg H.H., Barneveld A. 1999. The effect of orthopaedic shoeing on the force exerted by the deep digital flexor tendon on the navicular bone in horses. *Eq. Vet. J.* 31(1), 25-30.

Williams G. 1977. Measuring the effect of forces on the equine foot. *Anvil Mag.*, June, 30-32.

Williams G., Smith T. 1977. Measuring the effect of forces on the equine foot. *Anvil Mag.* Aug., 24-25.

Williams G.E. 2001. Locomotor characteristics of horses with navicular disease. *Am. J. Vet. Res.* 62(2), 206-210.

Williams M.A., Stowe H.D., Stickle R.L. 1989. Relationship of nutrition and management factors to the incidence of equine developmental orthopedic disease: A field study. Proc. 7th. Int. Conf. Product. *Dis. Farm. Anim.* 32-36.

Williams M.A., Pugh D.C. 1993. Developmental orthopedic disease: minimizing the incident of poorly understood disorders. *Comp. Contin. Educ. Pract. Vet.* 15(6).

Wilson A.M., Pardoe C.H. 1998. Equine hoof cracks: mechanical considerations and repair techniques. *Eq. Vet. Educ.* Manual No.4, 52-56.

Wilson A.M., Seelig T.J., Shield R.A., Silverman B.W. 1998. The effect of foot imbalance on point of forrce application in the horse. *Eq. Vet. J.* 30 (6), 540-545.

Wilson A.M., McGuigan M.P., Fouracre L., MacMahon L. 2001. The force and contact stress on the navicular bone during trot locomotion in sound horses and horses with navicular disease. *Eq. Vet. J.* 33(2), 159-165.

Wilson D.G., Calderwood Mays M.B., Colahan P.T. 1985. Equine canker: A prospective and retrospective study (abstr.) *Vet. Surg.* 14, 70.

Wilson D.G., Calderwood Mays M.B., Colahan P.T. 1989. Treatment of canker in horses. *JAVMA* 194 (12), 1721-1723.

Wintzer H.J. 1986. The effect of vitamin H substitution on the growth and condition of hooves. *Tierarztl Prax.* 14(4), 495-500.

Witte S.T., Will L.A., Olsen C.R., Kinker J.A., Miller-Graber P. 1993. Chronic selenosis in horses fed locally produced alfalfa hay. *JAVMA*, 202(3), 406-409.

Woodall P. 2002. The biology of equine foot decay. MSc thesis, Univ. of Central Lancashire, Preston.

Wright I.M., Douglas J. 1993. Biomechanical considerations in the treatment of navicular disease. *The Vet. Rec.* July. 133, 109-114.

Wright I.M. 1993. A study of 118 cases of navicular disease: clinical features. *Eq. Vet. J.* 25(6), 488-492.

Wright I.M., Phillips T.J., Walmsley J.P. 1999. Endoscopy of the navicular bursa: A new technique for the treatment of contaminated and septic bursa. *Eq. Vet. J.* 31(1), 5-11.

Yelle M. 1986. Clinicians guide to equine laminitis. *Eq. Vet. J.* 18(2), 156-158.

Young L.R., Monticello S. 1989. Hoof repair using high-resin fiberglass tape. *Proc. AAEP* 35, 451-456.

Young J.H. 1993. White line disease. In: *Proc. 3rd. Congress of Eq. Med. and Surg.* Swiss Review for Veterinary Medicine, Geneva pp 69-71.

Yovich J.V., Stashak T.S., DeBowes R.M. 1986. Fractures of the distal phalanx of the forelimb in eight foals. *JAVMA* 189, 550-554.

Zebarth B.J., Sheard R.W. 1985. Impact and shear resistance of turf grass racing surfaces for Thoroughbreds. *Am. J. Vet. Res.* 46(4), 778-784.

Zenker W., Josseck H., Geyer H. 1995. Histological and physical assessment of poor hoof horn quality in Lipizzaner horses and a therapeutic trial with biotin and a placebo. *Eq. Vet. J.* 27(3), 183.

Index

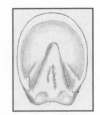

*Page numbers in **bold** indicate entries; page numbers in *italic* indicate figures; page numbers followed by **t** indicate tables.*

Therapeutic Farriery

Composed in Scala and Scala Sans, typefaces designed by
   Martin Majoor in 1994

Printed, Smyth sewn and bound by Thomson-Shore, Inc.,
   Dexter, Michigan

on 50# Nature's Natural text stock with 70# Fortune Matte insert
   and Rainbow Brick endsheets